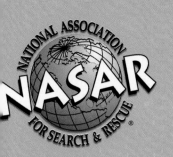

FUNDAMENTALS OF
Search
and
Rescue

Edited by
Donald C. Cooper

National Association for Search & Rescue, Inc.
Centreville, Virginia

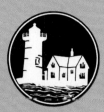

JONES AND BARTLETT PUBLISHERS
Sudbury, Massachusetts

BOSTON   TORONTO   LONDON   SINGAPORE

World Headquarters

Jones and Bartlett Publishers
40 Tall Pine Drive
Sudbury, MA 01776
978-44-5000
info@jbpub.com
www.jbpub.com

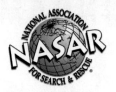

Executive Director: Megan Bartlett
Education Services Director: Janet Adere
Education Manager: Paul Burke
Research and Development
    Manager: Donald C. Cooper

National Association for Search and Rescue
P.O. Box 232020
Centreville, VA 20120-2020
703-222-6277
education@nasar.org
www.nasar.org

Jones and Bartlett's books and products are available through most bookstores and online booksellers. To contact Jones and Bartlett Publishers directly, call 800-832-0034, fax 978-443-8000, or visit our website www.jbpub.com. Substantial discounts on bulk quantities of Jones and Bartlett's publications are available to corporations, professional associations, and other qualified organizations. For details and specific discount information, contact the special sales department at Jones and Bartlett via the above contact information or send an email to specialsales@jbpub.com.

Production Credits

Chief Executive Officer: Clayton Jones
Chief Operating Officer: Donald W. Jones, Jr.
President, Higher Education and Professional Publishing:
Robert W. Holland, Jr.
V.P., Sales and Marketing: William J. Kane
V.P., Production and Design: Anne Spencer
V.P., Manufacturing and Inventory Control:
    Therese Connell
Publisher, Emergency Care: Lawrence D. Newell

Publisher, Public Safety: Kimberly Brophy
Associate Editor: Janet Morris
Associate Production Editor: Karen C. Ferreira
Photo Researcher: Kimberly Potvin
Marketing Director: Alisha Weisman
Interior and Cover Design: Anne Spencer
Composition and Illustration: Graphic World
Printing and Binding: RR Donnelley

ISBN-13: 978-0-7637-4807-4
ISBN-10: 0-7637-4807-2

6048

The procedures and protocols in this book are based on the most current recommendations of responsible sources. The Publisher and the National Association for Search and Rescue, however, make no guarantee as to, as assume no responsibility for, the correctness, sufficiency, or completeness of such information or recommendations. Other or additional safety measures may be required under particular circumstances.

Unless otherwise indicated, photographs have been supplied by Donald Cooper and NASAR. Illustrations were created by Graphic World.

Some images in this book feature models. These models do not necessarily endorse, represent, or participate in the activities represented in the images.

Library of Congress Cataloging-in-Publication Data

Fundamentals of search and rescue / edited by Donald C. Cooper.
    p. cm.
  Includes bibliographical references and index.
  ISBN 0-7637-4807-2
  1. Search and rescue operations. I. Cooper, Donald C.
  TL553.8.F86 2005
  363.34'81--dc22
                        2004026041
Printed in the United States of America
17 16 15   10 9 8 7

BRIEF CONTENTS

CONTENTS

RESOURCE PREVIEW

Fundamentals of Search and Rescue (FUNSAR) is the required text for anyone completing the FUNSAR course offered by the National Association for Search and Rescue (NASAR). FUNSAR provides a comprehensive and practical approach to the content presented in the FUNSAR course.

Written to provide an overview of all aspects of search and rescue procedures and policies, FUNSAR teaches the basic techniques employed by professional search and rescue personnel. This text is the core of the FUNSAR course with features that will reinforce and expand on the essential information. These features include:

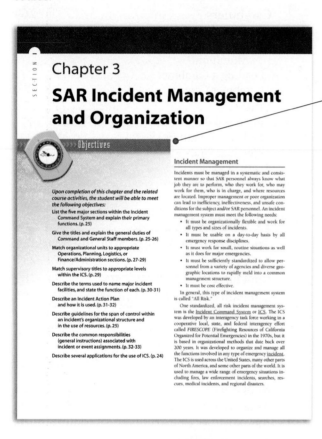

Knowledge Objectives outline the most important topics covered in the chapter.

SAR Tips provide advice from masters of the trade.

steps, locking each knee and synchronizing the breathing, to allow for a brief respite before taking the next small step. This technique is slow, but may be the only way to travel over difficult terrain, especially at high altitude. Think of it as steady, consistent, and slow travel, instead of erratic stop-and-go movement. A novice SAR hiker can virtually eliminate all long rest stops with this technique

OPERATIONS
The "rest step," adapted from mountaineering, is a method of allowing respite between steps. Lock each knee and synchronize the breathing in between each small step.

SAR Tips

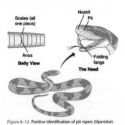
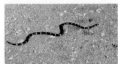

Figure 8–12 Positive identification of pit vipers (*Viperidae*).

Figure 8–13 Identification of coral snake (*Elapidae*). Note that coral snakes can vary greatly in color. In the United States, however, consider any red, black, and yellow banded snake a coral snake, especially if the red band touches the yellow (or white) band.

Full-color photographs and illustrations aid comprehension of difficult concepts.

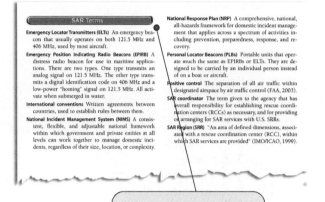

Search and rescue terms are easily identifiable within the chapter and define key terms the student must know. A comprehensive glossary of SAR Terms is found at the end of every chapter.

INSTRUCTOR RESOURCES

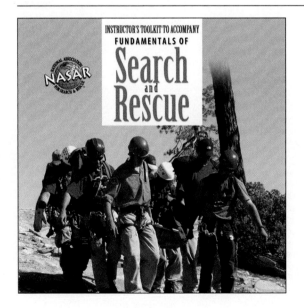

Instructor's ToolKit CD-ROM
ISBN: 0-7637-3630-9
Preparing for a FUNSAR course is easy with the resources on this CD-ROM, including:

- **Adaptable PowerPoint Presentations**—Provides you with a powerful way to make presentations that are educational and engaging to your students with slides that can be edited and modified to meet your needs. To save you time, we have incorporated the most important images into the slides to emphasize key points.

- **Instructor's Resource Manual**—Contains helpful teaching tips, lecture outlines, skill station scenarios, and additional coverage of key topics.

- **Image Bank**—Provides you with a selection of the most important images found in the text. Use them to incorporate more images into the PowerPoint presentations, make handouts, or enlarge a specific image for further discussion.

- **NASAR Exam Questions**—Contains multiple-choice and scenario-based questions, with page references to FUNSAR.

ACKNOWLEDGEMENTS

Contributors

Craig Bannerman
Donald C. Cooper
Frank Fire, Jr.
Steve Foster
John R. Frost
Mike Guzo
Patrick "Rick" LaValla
Jeff Lehman
Winnie Pennington
Timothy Provost
Robert "Skip" Stoffel
Susan J. Thrasher
Edward C. Wolff

The editor and contributors wish to thank the following individuals and groups for their gracious and enlightened review of, and assistance with, this resource:
American Meteorological Society
NASAR Education Committee
Cole Brown, III
Roger Bryant
Jacki Golike
Carol Iverson
Georges Kleinbaum
Chris Long
Dave Maynard
Tom Millen
James Newberry
Donald Patch
Larry Pugh
Matthew Scharper
Jim Stumpf
Frank Wysocki

Art and Graphics

CMC Rescue, Inc.
Donald C. Cooper
Graybeard Graphics
National Association for Search and Rescue
Pigeon Mountain Industries, Inc.

PREFACE

At the annual conference of the National Association for Search and Rescue (NASAR) in Reno, Nevada, in 1984, a special interest group meeting, chaired by Willis Larson, was held to discuss the potential development of a basic search and rescue (SAR) skills training program that could standardize such skills across the United States. Donald C. Cooper volunteered to coordinate the research and development of the program. Over the following year, research was conducted whereby many experts in the field of SAR were identified and asked to suggest what should be included in such a training program. Their input, combined with research from numerous other sources, was collected and collated to form the initial basis for the first version of this document and its related training program.

The following individuals were involved in the original research:

Betty J. Burke	John F. Hays	Mark Pennington
Stan Bush	Bob Hill	Bill Pierce
Donald C. Cooper	Steve Hudson	G. Wesley Reynolds
Bob Deckwa	Ernie Jesch	George Rice
Gene Fear	A.S.G. Jones	Jim Segerstrom
Udo Fischer	Willis Larson	Robert "Skip" Stoffel
John Gallagher	Patrick "Rick" LaValla	Adam Ustik
Rick Goodman	M.J. McCartor	Tom Vines
Hatch Graham	Lois Clark McCoy	J.W. "Bill" Wade
Paul Green	Greg McDonald	Jon Wartes
Dan Hawkins	Michael R. McEwan	

In 1985, the first prototype basic SAR program (later named FUNSAR for Fundamental Search and Rescue Skills Program) was taught at Cuyahoga Community College in Parma, Ohio. Soon thereafter, Western Piedmont Community College in western North Carolina, in cooperation with Burke County Emergency Management, sponsored the second program to train SAR personnel using the prototype developed.

Many programs were taught over the subsequent few years across the United States. Modifications were made to the program, and revisions in the course content made this SAR skills program the most widely accepted standard available at the time. The following gracious individuals and members of the SAR community helped revise and improve the program that ultimately made this textbook possible:

Duane Alire	Peter Goth, MD	Randy McKinney
Warren Bowman, MD	Jeff Harbour	Al Musgrove
Roger Bryant	John F. Hays	David Rodgers
Burke County EM	J. Hunter Holloway	Terry Shaeffer
Cuyahoga Valley National Park	David H. Hoover	J.W. Shiner
Ralph DeCunzo	Peter Howells	Albert "Ab" Taylor
Charles Erwin	E. Frank Kirk	William V. Vargas
Vikki Fenton	Steve Larakis	Kirk Waggoner
Steve Foster	Norman Lawson, Jr.	Nick Waters
Lloyd Gallagher	John McComas	Tim Woods

NASAR was interested in publishing the materials collected for use in the program but did not have the resources to do it at the time. So, Rick LaValla and Skip Stoffel offered to use their corporate identity (ERI, Inc.) to publish the material as a book, and the first edition was published in 1989. In the first two years of its use, the following people made valuable contributions to the improvement of the contents:

Paul Anderson	Steve Foster	David Rodgers
Michael Cooper	Dan Hawkins	John Stroup
Roger Bryant	Mark King	Ab Taylor
Peggy Fisher	Bill Ramsey, MD	Tom Vines

Since that early version of the book, certain individuals have offered support and help that far exceed the normal "call of duty." This support sometimes included editing, ideas, and suggestions for modifications. But, most often it simply involved moral support, simple kindness, logistical offerings, and a listening ear. To these individuals, special thanks are due on behalf of anyone who may ever benefit from the contents of this publication. It is individuals such as these that truly make involvement in SAR satisfying.

Paul Anderson	Bob Hill	Sally Santeford
Burke County Emergency	Peter Howells	David Schrader
Management, NC	A.S.G. Jones	Rick Tate
Roger Bryant	Logan County Public	Ab & Lillian Taylor
Julie Cooper	Rescue, WV	Bill Wade
Steve Foster	Willis Larson	Nick Waters
Dan Hawkins	Norman Lawson, Jr.	West Virginia SAR Network

In 2002, NASAR entered into an agreement with Jones and Bartlett Publishers and acquired the rights to the book that was previously published elsewhere. After hundreds of hours of work by dozens of individuals, the book evolved to its current state. It should be noted, however, that there is no way to mention every individual and group that participated in the research, development, and improvement of this material. So, for those of you who helped, and for those of you who will help expand, evolve, and convey this information to those who need it, we all thank you. You are all the reason for our energy, enthusiasm, and continuing participation in this important field.

—Donald C. Cooper, Ed.

PHOTO CREDITS

Chapter 1

Overview of Land Search and Rescue

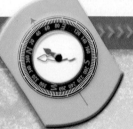

Objectives

Upon completion of this chapter and the related course activities, the student will be able to meet the following objectives:

Define "search and rescue." (p. 1)

Demonstrate awareness of national volunteer organizations including:
National Association for Search and Rescue (NASAR). (p. 3)
Citizen Corps. (p. 4-5)
Community Emergency Response Teams. (p. 5-6)

A Brief History of Search and Rescue (SAR)

One of the core human beliefs shared across many cultures is the desire to live a long, happy, and healthy life. Thus, applying equipment and technology to help people cheat death continues to be a significant goal for many contemporary societies. It is not surprising then that rescue—the act of saving another's life—has become an honorable, respected, and heroic vocation.

Searches and rescues have been carried out around the world for centuries, but it has only been recently that we have referred to these acts collectively as "search and rescue" or "SAR." Ever since humans began traveling into unknown terrain, they have encountered difficulties and required assistance. During these difficulties, others with the appropriate equipment and skill were often compelled, for one reason or another, to help out. In the mountains, the locals, often very knowledgeable about the territory and well equipped to deal with it, were called upon to assist when the less skilled and equipped found themselves in distress. In the deserts, oceans, jungles, and other environments around the globe, the same incidents often happened: those who possessed the proper equipment and skill were frequently called upon to search for, and rescue, others in distress.

As technology improved, human populations became more reliant on it and less reliant on the skills that had previously allowed them to help themselves. As populations expanded into previously isolated areas, the need for assisting people in distress became increasingly necessary. In the early part of the 20th century, several countries found it necessary to develop a specific capability to find and recover wartime marine and aircraft crews. This interest, and wartime funding, began what many consider to be the birth of organized government-supported SAR. During this era, the considerable wartime resources of the

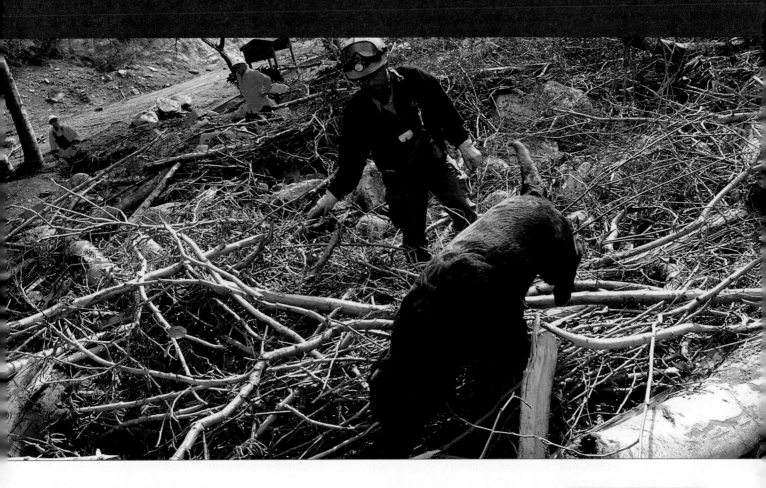

United States government were brought to bear on the problems of finding such things as downed aircraft, missing vessels, unexploded ordinance, and enemy locations, and rescuing, retrieving, or destroying that which was sought. This attention and funding as well as improved technology in general produced the basis for much of organized SAR as it is known today.

Contemporary SAR systems provide the response for overdue, lost, injured, or stranded people in many environments. One type of environment that is often associated with SAR is the wilderness. However, it is important to note that in SAR, wilderness can take on several meanings. For instance, most consider "wilderness" to be a region that is generally uninhabited and devoid of any synthetic ("manmade") amenities. While this certainly describes natural areas such as large parks and rural areas, it also describes many regions, even urban, which have been devastated by a disaster such as an earthquake or hurricane. This also makes it easy to see why SAR is an extremely important part of nearly every disaster, fire service, law enforcement, and emergency medical service (EMS) emergency. Because the majority of the world's population resides in urban areas and because disasters are common, emergency responders, including SAR personnel, are often just as likely to encounter an urban wilderness as they are a natural one (Figure 1–1).

Search and rescue programs, equipment, and personnel vary geographically in accordance to local needs and available resources. Therefore, SAR has many definitions and meanings. The first explicit definition of the term "search and rescue" in the context we use today was likely contained in the proceedings of the Provisional International Civil Aviation

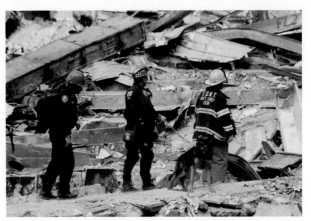

Figure 1–1 SAR personnel are often just as likely to encounter an urban wilderness as they are a natural one.

Organization (PICAO), circa 1946. In an article in the 1946 *Air Sea Rescue Bulletin* entitled, "Evolution of SAR: An Editorial," the (unknown) author noted that PICAO adopted the term "search and rescue" and recommended that it be defined as, "The act of finding and returning to safety the survivors from an emergency incident." Setnicka (1980) defined SAR as, "…any operation aimed at helping someone in trouble, someone who cannot solve his or her problem alone…." The same author uttered the classic line that SAR was essentially, "a *transportation* problem—of rescuers to the victim and the victim to safety." More contemporary references, such as *The International Aeronautical and Maritime Search and Rescue (IAMSAR) Manual* (1999), have found it useful to define "search" and "rescue" separately. Defined separately, <u>search</u> is an operation using available personnel and facilities to locate persons in distress, and <u>rescue</u> is an operation to retrieve persons in distress, provide for their initial medical or other needs, and deliver them to a place of safety.

Foundational Concepts in SAR

Beyond what is taught in the National Association for Search and Rescue's "Introduction to SAR" course, two concepts are important to grasp before discussing how one gets involved in search and rescue: the elements of SAR education and the SAR "tool" acquisition process.

SAR Education

Fundamental search and rescue skills are a diverse collection of topics that cover many areas. For the discussion in this text, all of these skills have been divided into three basic categories for organizational purposes. Those categories are:

- Search
- Rescue
- Survival/Support.

All of the skills and knowledge contained in this text can be grouped into one or more of these categories:

- Search training continues one's education in the area of searching only.
  - Specialties include land search, water search, air search, the application of search theory, search planning, and search dogs.
- Rescue training includes diverse specialties that differ in terrain and equipment.
  - Specialties are based in the environments in which they are required including mountain, wilderness, ice, water, and urban rescue as well as many others.

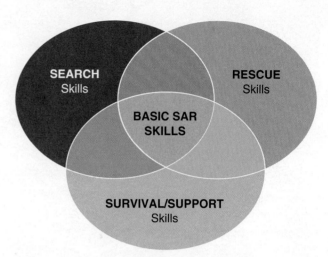

Figure 1–2 Basic SAR skills (the fundamentals) are an intersection of search, rescue, and survival/support skills.

  - Equipment differs greatly from rescue type to rescue type.
- Survival/Support training is an area of study that includes many skills that are also included in search and rescue, but are skills that may be required independent of both.
  - Such skills include wilderness survival, navigation, improvisation, fitness, and communication (Figure 1–2).

Tools for SAR

Search and rescue is an extremely diverse field that involves more art than science. Determining what will and what will not work is often based upon the educated opinions of those involved, and these opinions may vary greatly. What works in one situation may not work in others. Because of this, SAR is difficult to learn based on one source or the teachings of one instructor. It is important in SAR, therefore, to gain knowledge from many sources, tempering everything with practicality and experience.

SAR education is a "tool" acquisition process. Specific knowledge and skills are tools to the rescuer, as are hammer and nails to the carpenter. A specific skill (tool) may be used, but situations will occasionally require tools beyond the contents of one's existing tool chest. In SAR, the tools are collected from appropriate sources—through formal education and experience—and then used where necessary to meet an objective. Some tools work better than others in certain situations, but all may be of value at one time or another (Figure 1–3).

Every student or practitioner of SAR should acquire as many "tools" as possible. The more tools you have,

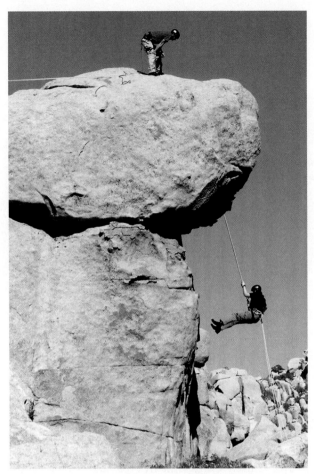

Figure 1–3 SAR education is a "tool" acquisition process.

the better the chances that you will have what it takes to perform safely and effectively. Specialization may be necessary, but not to the exclusion of a broad base of knowledge and skill. As in most pursuits, a single tool should not be expected to work perfectly for every job. Users vary, and so do the ways in which the tools can be applied to attain a goal; what works for one may not work for another. These tools may eventually serve as the only foundation on which to build a system that is expected to save a life. As such, they must be well chosen and skillfully applied.

Avoid anyone who claims to teach the only real truth in SAR. Nothing is more dangerous in SAR than an individual who lacks an open mind and thinks that he or she possesses the only true way. There are as many ways to perform any particular search or rescue as there are opinions on which is best. Every search and/or rescue can be improved upon. Learning how such improvements can be made is the key to advancing beyond basic tool application.

Getting Involved in SAR

There are a number of organizations through which individuals can get involved in search and rescue in the United States, including NASAR, the USA Freedom Corps, Community Emergency Response Teams, and other national, state, and local organizations.

National Association for Search and Rescue (NASAR)

The National Association for Search and Rescue (NASAR) is a not-for-profit membership organization of dedicated paid and unpaid SAR professionals. NASAR acts as an umbrella organization where people of all SAR specialties can meet, network, and coordinate their wide-ranging skills to establish maximum effectiveness in emergency situations. Since 1972, NASAR has provided its members with educational opportunities, timely publications, and a variety of conferences, workshops and symposia, the most well known being its own annual conference. NASAR offers formal training opportunities that have grown to include topics ranging from the most rudimentary SAR skills through sophisticated incident management.

In 1991, NASAR developed some of the first national certification criteria for search and rescue personnel. These criteria are referred to as SAR TECH™ III, SAR TECH™ II, and SAR TECH™ I/Crewleader III, and were developed to evaluate three levels of search responder so that a measurable level of individual and crew capability could be available for Incident Commanders. The criteria have also been adopted by several states in the U.S. and by a multitude of SAR teams nationwide; the development and acceptance of these criteria continue to grow. NASAR also participates in international standards making processes such as those of the National Fire Protection Association (NFPA) and American Society for Testing and Materials (ASTM) International (Figure 1–4). NASAR maintains a specialty bookstore that contains authoritative and often difficult to find texts, and has established an extensive web site.

As an umbrella organization, NASAR has close ties to the widest variety of SAR-related organizations, including all types of public safety agencies. Among the active partner organizations are the Mountain Rescue Association (MRA), Civil Air Patrol, approximately 300 search dog organizations, numerous local volunteer SAR units, dive rescue units, cave rescue groups, and other related organizations. In the United States, NASAR maintains a close relationship with the Federal Emergency Management Agency (FEMA), the United States Air Force Rescue Coordination Center (AFRCC), the National Park Service, the National Forest Service,

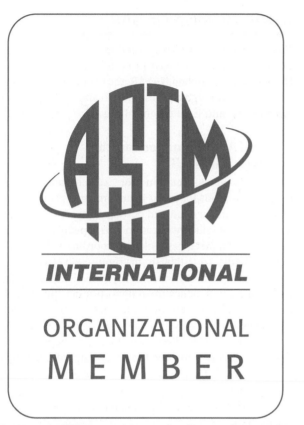

Figure 1–4 NASAR participates in the standards-setting process as a member of ASTM International.

Office of Foreign Disaster Assistance (USAID/OFDA), and the United States Coast Guard (USGC). NASAR also participates on the National SAR Committee (NSARC). Internationally, NASAR enjoys a close relationship with the Canadian SAR Secretariat and the Royal Canadian Mounted Police (RCMP), and has a growing member presence in countries all over the world.

USA Freedom Corps

Following the tragic events of September 11, 2001, state and local government officials have increased opportunities for U.S. citizens to become an integral part of protecting their country and supporting local first responders. Officials agree that the formula for ensuring a more secure and safer homeland consists of preparedness, training, and citizen involvement in supporting first responders.

During his 2002 State of the Union address, President George W. Bush called upon every American to get involved in strengthening the country's communities and sharing America's compassion around the world. He called on every American to dedicate at least two years

over the course of their lives to the service of others. He included all Americans because everyone can do something, and he created the USA Freedom Corps to help all Americans to answer his call.

The USA Freedom Corps is a Coordinating Council housed at the White House and chaired by the President of the United States. The organization is working to strengthen American culture of service and to help find opportunities for every American to start volunteering. Over the past thirty years, community involvement in the United States has been in decline. President Bush has challenged all Americans to foster a renewed culture of citizenship, service, and responsibility. The USA Freedom Corps was designed to bring together the resources of the federal government with the nonprofit, business, educational, faith-based, and other sectors to begin this process and to measure the results.

A comprehensive USA Freedom Corps Network has already been built where individuals can find service opportunities that match their interests and talents in their hometowns, across the country, or around the world. Service opportunities are being expanded to protect the U.S. homeland, to meet important community needs, and to extend American compassion around the world through partnerships with these and other organizations that create the volunteer service infrastructure. At the same time, the USA Freedom Corps is working to expand and strengthen federal service programs like the Peace Corps, Citizen Corps, AmeriCorps, and Senior Corps, and to raise awareness of and break down barriers to service opportunities with all federal government agencies.

Citizen Corps

After September 11, 2001, America witnessed a wellspring of selflessness and heroism. People in every corner of the country asked, "What can I do?" and "How can I help?" Citizen Corps was created to help all Americans answer these questions through public education and outreach, training, and volunteer service.

Citizen Corps, a vital component of USA Freedom Corps, was created to help answer these questions and coordinate volunteer activities that will make American communities safer, stronger, and better prepared to respond to any emergency situation. It provides opportunities for Americans to participate in a range of measures to make their families, their homes, and their communities safer from the threats of crime, terrorism, and disasters of all kinds. Citizen Corps programs build on the successful efforts that are in place in many communities around the country to prevent crime and respond to emergencies. Programs that began through local innovation are the foundation for Citizen Corps and this national approach to citizen participation in community safety.

Citizen Corps is coordinated nationally by FEMA. In this capacity, FEMA works closely with other federal entities, state and local governments, first responders and emergency managers, the volunteer community, and the White House Office of the USA Freedom Corps.

Citizen Corps Councils helps drive local citizen participation by coordinating Citizen Corps programs, developing community action plans, assessing possible threats, and identifying local resources.

- An expanded Neighborhood Watch Program (NWP) incorporates terrorism awareness and education into its existing crime prevention mission, and serves as a way to bring residents together to focus on disaster preparedness and training.
- Volunteers in Police Service (VIPS) provides support for resource-constrained police departments by incorporating civilian volunteers so that law enforcement professionals have more time for frontline duty.
- The Community Emergency Response Team (CERT) trains people in neighborhoods, the workplace, and schools in basic disaster response skills, such as fire suppression, urban search and rescue, and medical operations, and helps them take a more active role in emergency preparedness.
- The Medical Reserve Corps (MRC) coordinates volunteer health professionals as well as other citizens with an interest in health issues to provide ongoing support for community public health needs and resources during large-scale emergencies, such as assisting emergency response teams, providing care to victims with less serious injuries, and removing other burdens that inhibit the effectiveness of physicians and nurses.

Community Emergency Response Team (CERT)

First responders such as fire and EMS personnel arriving at the scene of a major disaster will not be able to meet the demand for their services. Large numbers of victims, communication difficulties, road blockages, and general infrastructure failures will prevent people from accessing the emergency services they have come to expect at a moment's notice through 9-1-1 (Figure 1–5). Instead of relying on emergency services, citizens will have to depend on each other in these situations to meet their immediate life-saving and life-sustaining needs. Research from large-scale disasters shows that "spontaneous volunteers"— friends, family, and neighbors, or people in the right place at the right time—will save more lives than all trained rescuers combined. During the Mexico City earthquake in

September 1985, untrained, impromptu rescuers were credited with saving over 800 lives. Unfortunately, 100 people lost their lives while attempting to save others. It is now thought that the loss of these citizen rescuers could have been prevented through training.

If it can be predicted that first responders will not be able to meet immediate needs following a major disaster, and spontaneous volunteering will occur, especially when there is no warning (such as in an earthquake), what can a government do to better prepare its citizens for this eventuality? FEMA makes the following recommendations:

> **INFO**
> The mission of Citizen Corps is to harness the power of every individual through education, training, and volunteer service to make communities safer, stronger, and better prepared to respond to the threats of terrorism, crime, public health issues, and disasters of all kinds.

1. Present citizens the facts about what to expect following a major disaster in terms of immediate services.
2. Give the message about their responsibility for mitigation and preparedness.
3. Train them in needed life-saving skills with emphasis on decision-making skills, rescuer safety, and doing the greatest good for the greatest number.
4. Organize teams so that they are an extension of first responder services offering immediate help to victims until professional services arrive.

These are the four elements of a Community Emergency Response Team (CERT) program. The CERT

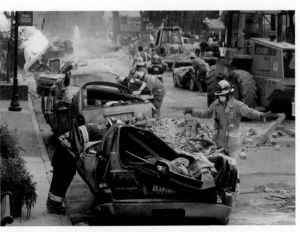

Figure 1–5 Major disasters can stress the EMS system to the point of breaking.

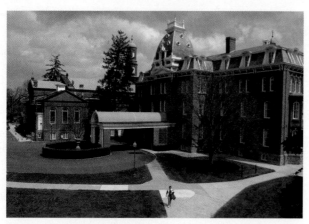

Figure 1–6 The National Fire Academy in Emmitsburg, Maryland trains many of today's leaders in disaster operations.

concept was developed and implemented by the Los Angeles City Fire Department (LAFD) in 1985. The Whittier Narrows earthquake in 1987 underscored the area-wide threat of a major disaster in California and confirmed the need for training civilians to meet their own immediate needs. As a result, the LAFD created the Disaster Preparedness Division with the purpose of training citizens, including private and government employees.

The LAFD program furthers the process of citizens understanding their responsibility in preparing for disaster. It also increases their ability to safely help themselves, their families, and their neighbors. These are the reasons FEMA was interested in the program and believed it applicable to all hazards. Today, the Emergency Management Institute (EMI) and the National Fire Academy have adopted and expanded the CERT materials to support a course taught nationwide (Figure 1–6).

The CERT course will benefit any citizen who takes it. This individual will be better prepared to respond to and cope with the aftermath of a disaster. Additionally, if a community wants to supplement its response capability after a disaster, civilians can be recruited and trained as neighborhood, business, and government teams that, in essence, will be auxiliary responders. These groups can provide immediate assistance to victims in their area, organize spontaneous volunteers who have not had the training, and collect disaster intelligence that will assist professional responders with prioritization and allocation of resources following a disaster. Since 1993 when this training was made available nationally by FEMA, communities in 28 U.S. states and Puerto Rico have conducted CERT training.

Other Organizations

There is no shortage of opportunities for Americans to help others through volunteering and getting involved with organizations that provide emergency assistance. The American Red Cross, AmeriCorps, and the Corporation for National and Community Service are all examples of organizations that can provide rewarding experiences for those wishing to get involved in emergency service and community support efforts.

SAR Terms

Rescue An operation to retrieve persons in distress, provide for their initial medical or other needs, and deliver them to a place of safety.

Search An operation using available personnel and facilities to locate persons in distress.

References

Air Sea Rescue Bulletin (July, 1946). *Evolution of SAR: An Editorial.*

Setnicka, T.J. (1980). *Wilderness Search and Rescue.* K. Andrasko, Ed. Boston, MA: Appalachian Mountain Club.

International Maritime Organization and International Civil Aviation Organization (IMO/ICAO). (1999). *International Aeronautical and Maritime Search and Rescue Manual, Vol. I. Organization and Management, Vol. II. Mission Co-ordination, Vol. III. Mobile Facilities.* London/Montreal: International Maritime Organization (IMO) and International Civil Aviation Organization (ICAO).

Chapter 2
Search and Rescue Systems

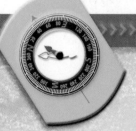

Objectives

Upon completion of this chapter and the related course activities, the student will be able to meet the following objectives:

As they relate to the SAR in the United States, describe the general roles of:
National SAR Committee (NSARC). (p. 13)
National SAR Plan. (p. 13)
National SAR Supplement to the IAMSAR Manual. (p. 14)

Describe the elements of the COSPAS-SARSAT system and the role an alerting personal locator beacon (PLB) plays in this system. (p. 11-12)

Demonstrate an understanding of the phrase, "All SAR is local." (p. 15)

List the major responsibilities for search and rescue for the following:
Federal SAR Authorities. (p. 13)
State SAR Authorities. (p. 15)
Local SAR Authorities. (p. 15)

Describe the general operational capabilities of a FEMA Urban SAR Task Force. (p. 17-18)

Describe three criteria for triggering an AMBER alert according to the National Center for Missing & Exploited Children. (p. 20)

Describe three steps a parent or childcare provider should take when a child is missing. (p. 21)

The Global SAR System

Working together, the International Civil Aviation Organization (ICAO) and the International Maritime Organization (IMO) coordinate, on a global basis, member countries' efforts to provide SAR services. The general goal of ICAO and IMO is to provide an effective, integrated, worldwide system that makes and keeps SAR services available wherever people travel. Pursuant to this goal, these organizations jointly developed the *International Aeronautical and Maritime Search and Rescue* (IAMSAR) *Manual*. A basic, practical, and humanitarian effect of having such a system is that it eliminates the need for each country to provide SAR services for its own citizens wherever they travel worldwide. Instead, the globe is divided into SAR regions (SRRs), each with a rescue coordination center (RCC) and associated SAR services, which assist anyone in distress within the SRR without regard to nationality or circumstances (IMO/ICAO, 1999).

International Stages of SAR Operations

The international SAR community has developed an approach to organizing operations not unlike that which has evolved in the land SAR community over the past several decades. This system is documented in the *IAMSAR Manual*. While SAR personnel working in an international environment may find this information useful, the land SAR community in general would do well to seriously consider adopting some or all of these internationally accepted and useful concepts and terms.

The *IAMSAR Manual* describes a series of five stages of a SAR operation through which most SAR events pass: Awareness, Initial Action, Planning, Operations, and Conclusion. The manual suggests that, "These stages should be interpreted with flexibility, as many of the actions described may be performed simultaneously or in a different order to suit specific circumstances"

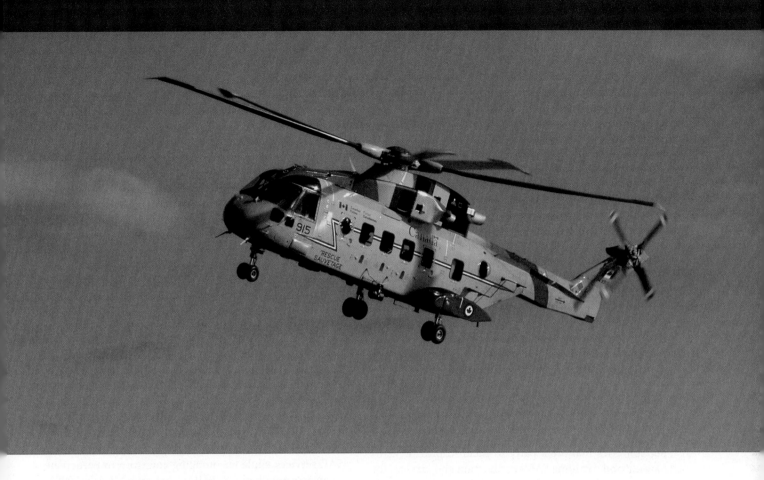

(IMO/ICAO, 1999). The reason the *IAMSAR Manual* does not have a "Preplanning" stage is twofold: First, the five stages of a SAR operation concern what happens in a specific incident. Preplanning can address types of incidents, but not specific incidents. Second, the preplanning function is addressed in what are called plans of operations or operations plans (OPLANs); see Appendix C of the *IAMSAR Manual* Volume II. These are "standing" plans for how to deal with various kinds of situations that may arise.

Awareness Stage

A SAR organization cannot respond to an incident until it becomes aware that someone is in need of assistance. At this stage, information is received that someone (or an aircraft or vessel) is, or will be, in distress. There may not be enough information to initiate action, or action may not be necessary, yet.

Initial Action Stage

When enough information is available, immediate action may be necessary. The first action is always to evaluate the information available, attempt to gain more, and determine the degree of the emergency. The "phase" of the emergency is used by the SAR authority to describe the level of confidence in the available information and the level of concern it raises about the safety of an aircraft or vessel and the person(s) on board. The

IAMSAR Manual describes three emergency phases: uncertainty, alert, and distress.

Uncertainty Phase – A situation wherein doubt exists as to the safety of an aircraft or vessel and the person(s) on board.

Alert Phase – A situation wherein apprehension exists as to the safety of an aircraft or vessel and the person(s) on board.

Distress Phase – A situation wherein there is reasonable certainty that a vessel or other craft, including an aircraft or person, is threatened by grave and imminent danger and requires immediate assistance.

An overdue aircraft, as an example, may be late for a wide range of reasons. The phases of the emergency allow those in charge to establish and communicate a summary of the available information that matches its validity, the urgency of action, and the extent of the response required. The *IAMSAR Manual* requires specific initial actions based on the established emergency phase.

Planning Stage

The planning stage is essential, especially when the location of the distress situation is unknown. "Proper and accurate planning is critical to SAR mission success; if the wrong area is searched, there is no hope that search personnel will find the survivors, regardless of the quality of their search techniques or the amount of their search effort" (IMO/ICAO, 1999). The *IAMSAR Manual* suggests the use of computers for operational planning, but also includes basic information on manual methods of planning searches.

Operations Stage

This stage encompasses all the physical activities involved in finding, providing assistance to, and rescuing people in distress. In short, this is the phase in which the plans are carried out.

Conclusion Stage

This stage is entered when it is determined that no one is in distress, when the search and/or rescue is concluded, or when nothing was found and the search is called off. This is the phase in which all SAR resources are notified that the mission is concluded.

International Agreements

International conventions, or written agreements between countries, are often what countries use to establish rules between them. The Convention on International Aviation, the International Convention on Maritime Search and Rescue, and the International Convention for the Safety of Life at Sea (SOLAS) all include rules requiring countries that are a party to them to provide aeronautical and maritime SAR coordination and services for their territories and territorial seas. Coverage of the high seas is apportioned among the member countries by these instruments as well. To carry out its SAR responsibilities, a country usually establishes a national SAR organization, or joins one or more other countries to form a regional SAR organization. In the United States, the national SAR organization is called the National Search and Rescue Committee (NSARC). NSARC is responsible for two documents: the U.S. *National SAR Plan* and the U.S. *National SAR Supplement to the IAMSAR Manual.*

While airborne, virtually all commercial aircraft on international routes are under positive control (i.e., followed by radar and in direct communication with air traffic controllers) by air traffic services (ATS) units. ICAO has linked ATS units into a worldwide system. Consequently, SAR agencies are usually notified very quickly when an international commercial flight has an emergency. Commercial aircraft on domestic routes and general aviation aircraft may not be under positive control, which can result in delayed reporting of their emergencies. 121.5 MHz is the international aeronautical distress frequency and is monitored by ATS, some commercial airliners, and other aeronautical facilities where needed to ensure immediate reception of distress calls. Emergency locator transmitters (ELTs) are carried in most aircraft and are required in most aircraft flown in the United States (see Cospas-Sarsat on page 11).

The IAMSAR Manual

To assist countries in meeting their obligations under certain international conventions as well as their own SAR needs, the three-volume *IAMSAR Manual* was developed jointly by ICAO and IMO (Figure 2–1). In short, the *IAMSAR* volumes provide guidelines for a common aviation and maritime approach to organizing and providing SAR services while encouraging countries to participate in an integrated, global SAR system (IMO/ICAO, 1999).

Each of the *IAMSAR Manual* volumes is written with specific SAR system duties in mind, and can be used as a stand-alone document, or in conjunction with the other two volumes, as a means to attain a full view of the SAR system. Volume 1, *Organization and Management*, discusses the global SAR system concept, establishment and improvement of national and regional SAR systems, and cooperation with neighboring countries to provide effective and economical SAR services. Volume II, *Mission Co-*

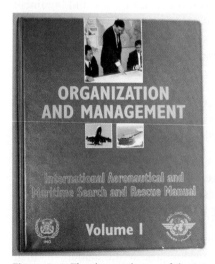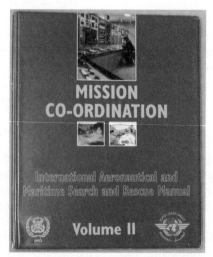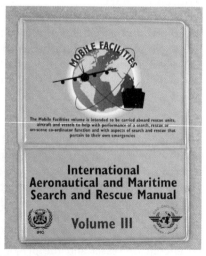

Figure 2–1 The three volumes of the *International Aeronautical and Maritime Search and Rescue Manual.*

ordination, assists personnel who plan and coordinate SAR operations and exercises. Volume III, *Mobile Facilities*, is intended to be carried aboard rescue units, aircraft, and vessels to help with performance of a search, rescue, or on-scene coordinator functions, and with aspects of SAR that pertain to their own emergencies.

Although no more details of the *IAMSAR Manual* will be offered here, it should be clear that this internationally accepted document has a great deal to offer those interested in all types of SAR, including land SAR. This manual describes concepts and methods that have wide applicability to SAR and makes an outstanding contribution to any serious SAR library. The three-volume *IAMSAR Manual* is available for purchase from ICAO and IMO.

Cospas-Sarsat

Cospas-Sarsat is an international humanitarian SAR system that uses satellites to detect and locate emergency beacons carried by ships, aircraft, or individuals. The system consists of a network of satellites, ground stations, mission control centers, and rescue coordination centers. When an emergency beacon is activated, the signal is received by a satellite and relayed to the nearest available ground station. The ground station, called a Local User Terminal (LUT), processes the signal and calculates the position from which it originated. This position is transmitted to a Mission Control Center (MCC) where it is joined with identification data and other information on that beacon. The Mission Control Center then transmits an alert message to

the appropriate rescue coordination center (RCC) based on the geographic location of the beacon. If the location of the beacon is in another country's service area, then the alert is transmitted to that country's MCC (**Figure 2–2**).

The SARSAT system was developed in a joint effort by the United States, Canada, and France. The COSPAS system was developed by Russia. These four nations banded together in 1979 to form Cospas-Sarsat. In 1982, the first satellite was launched and the first life was saved using the system. By 1984, the system was declared fully operational.

In the United States, the SARSAT system was developed by NASA. Once the system was functional, its operation was turned over to the National Oceanic and Atmospheric Administration (NOAA) where it remains today.

As the system began to take hold, more and more emergency beacons found their way onto the market. ELTs continued to operate exclusively on 121.5 MHz, but maritime beacons (Emergency Position Indicating Radio Beacons, or EPIRBs) were being built that operated on 406 MHz. The U.S. Coast Guard in its role as maritime search and rescue coordinator immediately began to see the benefits of 406 MHz, and in 1990, took proactive steps to bring it into widespread usage.

The Cospas-Sarsat organization also continued to grow. The four original member nations have, as of this writing, been joined by 31 other nations that operate 47 ground stations and 25 Mission Control Centers worldwide or serve as Search and Rescue Points of Contact (SPOCs).

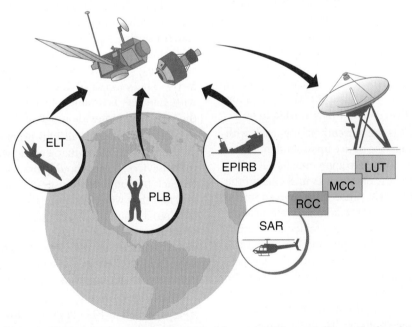

Figure 2–2 When a distress radio beacon is activated, the signal is received by a satellite and relayed to the nearest available ground terminal or LUT, which calculates the position from which the signal originated. This position is transmitted to a Mission Control Center (MCC) where it is joined with identification data and transmitted to the appropriate rescue coordination center (RCC) based on the geographic location of the beacon. The RCC then notifies the appropriate SAR response organization(s).

INFO
- COSPAS – (in Russian) Cosmicheskaya Sistyema Poiska Avariynich Sudov (in English, Space System for the Search of Vessels in Distress)
- ELT – Emergency Locator Transmitter
- EPIRB – Emergency Position Indicating Radio Beacon
- PLB – Personal Locator Beacon
- SARSAT – Search and Rescue Satellite-Aided Tracking

Distress Radio Beacons

The most recognizable component of the SARSAT system is the distress radio beacon, also known as a "beacon." There are generally three types of beacons used to transmit distress: EPIRBs designed for maritime use, ELTs designed for aviation use, and PLBs designed for use by individuals and land-based applications. Although the three types of devices are physically different due to the differing environments in which they must operate, they all work on the same principle and in the same way. When turned on, these devices transmit alert signals on specific frequencies that are intended to be received by Cospas-Sarsat satellites.

Emergency Position Indicating Radio Beacons (EPIRB) EPIRBS are for use in maritime applications and there are two types. One type transmits an analog signal on 121.5 MHz. The other type transmits a digital identification code on 406 MHz and a low-power "homing" signal on 121.5 MHz. All activate when submerged in water.

Emergency Locator Transmitters (ELTs) Emergency Locator Transmitters were the first emergency beacons developed and most aircraft are required to carry them. ELTs were intended for use on the 121.5 MHz frequency to alert aircraft flying overhead. A major limitation to these is that another aircraft must be within range and listening to 121.5 MHz to receive the signal. One of the reasons the Cospas-Sarsat system was developed was to provide a better receiving source for these signals. Another reason was to provide location data for each activation (something that over-flying aircraft were unable to do).

Different types of ELTs are currently in use, each with a "G" switch that activates the device upon sudden impact (high forces of gravity). There are approximately 170,000 of the older generation 121.5 MHz ELTs in service in the United States. Unfortunately, these have proven to be highly ineffective. They have a 99% false alert rate, activate properly in only 12% of crashes, and provide no identification data. In order to fix this problem, 406 MHz ELTs were developed to work specifically with the Cospas-Sarsat system. These newer ELTs dramatically reduce the false alert impact on SAR resources, have a higher accident survivability success rate, and decrease the time required to reach accident victims by an average of six hours.

Presently, most aircraft operators are required to carry an ELT and have the option to choose either a 121.5 MHz or a 406 MHz version. A 1996 U.S. Govern-ment study concluded that 134 extra lives and millions of dollars in SAR resources could be saved per year if only 406 MHz ELTs were used. Unfortunately, because 406 MHz ELTs currently cost nearly three times as much as 121.5 MHz ELTs, convincing aircraft owners to upgrade has been a slow process.

On the recommendation of the ICAO and the IMO, the Cospas-Sarsat Council announced in 2000 that it will be phasing out 121.5/243 MHz satellite alerting from the system. Users of 121.5/243 MHz beacons will have until February 1, 2009 to switch over to the generally superior 406 MHz models.

Personal Locator Beacons PLBs are portable units that operate much the same as EPIRBs or ELTs. These beacons are designed to be carried by an individual person instead of on a boat or aircraft. Unlike ELTs and some EPIRBs, they can only be activated manually and operate exclusively on 406 MHz in the United States. Similar to EPIRBs and ELTs, all PLBs also have a built-in, low-power homing beacon that transmits on 121.5 MHz. This allows rescue forces to home in on a beacon once the 406 MHz satellite system has put them within two to three miles. Some newer PLBs also allow GPS units to be integrated into the distress signal. This GPS-encoded position dramatically improves the location accuracy—down to the 100-meter level.

In the United States, PLBs were in limited use until July 1, 2003, after which PLBs were fully authorized for nationwide use. Prior to that date, only residents of Alaska in the United States could operate PLBs legally. The Alaska PLB Program was set up to test the capabilities of PLBs and their potential impact on SAR resources during public usage. Since March of 1995, the experiment has proven very successful and has helped save nearly 400 lives while generating only a few false alerts. The success of the Alaska PLB Program along with Canada's favorable experience undoubtedly paved the way for nationwide usage of these devices.

NOAA encourages all PLB users to be acutely aware of the responsibility that comes with owning one of these devices. Users should contact the NOAA to register each beacon prior to use. PLBs are a distress alerting tool and they work exceptionally well. PLB users should familiarize themselves with proper testing and operating procedures to prevent false activation and be careful to avoid their use in non-emergency situations. The proper use of PLBs is also an outstanding opportunity for SAR personnel to get involved in preventive SAR.

The Cospas-Sarsat specifications for 406 MHz beacons were amended in 1995 to provide for optionally encoding position information in the transmitted beacon message. Beacons with this capability are referred to as "location protocol beacons." Location protocol coding schemes are available to all user categories—maritime EPIRBs, aviation ELTs, and PLBs—and are compatible with all Cospas-Sarsat system components. Because location protocol beacons determine and transmit their location in the beacon message, they are able to provide rapid alerting and location information using the Global Positioning System (GPS) or other global navigation satellite systems.

SAR in the United States

A well-tested, comprehensive federal search and rescue system exists in the United States. An overview of this system and the documents that provide the foundation for it is necessary for a full understanding of where one fits into the bigger picture of SAR in the United States.

The United States National Search and Rescue Plan (1999)

The U.S. *National Search and Rescue Plan* (NSP) was developed primarily to provide guidance to signatory federal agencies (agencies who participate in the plan) for coordinating civil SAR services to meet domestic needs and international commitments (Figure 2–3). The federal government assists with the coordination of certain SAR services, including the coordination of any federal or military resources which may be requested by local or state agencies. Guidance for implementing the NSP is provided in the *IAMSAR Manual*, the *National Search and Rescue Supplement* (NSS, a domestic interagency supplement to the *IAMSAR Manual*), and other relevant directives of the plan participants (NSARC, 1999).

The National SAR Committee (NSARC) is responsible for coordinating and improving federal involvement in civil SAR for the aeronautical, maritime, and land communities within the United States. NSARC is also the federal-level committee formed to sponsor and oversee the U.S. NSP. Member agencies of NSARC are the signatories of the NSP.

Many U.S. states have chosen to retain established SAR responsibilities within their boundaries for incidents primarily local or intrastate in character. In such cases, agreements have been made between SAR coordinator(s) and relevant state organizations. For land SAR, the federal SAR Coordinator is the U.S. Air Force, which maintains a rescue coordination center (AFRCC) at Langley Air Force Base in Virginia. The relevant state organizations vary from state to state, but agreements exist between each state and the AFRCC.

The *IAMSAR Manual* and the NSP define a <u>SAR Region</u> (or SRR) as "an area of defined dimensions, associated with a rescue coordination center (RCC), within which SAR services are provided" (IMO/ICAO, 1999). An RCC is a unit responsible for promoting efficient organization of SAR services and for coordinating

United States
National Search and Rescue Plan--1999

POLICY

1. It is the policy of the signatory federal agencies to provide a National Search and Rescue Plan for coordinating civil search and rescue (SAR) services to meet domestic needs and international commitments. Implementing guidance for this Plan is provided in the *International Aeronautical and Maritime Search and Rescue Manual* (IAMSAR Manual discussed below), the *National Search and Rescue Supplement* (a domestic interagency supplement to the IAMSAR Manual), and other relevant directives of the Participants to this Plan.

PURPOSE

2. This Plan continues, by interagency agreement, the effective use of all available facilities in all types of SAR missions. The National Search and Rescue Plan-1986 is superseded by this Plan.

TERMS AND DEFINITIONS

3. The following terms and definitions are based on international usage for civil SAR. For more information about these terms and others commonly used for civil SAR, refer to the IAMSAR Manual, which is jointly published by the International Civil Aviation Organization (ICAO) and the International Maritime Organization (IMO).

Search and rescue coordinator. A federal person or agency with overall responsibility for establishing and providing civil SAR services for a search and rescue region(s) for which the U.S. has primary responsibility.

Search and rescue region (SRR). An area of defined dimensions, recognized by ICAO, IMO or other cognizant international body, and associated with a rescue coordination center within which SAR services are provided.

Search and rescue services. The performance of distress monitoring, communication, coordination and SAR functions, including provision of medical advice, initial medical assistance, or medical evacuation, through the use of public and private resources including cooperating aircraft, vessels and other craft and installations.

Rescue coordination center (RCC). A unit, recognized by ICAO, IMO or other cognizant international body, responsible for promoting efficient organization of civil SAR services and for coordinating the conduct of SAR operations within an SRR.

Rescue sub-center (RSC). A unit subordinate to an RCC established to complement the latter according to particular provisions of the responsible authorities.

Joint rescue coordination center (JRCC). An RCC responsible for more than one primary type of SAR services, e.g., both aeronautical and maritime SAR incidents. *NOTE: The term "JRCC" will not be used for civil SAR purposes solely on the basis that an RCC is staffed by personnel from, or is sponsored by, more than one organization.*

Figure 2–3 Page 1 of the U.S. *National Search and Rescue Plan.*

the conduct of SAR operations within an SRR. For every SRR, there is one RCC, and the goal is to have no overlaps or gaps between SRRs around the world.

In the United States, there are two types of SRRs: maritime and aeronautical. Although only the ocean areas surrounding the United States and its territories fall within the maritime SRRs, both the ocean and land areas of the United States fall within aeronautical SRRs (aircraft can fly over both water and land). The maritime SRRs surrounding the United States include, in the Pacific, Juneau, Honolulu, Seattle, and Alameda; and in the Atlantic, Boston, Norfolk, Miami, New Orleans, and San Juan. The oceans surrounding the United States and its territories also fall within aeronautical SRRs whose names and limits coincide with their maritime counterparts. However, with the exception of U.S. islands (Hawaiian, Puerto Rico, etc.) that are contained entirely within maritime SRRs and the Great Lakes (Cleveland Maritime SRR), all U.S. land falls within either the Elmendorff Aeronautical SRR (Alaska) or the Langley Aeronautical SRR (continental United States).

According to the NSP, a <u>SAR coordinator</u> has overall responsibility for establishing RCCs as necessary, and for providing or arranging for SAR services with U.S. SRRs (NSARC, 1999). The SAR Coordinators for the United States are as follows:

- The U.S. Air Force for the recognized U.S. aeronautical SRR corresponding to the continental United States other than Alaska

- The U.S. Pacific Command for the recognized U.S. aeronautical SRR corresponding to Alaska
- The U.S. Coast Guard for the recognized U.S. aeronautical and maritime SRRs that coincide with the ocean environments, and including Hawaii.

Although not considered a national SAR Coordinator, the National Park Service (NPS) is the lead agency that provides SAR and other emergency services within national parks. In small parks, this is often achieved through agreements with surrounding emergency service providers. Outside national parks, state and local authorities or SAR units often accept responsibility for providing domestic land SAR services.

Because of the unique scale and SAR challenges in Alaska, the U.S. Coast Guard is the lead federal agency for inland SAR in certain areas of the state, including the Alaska Peninsula (south of 58N), the Aleutian Islands, and all other coastal islands. The reason for this is simple: U.S. Coast Guard assets can respond much quicker than the U.S. Air Force Anchorage RCC to these areas. A division of the Alaska State Troopers is the state agency responsible for land SAR in Alaska. Due to the unforgiving environment, all federal, state, and local agencies work closely together in response to SAR missions in Alaska.

In addition to the specific assignments of SAR Coordinators, the NSP allows, "…local and state authorities to designate a person to be a SAR Coordinator within their respective jurisdictions" (NSARC, 1999). These local and state SAR Coordinators, if they are established, become important contacts for the national SAR Coordinators.

Participating Federal Agencies

The following federal agencies are signatories to the NSP and members of the National Search and Rescue Committee (NSARC, 1999):

- The agencies of the Department of Transportation (DOT)
- The Department of Defense (DOD)
- The Department of Commerce (DOC)
- The Federal Communications Commission (FCC)

- The National Aeronautics and Space Administration (NASA)
- Land management components of the Department of the Interior (DOI)

The National SAR Supplement (NSS)

NSARC also directs the preparation of the *National SAR Supplement* (NSS) (Figure 2–4), which provides guidance to federal agencies concerning implementation of the NSP. The NSS provides specific additional national standards and guidance that build upon the baseline established by the *IAMSAR Manual*. The NSS provides guidance to all federal forces, military and civilian, that support civil SAR operations.

Specifically, the NSS is designed to serve as both a training and operational tool for civil SAR operations. SAR planning is both an art and a science, relying greatly on the creativity and experience of the personnel involved. Because of the many variables encountered during SAR operations and the individuality of each SAR case, the guidance provided in the NSS must be tempered with sound judgment, having due regard for the individual situation. Very little in the NSS is mandatory because it is not intended to relieve SAR personnel of the need for initiative and sound judgment.

Each of the signatory agencies of the NSARC (and NSP) may also develop an addendum to the NSS for their agency. Such documents could include policies, information, and procedures on civil SAR matters applicable to the agency concerned, and consistent with both the *IAMSAR Manual* and NSS.

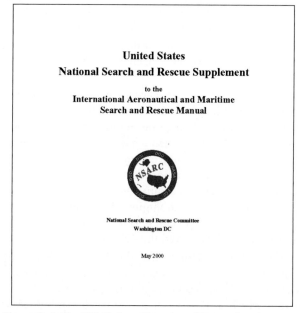

Figure 2–4 The U.S. *National Search and Rescue Supplement to the IAMSAR Manual.*

The U.S. National Search and Rescue School

The U.S. National Search and Rescue School is operated jointly by the U.S. Air Force and the U.S. Coast Guard at the U.S. Coast Guard Training Center in Yorktown, Virginia (Figure 2–5). The school provides two main search and rescue planning courses for the maritime and inland environments.

The maritime course provides training in oceanic and coastal search planning techniques and in the performance of duties as SAR Mission Coordinators. Instruction parallels the sequential stage and supporting components of the SAR system as organized by the *IAMSAR Manual* and NSS. The course is three weeks in length and upon successful completion, the student has the ability to manage and coordinate maritime/aeronautical SAR responses efficiently and effectively, including international coordination if/when required, and possesses a comprehensive understanding of the international SAR system. The program also teaches enough about search theory to provide the student with an excellent working knowledge of its application in the maritime and aeronautical environments. Attendance is generally limited to students requiring this specific formal training for their duties in RCCs in the maritime environment, and thus is not open to the public.

The five-day Inland SAR Planning course is advertised as a comprehensive, graduate-level look at search theory and its application to land and air searches for missing persons and aircraft with a focus on wilderness, not urban, searches. The course consists of classroom lessons and practical, tabletop exercises, and does not include field training. Emphasis is on the planning necessary for effective area-type searching during an extended search using specific elements of search theory to allocate limited resources to their best effect—in essence, what to do after initial tactics and resources have not found the

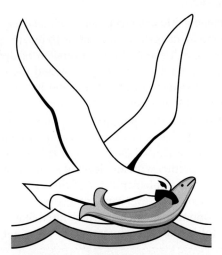

Figure 2 5 The National SAR School Emblem depicts an albatross rescuing a dolphin from the perils of the sea.

missing person. Additional topics include search area development, effort allocation, an overview of the Incident Command System (ICS), the federal role in SAR, and related subjects. The course does not teach search tactics or technical procedures and is directed toward federal, state, and local SAR leaders in emergency services and law enforcement, as well as Civil Air Patrol, and international and volunteer SAR agencies. In short, the course is meant for those few individuals who are responsible for the planning and overall conduct of inland search missions. The target audience includes on-scene incident commanders and their planners, operations leaders, and supervisors. The general searcher or search team leader, while arguably the most important part of the SAR team, would likely not find this course useful. Classes are held at various locations around the United States approximately ten to twelve times per year.

Comprehensive Emergency Management and Disaster Response

No discussion of any type of emergency service, including SAR, would be complete without at least a mention of the idea of comprehensive emergency management. In this concept, "emergency management" is an umbrella system that incorporates all aspects of dealing with emergencies and disasters.

Routine emergencies are daily situations faced by citizens and local emergency services personnel. For example, when fire fighters respond to a call, they are managing an emergency. When the EMS unit responds to a home or arrives at the scene of a traffic accident, the EMS unit is managing an emergency.

Emergency management programs at the local level are responsible for providing overall pre-disaster planning and other programs such as training and exercises for natural and human-caused disasters that can affect a community. They are the first line of defense in coordinating a large-scale event, such as a hurricane or an earthquake, in any community to ensure an effective response to, and recovery from, such events.

While responsibility for responding to emergencies and disasters begins at the local level, the next higher level of response (county, state, or national) is activated when resources and capabilities are exhausted. At the most basic level, if a homeowner cannot extinguish a fire, the homeowner will call the local fire department. If a local community is overwhelmed and cannot respond to a disaster, it asks the state for assistance. Similarly, when the state's resources are exhausted it will turn to the federal government for assistance. In the United States, this relationship is spelled out in the *Robert T. Stafford Disaster Relief and Emergency Assistance Act,* as amended (2000).

The concept used for handling all types of disasters and their consequences is called comprehensive emergency management (CEM). CEM was institutionalized in the United States with the creation of the Federal Emergency Management Agency (FEMA) in 1979. FEMA emerged from the consolidation of five federal agencies, each dealing separately with an aspect of large-scale emergencies. Since that time many state, local, and tribal governments have accepted CEM and changed the names of their organizations to include the words "emergency management." More importantly, the name change reflects a switch in orientation from preparedness for single hazards or narrowly defined categories of hazards toward an all-hazards approach—attack, natural, and man-made—to potential threats to life and property. The commonalities among all types of man-made and natural disasters suggest strongly that many of the same management strategies will apply to all such emergencies. In a real sense, planning for one means planning for all.

Homeland Security Presidential Directive/HSPD-5

On February 28, 2003, President George W. Bush signed Homeland Security Presidential Directive/HSPD-5. This directive established a single, comprehensive national management system to prevent, prepare for, respond to, and recover from terrorist attacks, major disasters, and other domestic emergencies. To achieve this directive, the Department of Homeland Security (DHS) was charged with two things. First, they were to develop a National Incident Management System (NIMS) to provide a consistent nationwide approach for federal, state, and local governments to work effectively and efficiently together to prepare for, respond to, and recover from domestic incidents, regardless of cause, size, or complexity. Second, the DHS was to develop a National Response Plan (NRP) to integrate federal government domestic prevention, preparedness, response, and recovery plans into one all-discipline, all-hazards, unclassified plan.

NIMS is intended to provide a consistent, flexible, and adjustable national framework within which government and private entities at all levels can work together to manage domestic incidents, regardless of their size, location, or complexity. This flexibility applies across all phases of incident management: prevention, preparedness, response, recovery, and mitigation. NIMS is also intended to provide a set of standardized organizational structures—such as the ICS, multi-agency coordination systems, and public information systems—as well as requirements for processes, procedures, and systems designed to improve interoperability among jurisdictions and disciplines in various areas.

There are six major components of NIMS that are intended to integrate existing best practices into a consistent, nationwide approach to domestic incident management that is applicable at all jurisdictional levels and across functional disciplines in an all-hazards context. These components are:

- *Command and Management* – NIMS standard incident management command structures are based on three key organizational systems: the ICS (organizational structure throughout an incident); multi-agency coordination systems (organizational structure of outside entities through assistance arrangements); and public information systems (systems for communicating during emergencies).

- *Preparedness* – This involves an integrated combination of planning, training, exercises, personnel qualifications and certification standards, equipment acquisition and certification standards, and publication management processes and activities.

- *Resource Management* – NIMS defines standardized mechanisms and establishes requirements for processes to describe, inventory, mobilize, dispatch, track, and recover resources over the life cycle of an incident.

- *Communications and Information Management* – NIMS identifies the requirement for a standardized framework for communications, information management (collection, analysis, and dissemination), and information sharing at all levels of incident management.

- *Supporting Technologies* – Technology and technological systems provide supporting capabilities essential to implementing and continuously refining the NIMS. These include voice and data communications systems, information management systems (i.e., record keeping and resource tracking), and data display systems. Also included are specialized technologies that facilitate ongoing operations and incident management activities in situations that call for unique technology-based capabilities.

- *Ongoing Management and Maintenance* – This component establishes an activity to provide strategic direction for and oversight of the NIMS, supporting both routine review and the continuous refinement of the system and its components over the long term.

HSPD-5 has the potential to cause significant changes to all phases of emergency response and management in the United States. As of this writing, it is too early to predict with any level of accuracy what the impact of a full implementation of this directive might look like. However, everyone interested in emergency response and management in the United States should closely follow the development of these important issues.

The National Response Plan

In Homeland Security Presidential Directive (HSPD)-5, the President directed the development of a new U.S. National Response Plan (NRP) to align Federal coordination structures, capabilities, and resources into a unified, all-discipline, and all-hazards approach to domestic incident management. This approach ties together a complete spectrum of incident management activities to include the prevention of, preparedness for, response to, and recovery from terrorism, major natural disasters, and other major emergencies. The NRP was published in November of 2004 and its full text can be found at www.au.af.mil/au/awc/awcgate/nrp/nrp.pdf. Excerpts from the NRP follow.

The purpose of the NRP is to establish a comprehensive, national, all-hazards framework for domestic incident management across a spectrum of activities including prevention, preparedness, response, and recovery. The NRP incorporates best practices and procedures from various incident management disciplines—homeland security, emergency management, law enforcement, firefighting, hazardous materials response, public works, public health, emergency medical services, and responder and recovery worker health and safety—and integrates them into a unified coordinating structure.

The NRP incorporates relevant portions of and, upon full implementation, supersedes the Initial National Response Plan (INRP), Federal Response Plan (FRP), U.S. Government Interagency Domestic Terrorism Concept of Operations Plan (CONPLAN), and Federal Radiological Emergency Response Plan (FRERP). The NRP, as the core operational plan for national incident management, also establishes national-level coordinating structures, processes, and protocols that will be incorporated into certain existing Federal interagency incident- or hazard-specific plans (such as the National Oil and Hazardous Substances Pollution Contingency Plan) that are designed to implement the specific statutory authorities and responsibilities of various departments and agencies in particular contingency scenarios. These plans are linked to the NRP in the context of Incidents of National Significance, but remain as stand-alone documents in that they also provide detailed protocols for responding to routine incidents that normally are managed by Federal agencies without the need for Department of Homeland Security (DHS) coordination.

The NRP consists of five primary components:

1. The "Base Plan" describes the structure and processes comprising a national approach to domestic incident management designed to integrate the efforts and resources of Federal, State, local, tribal, private-sector, and nongovernmental organizations. The Base Plan includes planning assumptions, roles and responsibilities, concept of operations, incident management actions, and plan maintenance instructions.

2. "Appendixes" provide other relevant, more detailed supporting information, including terms, definitions, acronyms, authorities, and a compendium of national interagency plans.

3. The fifteen "Emergency Support Function (ESF) Annexes" detail the missions, policies, structures, and responsibilities of Federal agencies for coordinating resource and programmatic support to States, tribes, and other Federal agencies or other jurisdictions and entities during Incidents of National Significance. The introduction to the ESF Annexes summarizes the functions of ESF coordinators and primary and support agencies.

4. The "Support Annexes" provide guidance and describe the functional processes and administrative requirements necessary to ensure efficient and effective implementation of NRP incident management objectives.

5. The "Incident Annexes" address contingency or hazard situations requiring specialized application of the NRP. The Incident Annexes describe the missions, policies, responsibilities, and coordination processes that govern the interaction of public and private entities engaged in incident management and emergency response operations across a spectrum of potential hazards (e.g., terrorism, catastrophic incidents, nuclear/radiological incidents, etc).

Implementation of the NRP and its supporting protocols will require extensive cooperation, collaboration, and information-sharing across jurisdictions, as well as between the government and the private sector at all levels. Much like with NIMS, the evolution and implementation of the NRP must be watched closely and has great potential to forever change the face of emergency management and response in the United States.

FEMA Urban Search and Rescue (USAR)

FEMA serves as the lead agency for National Response Plan's ESF-9 (Urban Search and Rescue) and, as such, coordinates the National Urban Search and Rescue Response System. As of this writing, the system comprises a network of 28 specially equipped and trained USAR task forces from locations across the United States that can be requested to provide assistance at large-scale, usually regional, disasters.

Anatomy of a USAR Mission (courtesy of FEMA)

While every USAR assignment is unique, a mission might go something like this:

1. Response always begins at the local level. Local rescuers always respond first. If the emergency is great enough, the state can request support from the FEMA task force.

2. Following the disaster the local emergency manager requests assistance from the state, the state in turn requests federal assistance, and FEMA deploys the three closest task forces.

3. After arriving at the site, structural specialists, who are licensed professional engineers, provide direct input to FEMA task force members about structural integrity of the building and the risk of secondary collapses.

4. The search team ventures around and into the collapsed structure shoring up structures and attempting to locate trapped victims. The team uses electronic listening devices, search cameras, and specially trained search dogs to locate victims.

5. Once a victim is located, the rescue group begins the daunting task of breaking and cutting through thousands of pounds of concrete, metal, and wood to reach the victims. They also stabilize and support the entry and work areas with wood shoring to prevent further collapse.

6. Medical teams, composed of trauma physicians, emergency room nurses, and paramedics, provide medical care for the victims as well as the rescuers, if necessary. A fully stocked mobile emergency room is part of the task force equipment cache. Medics may be required to enter the dangerous interior of the collapsed structure to render immediate aid.

7. Throughout the effort hazardous materials specialists evaluate the disaster site, and decontaminate rescue and medical members who may be exposed to hazardous chemicals or decaying bodies.

8. Heavy rigging specialists direct the use of heavy machinery, such as cranes and bulldozers. These specialists understand the special dangers of working in a collapsed structure, and help to ensure the safety of the victims and rescuers inside.

9. Technical information and communication specialists ensure that all team members can communicate with each other and the task force leaders, facilitating search efforts and coordinating evacuation in the event of a secondary collapse.

10. Logistics specialists handle the more than 16,000 pieces of equipment to support the search for and extrication of the victims. The equipment cache includes such essentials as concrete cutting saws, search cameras, medical supplies, and tents, cots, food, and water to keep the task force self-sufficient for up to four days.

The FEMA USAR Response System is designed to provide a coordinated response to disasters in the urban environment. Special emphasis is placed on the capability to locate and extricate victims trapped in collapsed structures, primarily of reinforced concrete construction. Typically, the following operations are conducted by FEMA USAR teams:

- Physical and technical search and rescue operations in damaged collapsed structures
- Emergency medical care to both task force response personnel and entrapped victims
- Reconnaissance to assess damage and provide feedback to local, state, and federal officials
- Assessment/shut off of utilities to buildings
- Hazardous materials surveys/evaluations
- Structural/hazard evaluations of buildings needed for immediate occupancy to support disaster relief operations
- Stabilizing damaged structures, including necessary shoring and cribbing.

Prior to the weapons of mass destruction (WMD) upgrade after September 11, 2001, the minimum personnel complement of a USAR type I task force would have been 62. With the addition of eight hazardous materials specialists (whose role is primarily detection and identification, not mitigation), this total is now up to 70 (this number assumes that one or more of the logistics specialists hold commercial drivers licenses, eliminating the need for separate driver positions; Figure 2–6).

To be sure a full team can respond to an emergency, task forces must staff all positions with more than one individual, and many staff three or four deep. So, each task force may include more than 150 highly trained members. These members are drawn from a combination of local fire departments, law enforcement agencies, federal and local governmental agencies, and private companies—a true partnership of local, state, federal, and private organizations. Each member of the task forces must be at least an Emergency Medical Technician-Basic (EMT-B) and complete hundreds of hours of specialized, intensive training. Specialties such as canine search, rescue, and rigging require training in addition to the cross training all team members must undergo.

A task force is designed to be self-sufficient for the first 72 hours of operation and to be able to function for up to ten days before being replaced. Members of the task force divide into two groups and operate in twelve-

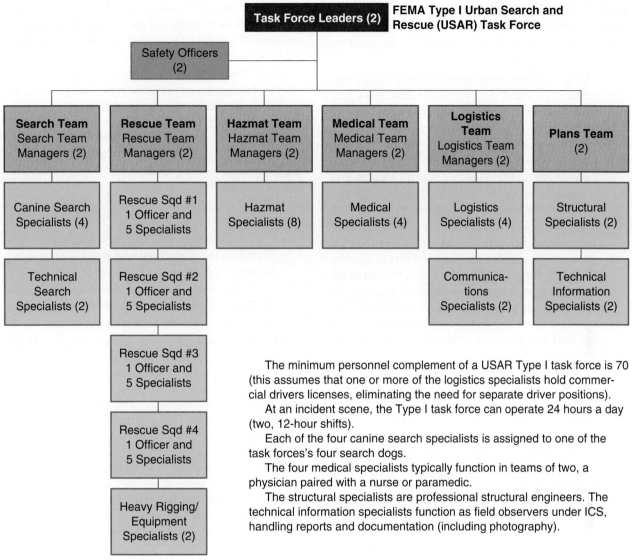

The minimum personnel complement of a USAR Type I task force is 70 (this assumes that one or more of the logistics specialists hold commercial drivers licenses, eliminating the need for separate driver positions).

At an incident scene, the Type I task force can operate 24 hours a day (two, 12-hour shifts).

Each of the four canine search specialists is assigned to one of the task forces's four search dogs.

The four medical specialists typically function in teams of two, a physician paired with a nurse or paramedic.

The structural specialists are professional structural engineers. The technical information specialists function as field observers under ICS, handling reports and documentation (including photography).

Figure 2–6 FEMA Type I Urban SAR Task Force organization (with WMD upgrade).

hour shifts on the scene. One group works while the other group rests. All task force members must be sufficiently cross-trained in their skill areas to ensure depth of capability and integrated task force operations. By design, there are two personnel assigned to each identified task force position for the rotation and relief of personnel. This allows for round-the-clock task force operation.

The equipment cache used to support this capability weighs nearly 60,000 pounds, includes more than 16,400 pieces of equipment, is worth about $1.4 million, and fills (including personnel) a military C-141 or two C-130 transport aircraft. The equipment cache consists of five types of equipment: medical, rescue, communications, technical support (over 500 items including fiber-

based cameras and electronic listening devices), and logistics (e.g., food, water, cold weather clothing, etc).

Each task force is designed to be able to be rapidly deployed in an emergency; hence all members must meet a six-hour window for mobilization. Depending on the location of the disaster, a task force will respond to the scene either by ground using its own trucks, or via a military or civilian aircraft. In general, an initial task force can be at the scene of a disaster within twenty-four hours anywhere in the contiguous United States.

When the task forces are not on a FEMA-requested response, they function as technical rescue teams in their own communities and, in many cases, serve as regional or statewide rescue teams.

USAR Canine (K-9) Team Evaluation/Certification

- Each FEMA USAR canine/handler team must be certified in search and rescue.

- For the handler, certification includes written and verbal tests regarding search and rescue strategies, briefing and debriefing skills, and canine handling skills.

- For the search and rescue canine, certification includes proper command control, agility skills, barking alert skills to notify rescuers of a find, and willingness to overcome innate fears of tunnels and wobbly surfaces under the guidance of the handler.

- There are two levels of certification for search and rescue canine/handler teams. Basic certification requires the search animal to perform to specific standards under the handler's direct supervision and guidance. Advanced certification requires the search animal to perform to those standards outside the direct supervision and guidance of the handler, and to successfully search more difficult rescue simulation courses.

- Canine/handler teams must be re-certified at least every two years in order to participate in FEMA search and rescue operations.

Miscellaneous SAR Tools

Two private initiatives can be of great value to SAR personnel when children are the subject of a search: The AMBER Plan and The National Center for Missing & Exploited Children.

The Amber Plan

The AMBER Plan is a voluntary partnership between law-enforcement agencies and broadcasters to activate an urgent bulletin in the most serious child-abduction cases. AMBER refers to *America's Missing: Broadcast Emergency Response*. Broadcasters use the Emergency Alert System (EAS), formerly called the Emergency Broadcast System, to air a description of the abducted child and suspected abductor. This is the same concept used during severe weather emergencies. The goal of the AMBER Alert is to instantly galvanize the entire community to assist in the search for and safe return of the child.

The AMBER Plan was created in 1996 as a legacy to 9-year-old Amber Hagerman, a little girl who was kidnapped while riding her bicycle and brutally murdered in Arlington, Texas. The tragedy shocked and outraged the entire community. Residents contacted radio stations in the Dallas area and suggested they broadcast special "alerts" over the airwaves so that they could help prevent such incidents in the future. In response to the community's concern for the safety of local children, the Dallas/Fort Worth Association of Radio Managers teamed up with local law-enforcement agencies in northern Texas and developed this innovative early warning system to help find abducted children. Statistics show that when a child is abducted, time is critical.

Once law enforcement has been notified about an abducted child, it must first determine if the case meets the AMBER Plan's criteria for triggering an alert. Each state program establishes its own AMBER Plan criteria; however, the National Center for Missing & Exploited Children suggests three criteria that should be met before an AMBER Alert is activated:

- Law enforcement confirms a child has been abducted

- Law enforcement believes the circumstances surrounding the abduction indicate that the child is in danger of serious bodily harm or death

- There is enough descriptive information about the child, abductor, and/or suspect's vehicle to believe an immediate broadcast alert will help.

If these criteria are met, alert information must be put together for public distribution. This information can include descriptions and pictures of the missing child, the suspected abductor, a suspected vehicle, and any other information available and valuable to identifying the child and suspect. The information is then faxed to radio stations designated as primary stations under the Emergency Alert System (EAS). The primary stations send the same information to area radio and television stations and cable systems via the EAS, and a message is immediately broadcast by participating stations to millions of listeners. Radio stations interrupt programming to announce the AMBER Alert, and television stations and cable systems run a "crawl" on the screen along with a picture of the child. Some states are also incorporating electronic highway billboards in their AMBER Plans. The billboards, typically used to disseminate traffic information to drivers, now alert the public of abducted children, displaying pertinent information about the child, abductor, or suspected vehicle that drivers might look for on highways.

National Center for Missing & Exploited Children

The National Center for Missing & Exploited Children (NCMEC) calls itself "The Nation's Resource Center for Child Protection." NCMEC provides services nationwide for families and professionals in the prevention of abducted, endangered, and sexually exploited children. NCMEC also assists law enforcement in the prosecution of the criminals who perpetrate these terrible crimes.

NCMEC is a more than 200-person, high-tech organization with global reach and, most importantly, success. Most NCMEC work is conducted, developed, analyzed, and completed on-site at its headquarters in Alexandria, Virginia, using state-of-the-art technology, highly trained professionals, and committed staff, interns, and volunteers. Two of the many services proved by NCMEC are Team Adam and LOCATER™.

Team Adam Named after Adam Walsh, the 6-year-old abducted and murdered son of John and Revé Walsh, Team Adam is a new resource for law enforcement provided by the National Center for Missing & Exploited Children. Patterned after the National Transportation Safety Board's system for sending trained specialists to the site of serious transportation incidents, Team Adam does the same thing in serious child-abduction and child-sexual-victimization cases. It is an on-site response and support system that provides assistance to local law-enforcement agencies.

NCMEC has identified an initial team of 20 specialists who are on call to respond directly to the scene of these incidents. The specialists are chosen based on their expertise and geographic home base to minimize response time and travel costs. Included in the initial team are retired FBI Agents and retired police officers from agencies around the country. NCMEC provides intensive training to ensure that each specialist is prepared to perform the tasks required in a uniform and consistent manner. The specialists work in full coordination with federal, state, and local law enforcement agencies. They advise, assist, and offer NCMEC's extensive resources, including direct access to NCMEC's case-management and case-analysis systems, lead analysis, and data-mining services. If needed, NCMEC also equips the law-enforcement agency with computer and communications technology to enable rapid distribution of key information to other agencies and personnel. They are prepared and authorized to provide additional assistance to the investigators, the victim's family, and the media as appropriate.

Team Adam is necessary because time is the enemy in missing-child cases. According to a study by the State of Washington's Office of the Attorney General, in 74% of child abduction-homicides the homicides occurred within the first three hours after the abduction (Hanfland, Keppel, & Weiss, 1997). Offenders who sexually assault and murder children can do so repeatedly. Rapid capture and prosecution is the best possible remedy. Rapid response is a key factor that correlates directly to the recovery of a child, who is still alive, after being taken by non-family abductors.

With 18,000 state and local law-enforcement agencies in the United States, some agencies may not be familiar with all of the available resources. Team Adam helps to ensure a quick and thorough response to these cases, helps to ensure that law enforcement knows of and has access to the best tools and latest technology, and greatly improves the odds of a successful recovery of the victim and prosecution of the assailant.

LOCATER™: The Lost Child Alert Technology Resource LOCATER (Lost Child Alert Technology Resource), is a cutting-edge software program that enables law-enforcement agencies to rapidly distribute critical images and information about missing-child cases. Using LOCATER, law-enforcement agencies create their own missing-person posters. High-quality copies can then be printed for distribution at roll calls, at incident command posts, and for distribution to the community. Posters can be transmitted electronically to other agencies, the media, and the public via the Internet or through a broadcast fax service.

LOCATER, including the software and help-desk technical support, is provided to law enforcement agencies free of charge. A limited supply of computer hardware and Internet services is also available for agencies that lack adequate equipment to properly run the software.

If My Child is Missing: Advice from The National Center for Missing & Exploited Children

Act immediately if you believe that your child is missing.

If your child is missing from home, search the house, checking closets, piles of laundry, in and under beds, inside old refrigerators—wherever a child may crawl or hide.

If you still cannot find your child, **immediately call your local law-enforcement agency.**

If your child disappears in a store, notify the store manager or security office. Then **immediately call your local law-enforcement agency.** Many stores have a Code Adam plan of action—if a child is missing in the store, employees immediately mobilize to look for the missing child. Some stores lock all outside doors until the child is located.

When you call law enforcement, provide your child's name, date of birth, height, weight, and any other unique identifiers such as eyeglasses and braces. Tell them when you noticed that your child was missing and what clothing he or she was wearing. Request that your child's name and identifying information be immediately entered into the **National Crime Information Center (NCIC) Missing Person File.**

After you have reported your child missing to law enforcement, call the **National Center for Missing & Exploited Children** on their toll-free telephone number, **1-800-THE-LOST (1-800-843-5678).** If your computer is equipped with a microphone and speakers you may talk to one of the Hotline operators via the Internet.

SAR Terms

Emergency Locator Transmitters (ELTs) An emergency beacon that usually operates on both 121.5 MHz and 406 MHz, used by most aircraft.

Emergency Position Indicating Radio Beacons (EPIRB) A distress radio beacon for use in maritime applications. There are two types. One type transmits an analog signal on 121.5 MHz. The other type transmits a digital identification code on 406 MHz and a low-power "homing" signal on 121.5 MHz. All activate when submerged in water.

International conventions Written agreements between countries, used to establish rules between them.

National Incident Management System (NIMS) A consistent, flexible, and adjustable national framework within which government and private entities at all levels can work together to manage domestic incidents, regardless of their size, location, or complexity.

National Response Plan (NRP) A comprehensive, national, all-hazards framework for domestic incident management that applies across a spectrum of activities including prevention, preparedness, response, and recovery.

Personal Locator Beacons (PLBs) Portable units that operate much the same as EPIRBs or ELTs. They are designed to be carried by an individual person instead of on a boat or aircraft.

Positive control The separation of all air traffic within designated airspace by air traffic control (FAA, 2003).

SAR coordinator The term given to the agency that has overall responsibility for establishing rescue coordination centers (RCCs) as necessary, and for providing or arranging for SAR services with U.S. SRRs.

SAR Region (SRR) "An area of defined dimensions, associated with a rescue coordination center (RCC), within which SAR services are provided" (IMO/ICAO, 1999).

References

Federal Aviation Administration [FAA]. (2003). *Aeronautical Information Manual* (AIM). Newcastle, Washington: Aviation Supplies and Academics, Inc.

Hanfland, K.A., Keppel, R.D., & Weiss, J.G. (1997). *Case management for missing children homicide investigation: Executive summary.* Olympia, Washington: Office of the Attorney General, State of Washington, and U.S. Department of Justice's Office of Juvenile Justice and Delinquency Prevention, May 1997.

Homeland Security, Department of [DHS]. (2004). *National Response Plan.* Washington, D.C.: U.S. Department of Homeland Security.

International Maritime Organization and International Civil Aviation Organization (IMO/ICAO). (1999). *International Aeronautical and Maritime Search and Rescue Manual: Vol. I. Organization and Management, Vol. II. Mission Co-ordination, Vol. III. Mobile Facilities.* London/Montreal: the International Maritime Organization (IMO) and the International Civil Aviation Organization (ICAO).

National Search and Rescue Committee (NSARC). (1999). *United States National Search and Rescue Plan.* Washington, D.C.: U.S. Superintendent of Documents.

National Search and Rescue Committee (NSARC). (2000). *United States National Search and Rescue Supplement to the International Aeronautical and Maritime Search and Rescue Manual.* Washington, D.C.: U.S. Superintendent of Documents.

Reaves, B.A., & Hickman, M.J. (2002). Census of state and local law enforcement agencies, 2000. *Bureau of Justice Statistics and Bulletin,* October 2002.

Robert T. Stafford Disaster Relief and Emergency Assistance Act. (2000). 42 U.S.C. 5121, et seq., as amended by the *Disaster Mitigation Act of 2000,* Public Law No. 106-390, 114 Stat. 1552 (the Stafford Act).

Chapter 3

SAR Incident Management and Organization

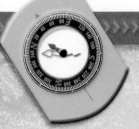

Objectives

Upon completion of this chapter and the related course activities, the student will be able to meet the following objectives:

List the five major sections within the Incident Command System and explain their primary functions. (p. 25)

Give the titles and explain the general duties of Command and General Staff members. (p. 25-26)

Match organizational units to appropriate Operations, Planning, Logistics, or Finance/Administration sections. (p. 27-29)

Match supervisory titles to appropriate levels within the ICS. (p. 29)

Describe the terms used to name major incident facilities, and state the function of each. (p. 30-31)

Describe an Incident Action Plan and how it is used. (p. 31-32)

Describe guidelines for the span of control within an incident's organizational structure and in the use of resources. (p. 25)

Describe the common responsibilities (general instructions) associated with incident or event assignments. (p. 32-33)

Describe several applications for the use of ICS. (p. 24)

Incident Management

Incidents must be managed in a systematic and consistent manner so that SAR personnel always know what job they are to perform, who they work for, who may work for them, who is in charge, and where resources are located. Improper management or poor organization can lead to inefficiency, ineffectiveness, and unsafe conditions for the subject and/or SAR personnel. An incident management system must meet the following needs:

- It must be organizationally flexible and work for all types and sizes of incidents.
- It must be usable on a day-to-day basis by all emergency response disciplines.
- It must work for small, routine situations as well as it does for major emergencies.
- It must be sufficiently standardized to allow personnel from a variety of agencies and diverse geographic locations to rapidly meld into a common management structure.
- It must be cost effective.

In general, this type of incident management system is called "All Risk."

One standardized, all risk incident management system is the Incident Command System or ICS. The ICS was developed by an interagency task force working in a cooperative local, state, and federal interagency effort called *FIRESCOPE* (Firefighting Resources of California Organized for Potential Emergencies) in the 1970s, but it is based in organizational methods that date back over 200 years. It was developed to organize and manage all the functions involved in any type of emergency incident. The ICS is used across the United States, many other parts of North America, and some other parts of the world. It is used to manage a wide range of emergency situations including fires, law enforcement incidents, searches, rescues, medical incidents, and regional disasters.

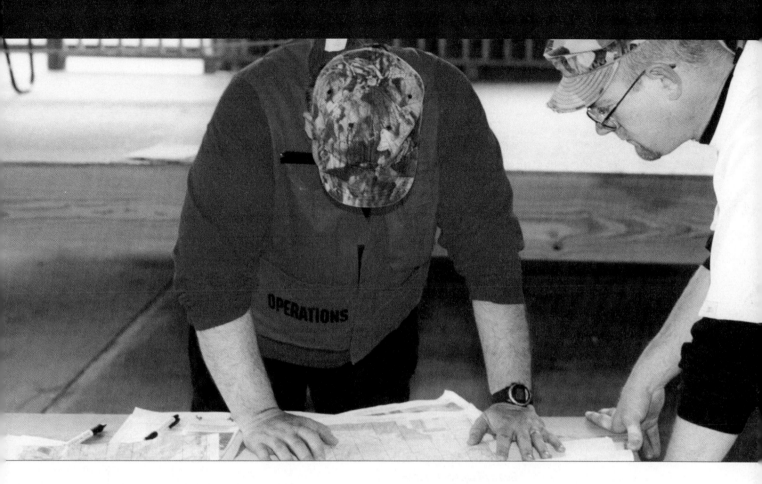

Primary ICS Management Functions

Every incident has certain similar activities or tasks that must be performed. The Incident Command System (ICS) refers to these as functions. The organization of the ICS is built around five major functional areas or sections:

1. Command
2. Operations
3. Planning
4. Logistics
5. Finance/Administration

All of these functions are usually performed at every incident, and a qualified person may perform multiple functions (Figure 3–1). At a small incident, or in the early stages of any incident, one person may perform all of these functions. Then, as the needs, size, and complexity of the incident grow, the organization can expand to adapt as necessary. In addition, each of the primary ICS sections may be subdivided as needed. As important management functions must be delegated in order to maintain a manageable span of control (3 to 7 persons according to ICS, but 5 or less is preferred), specific duties can be assigned to properly qualified individuals (Figure 3–2). However, a basic ICS operating premise is that the person at the top of the organization is responsible until the authority is delegated to another person.

Command Function

The command function provides overall management of an incident. In ICS, this function is carried out by the Incident Commander (IC) and the Command Staff (Figure 3–3). The Command Staff is made up of the Safety Officer, the Liaison Officer, and the Information Officer. Although these functions may be performed by a single person in a small incident, the IC may have to delegate these roles should a comfortable span of control be exceeded.

Usually, the person in charge of the first arriving units at the scene of an incident assumes the IC role. That person will remain in charge until formally relieved or until transfer of command is accomplished. As incidents grow in size or become more complex, a more highly qualified IC may be assigned by the responsible jurisdiction or agency. Even if other functions are not filled, an IC will always be designated. Initially, assigning tactical resources and overseeing operations will be under the direct supervision of the IC. As incidents grow, the IC may delegate authority for performance of certain activities to other qualified individuals as required.

> **INFO**
> ICS is the system used throughout the United States and many places around the world to manage all of the functions of an emergency incident.
>
> SARTips

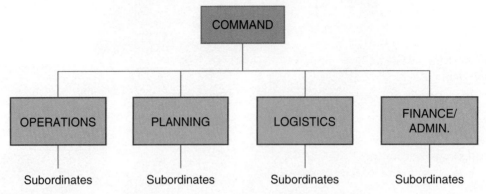

The Five ICS Sections
All of these activities are performed at most incidents

Figure 3–1 The five ICS Sections. All of these activities are performed at most incidents.

Maintain Span of Control at 1 to 5 or less

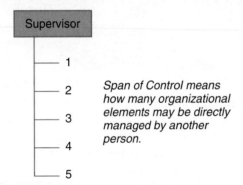

Figure 3–2 Important management functions must be delegated in order to maintain a manageable span of control: five or less is preferred.

The Incident Commander:

- Ensures effective management of the incident
- Selects an overall strategy
- Establishes incident objectives
- Approves the Incident Action Plan
- Coordinates and approves requests for resources.

Command Staff

In addition to the primary incident response activities of Operations, Planning, Logistics, and Finance/Administration, the IC has responsibility for several other important management activities and services. Depending on the size and type of an incident or event, it may be necessary to designate personnel to handle these additional activities.

Persons filling these positions are designated as the Command Staff and are called Officers. Each of these po-

Functional Hierarchy Including the Command Section and Command Staff

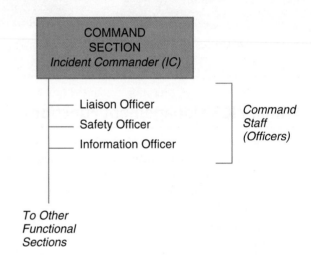

Figure 3–3 Functional hierarchy including the Command Section and Command Staff.

sitions may have one or more assistants if necessary. In large incidents or events it is not uncommon to see several assistants working under Command Staff Officers.

Safety Officer – This function monitors safety conditions and develops measures for assuring the safety of all assigned personnel.

Liaison Officer – On larger incidents or events, representatives from other agencies (usually called Agency Representatives) may be assigned to the incident to coordinate their agency's involvement. The Liaison Officer will be their primary contact.

Information Officer – The Information Officer will be the point of contact for the media or other organizations seeking information directly from the incident or event. Although several agencies may assign personnel to an incident or event as Information Officers, there will only be one incident Information Officer. Others will serve as assistants.

An agency or jurisdiction will often send tactical resources to assist at an incident. In ICS these are called assisting agencies. These outside agencies may also send an Agency Representative to work with the incident management team to coordinate between agencies or jurisdictional considerations. Agency Representatives report to the Liaison Officer. Other agencies such as the Red Cross or utility companies may also be involved in the incident, and are called cooperating agencies. Their Agency Representatives would also report to the Liaison Officer.

Operations Function

Operations is the term used to define all actions necessary to carry out the Incident Action Plan. In ICS, these tactical actions are performed collectively under one overall function that is carried out by the Operations section. As an incident grows in complexity and size, the Operations function is often the first function to be delegated. However, until Operations is established as a separate section led by a qualified Operations chief, the IC will retain direct control of tactical resources. The Operations Section Chief develops and manages the Operations section to accomplish the incident objectives.

There may be only one Operations Section Chief for each operational period. Except for the first one, an operational period is usually either an 8- or 12-hour portion of an incident. The Operations Section Chief is usually from the jurisdiction or agency that has the greatest involvement either in terms of resources assigned or area of concern.

Under ICS, medical care for the subject of a search and/or rescue is carried out by the Operations section, but medical care for personnel involved in the incident (e.g., SAR personnel) is carried out by the Logistics section.

The organization of the Operations section usually develops from the bottom up and may expand or contract based upon the existing and projected needs of the incident. For example, the IC or the Operations Section Chief may initially work with only a few single resources (Figure 3–4). As more resources are added to the incident, layers of organization may be needed within the Operations section to maintain proper span of control.

The first organizational layer used to maintain the span of control combines single resources into Strike Teams or Task Forces. A Strike Team is a combination of

Single Resources in the Operations Section

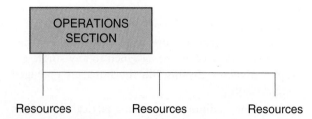

Figure 3–4 Single resources in the Operations Section. The IC or the Operations Section Chief may initially work with only a few single resources.

One Example of the Model ICS Functional Hierarchy

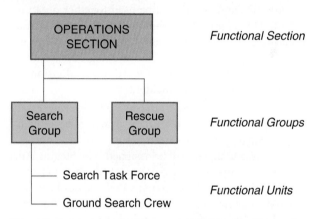

Figure 3–5 An example of the model ICS functional hierarchy. Functional groups are established to describe functional areas of operation.

a designated number of the same kind and type of resources with common communications and a leader. A Task Force is any combination of single resources within span of control guidelines, with common communications and a leader. During day-to-day SAR Operations this is the most commonly used organizational layer of management added. The goal is to keep the organization as simple and as streamlined as possible, and not to overextend the span of control.

The second layer of organization is accomplished by the Operations Section Chief who combines the single resources, Strike Teams, and/or Task Forces into functional groups and/or geographic divisions.

Functional groups are established to describe functional areas of operation (Figure 3–5). As the name implies, this form of organization deals not with geographic areas, but with functional activity. The kind of group to be established will be determined by the needs of an incident. For example, a medical group may be formed to respond to any injured person within an earthquake incident, or a rescue group may be used at a building fire scene. Groups will work wherever they are needed, and will not be assigned to any single geographic division. Groups, like divisions, are managed by supervisors.

A common method of organizing tactical operations at an incident where the incident covers a large area or is divided by a barrier is to subdivide it based on geography. When incident operations are broken down by geography, the resulting areas are called divisions. Divisions always refer to geographically defined areas, such as the area around a stadium, the inside or floors of a building, the east side of a river, or segments of a search area.

Divisions and groups can be used together on an incident. This approach is commonly used when a functional activity operates across divisional lines. For example, a specialized medical or rescue group would be used wherever required and moved across divisions as needed at an earthquake incident.

Staging Areas may be established wherever necessary to temporarily locate resources awaiting assignment. Once a Staging Area has been designated and named, a Staging Area Manager will be assigned. The Staging Area Manager reports to the Operations Section Chief or to the IC if the Operations Section Chief has not been designated. Staging areas and the resources within them will always be under the control of the Operations Section Chief.

While there may not be one "best" way to organize an incident, the organization should develop to meet the needs of the incident. The characteristics of the incident and the management needs of the IC will determine what organization elements should be established. The least number of management personnel possible should be used to effectively manage the incident.

Planning Function

The Planning section carries out the incident planning function. This section is responsible for the collection and evaluation of incident situation information, preparing situation status reports, displaying situation information, maintaining status of resources, developing a written Incident Action Plan, providing search investigation and planning, and preparing required incident related documentation. This is done under the direction of the Planning Section Chief if the IC has staffed this position. If a Planning Section Chief has not been assigned, the IC performs these functions.

The Planning section, if established by the IC, will have responsibility for several important functions (Figure 3–6):

- Maintaining resource status
- Maintaining and displaying situation status
- Preparing the written Incident Action Plan
- Providing documentation services
- Preparing the Demobilization Plan (large incidents)
- Providing search investigation and planning
- Providing a primary location for technical specialists assigned to an incident.

One of the most important functions of the Planning Section is to look beyond the current and next operational period, and anticipate potential problems or events. The Planning Section is also where any Technical Specialists assigned to the incident would report. Technical Specialists are advisors with special skills required at the incident such as map analysts, lost person behavior specialists, hazardous materials technicians, structural engineers, and the like.

Logistics Function

The Logistics Section is responsible for all of the services and support needs of an incident, including obtaining and maintaining essential personnel, facilities, equipment, and supplies (Figure 3–7).

The Logistics section, if established by the IC, will have responsibility for several important functions:

- Requesting all personnel and equipment
- Identifying and maintaining Staging Areas
- Providing all incident related receiving and stores
- Distributing all personnel, equipment and supplies

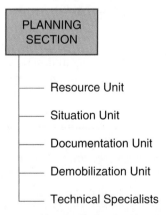

Functional Hierarchy for the Planning Section

Figure 3–6 Functional hierarchy for the Planning Section.

- Providing facilities for rest, feeding, and maintenance
- Supplying fuels, transportation, and repair service
- Providing and maintaining incident communications including providing equipment and personnel and managing a communications center if one is required
- Providing medical services for incident personnel (medical services for patients are provided by the Operations section)

Most incidents require much less than the full capability of the Logistics section. However, the Logistics Section Chief may establish separate subordinate units for one or more of the logistics support or service activities should the incident require it.

Logistics unit functions, with the exception of the Supply Unit, are geared toward supporting personnel and resources directly assigned to the incident. For example, the Logistics Section Food Unit does not provide feeding for people who have been sent to shelters during a flood. Under ICS, feeding at shelters would be handled as a part of an Operations Section activity. Food supplies would be ordered through the Logistics Section Supply Unit.

Finance/Administration Function

The Finance/Administration Section is responsible for financial activities that are required on site, and is usually only established in larger, more complex incidents. In shorter, simpler incidents, financial functions are usually carried out by financial personnel from the organizations represented at the incident. In incidents where no Finance/Administration section is established, the IC performs all finance functions.

In larger, more complex incidents, the Finance Section Chief will have responsibility for these important functions:

- Tracking payroll information (personnel hours)
- Investigating and processing claims for damage or injury to incident resources and personnel
- Maintaining cost records for purchased and leased equipment

Smaller incidents may also require certain Finance/Administration functions. For example, the IC may establish one or more units of the Finance/Administration Section for such things as procuring special equipment, contracting with a vendor, or for making cost estimates of alternative strategies.

Organization Terminology

At each level in the ICS organization, individuals with primary responsibility positions have distinctive titles (Figure 3–8).

PRIMARY POSITION	ICS TITLE	SUPPORT POSITION
Incident Commander	Incident Commander	Deputy
Command Staff	Officer	Assistant
Section	Chief	Deputy
Branch	Director	Deputy
Division/ Group	Supervisor	N/A
Strike Team/ Task Force	Leader	N/A
Unit	Leader	Manager
Single Resource	Use Unit Designation	N/A

Figure 3–8 At each level in the ICS organization, individuals with primary responsibility positions have unique and specific titles.

Branches and Units in the Logistics Section

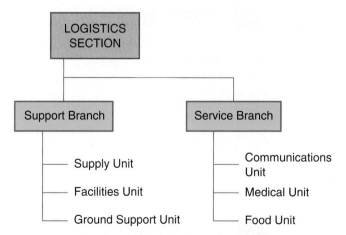

Figure 3–7 Branches and units in the Logistics Section. The Logistics Section is responsible for all of the services and support needs of an incident.

The use of position titles in ICS serves three important purposes:

1. Titles provide a common standard for multi-agency use at an incident. For example, if one agency uses the title "Branch Chief," another uses "Branch Manager," and another uses "Branch Officer," all for the same position, this can cause confusion and reflect the lack of standardization on the scene.

2. The use of distinctive titles for ICS positions allows for filling ICS positions with the most qualified individuals independent of their rank within their own organization.

3. The lack of standardization of position titles can also confuse the ordering process when requesting qualified personnel. For example, when ordering additional personnel to fill unit positions, it is important for proper communications between the incident and the agency dispatch facilities to know if they will be Unit Leaders, Unit Officers, supervisors, etc.

Common Terminology

In the ICS, common terminology should always be used for:

- Organizational elements
- Position titles
- Resources
- Facilities

Organizational Elements – There is a consistent pattern for designating each level of the organization (e.g., sections, branches, etc.).

Position Titles – Those charged with management or leadership responsibility in ICS are referred to by position title such as Officer, Chief, Director, Supervisor, Leader, etc. This is done to provide a way to place the most qualified personnel in organizational positions on multi-agency incidents without confusion caused by various multi-agency rank designations. It also provides a standardized method for ordering personnel to fill positions.

Resources – Common designations are assigned to various kinds of resources. Many kinds of resources may also be classified by type, which will indicate their capabilities (e.g., types of helicopters, patrol units, engines, etc.). For example, in ICS a vehicle that is used in fire suppression is called an engine. Recognizing that there are a variety of engines, a type classification is given based on tank capacity, pumping capability, staffing, and other factors.

SAR resources are also typed by their level of training, knowledge, skills and experience. (See Appendix 9 for the ICS glossary.)

Facilities – Each ICS incident facility serves a unique purpose and function, and has a specific designation.

Incident Facilities

Facilities will be established depending on the type and complexity of the incident or event. It is important to know and understand the names, functions, and unique purposes of the principal ICS facilities. These six facilities should be able to fulfill almost all incident facility requirements (Figure 3–9). Not all incidents, however, will use all facilities. An Incident Base, Camps, and Helibases are primarily used on larger incidents. However, specific applications may make use of other facilities, such as a triage center or temporary morgue.

Incident Command Post (ICP)

The location from which the Incident Commander oversees all incident operations and where the primary command functions are performed is called the Incident Command Post or ICP. All incidents must have a designated location for the ICP, and it can be located with other incident facilities. There will only be one ICP for each incident, including multi-agency or multi-jurisdictional incidents operating under a single or a unified command.

Some incidents may be large enough to have an on-site communications center to dispatch assigned resources. The communications center is often associated with or adjacent to the ICP. Also, some incidents will require space at the ICP to allow for various Command Staff and Planning Section functions.

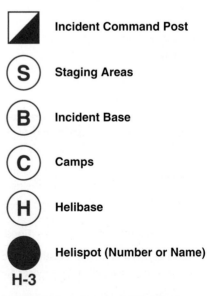

Figure 3–9 Map designations for ICS facilities.

Staging Areas

Staging Areas are temporary locations where resources are kept while awaiting incident assignment. Most large incidents will have a Staging Area, and some incidents may have several. All Staging Areas will be managed by a Staging Area Manager who reports to the Operations Section Chief or to the Incident Commander if an Operations Section has not been established.

There are many reasons for the use of Staging Areas. They provide locations for immediately available resources to await active assignments, and for greater accountability by having available personnel and resources together in one safe location. In addition, Staging Areas minimize excessive communications of resources calling for assignments, and allow the Operations Section Chief or IC to properly plan for resource use and to provide for contingencies.

Resources in a Staging Area are always in an "available" status, which means they are ready for assignment within three minutes. This is an important consideration for resource use planning and should be closely adhered to.

Incident Base

The Incident Base is the location at the incident at which primary service and support activities, including Logistics Section activities, are performed. Not all incidents will have one, but there will only be one Incident Base for each incident and it will not be relocated.

Typically, the Incident Base is the location where all uncommitted (out-of-service) equipment and personnel support operations are located. Therefore, tactical resources assigned to the Incident Base will normally be out-of-service.

Camps

Camps are temporary incident locations, within the general incident area, which are equipped and staffed to provide sleeping, food, water, and sanitary services to incident personnel. Camps differ from Staging Areas in that essential support operations are done at Camps, and resources at Camps are not always immediately available for use. Not all incidents will have Camps. In fact, very few search incidents ever need to establish a Camp.

Camps are separate facilities, and are not located at the Incident Base. They may be in place for several days, and may be moved depending upon incident needs. Very large incidents may have one or more Camps located in strategic areas. Camps are used when resources are required to travel long distances from their assignments to the Incident Base. All ICS functional unit activities performed at the Incident Base may also be performed at Camps. Each Camp will have a Camp Manager assigned.

Helibase

An area at which helicopters may be parked, maintained, and fueled is called a Helibase and is often located at an airport near the incident. It is very difficult, if not impossible, to construct a Helibase outside of an airport because of the many safety and environmental regulations.

Helispots

Helispots are temporary locations where helicopters can safely land to perform work supporting the incident. Large incidents may have several Helispots.

Incident Action Plan

Every incident needs a general outline or strategy that covers how the incident will be conducted. In ICS vernacular, this is called an Incident Action Plan or IAP. As a minimum, the IAP should provide incident objectives, guide operations, establish priorities for action, and describe the number and types of resources required. In shorter, less complex incidents, the IC may develop the IAP by him- or herself and never reduce it to writing. However, longer, more complex incidents may require that the IAP be written so that everyone knows the strategy and tactics being used. Although there may be several incident actions for each operational period, there should only be one Incident Action Plan per incident.

Essential elements in any written or oral Incident Action Plan are:

- *Statement of Objectives* – Appropriate to the overall incident.
- *Organization* – Describes what parts of the ICS organization will be in place for each Operational Period.
- *Assignments to Accomplish the Objectives* – These are normally prepared for each Division or Group and include the strategy, tactics, and resources to be used.
- *Supporting Material* – Examples can include a map of the incident, communications plan, medical plan, traffic plan, etc.

As part of the IAP, the IC should establish incidents objectives. Objectives are used to evaluate results and must be measurable (possess specific criteria for verification), "deadlineable" (time-specific), and describable (clear statement of exactly what is to be achieved). An example of an appropriate objective is, "Search segment 1 once with a dog team by 2100 hours." If these objectives are written, ICS form 202 may be used (see Appendix 7).

IAPs that include the measurable tactical operations to be achieved are always prepared around a time-frame called an operational period. Operational periods can be of various lengths, but should be no longer than 24 hours and no less than eight hours. Twelve-hour operational periods are common on many large incidents. The length of an operational period will be based on the needs of the incident, and these can change over the course of the incident. The planning for an operational period must also be done far enough in advance to ensure that requested resources are available when the operational period begins.

In ICS, an Incident Briefing Form (ICS 201) may be used on smaller incidents to record initial actions and list assigned and available resources. As incidents grow in complexity and/or size, ICS provides a format for a written Incident Action Plan.

Several ICS forms have been developed to help in preparing the Incident Action Plan. They are available in the *ICS National Training Curriculum* (1994) and a few examples are provided in Appendix 7.

Integrated Communications

The ability to communicate within ICS is absolutely essential. Just as every incident requires an Incident Action Plan, every incident also needs a communications plan. Like the action plan, it can be very simple and stated orally, or it can be quite complex, and form a part of a written Incident Action Plan.

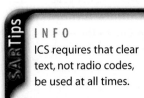

INFO
ICS requires that clear text, not radio codes, be used at all times.

An essential part of an effective multi-agency incident management system is for all communications to be in clear text. That is, ICS requires that clear text, not radio codes, be used at all times.

Resources Management

Resources assigned to an incident are managed in one of the following ways:

Single Resources – Single resources include both personnel and their required equipment.

Task Forces – A Task Force is any combination of single resources within span of control guidelines. They are assembled for a particular tactical need, with common communications and a leader. Task forces can be predetermined or assembled at an incident from available single resources.

Strike Teams – A Strike Team is a combination of a designated number of the same kind and type of resources with common communications and a leader. The number of resources to be used in the team will be based on what is needed to perform the function. Span of control guidelines should apply. Strike teams can be predetermined or assembled at an incident from available single resources.

The use of Task Forces and Strike Teams maximizes the effective use of resources, reduces span of control, and reduces communications traffic.

Tactical resources assigned to an incident will always be in one of three status conditions:

- *Assigned* – Resources performing an active assignment.
- *Available* – Resources ready for deployment.
- *Out of Service* – Resources not assigned and not available.

Common Responsibilities

There are certain common responsibilities or instructions associated with an incident assignment that everyone assigned to an incident should follow (**Figure 3–10**). Following these simple guidelines will make your job easier and result in a more effective operation.

1. Receive your incident assignment from your organization. This should include, at a minimum: a reporting location and time, likely length of assignment, brief description of assignment, route information, and a designated communications link if necessary. Different agencies may have additional requirements.

2. Bring any specialized supplies or equipment required for your job. Be sure you have adequate personal supplies to last you for the expected stay.

3. Upon arrival, follow the Check-in procedure for the incident. Check-in locations may be found at:
   – Incident Command Post (at the Resources Unit)
   – Staging Areas
   – Incident Base or Camps
   – Helibases
   – Division or Group Supervisors (for direct assignments)

4. Radio communications on an incident should use clear text, not radio codes. Refer to incident facilities by the incident name, for example, "Tallmadge Command Post," or "Main Street Staging Area." Refer to personnel by ICS title, for example, "Division C," and not a numeric code or name.

5. Obtain a briefing from your immediate supervisor. Be sure you understand your assignment.

6. Acquire necessary work materials. Locate and set up your work area.

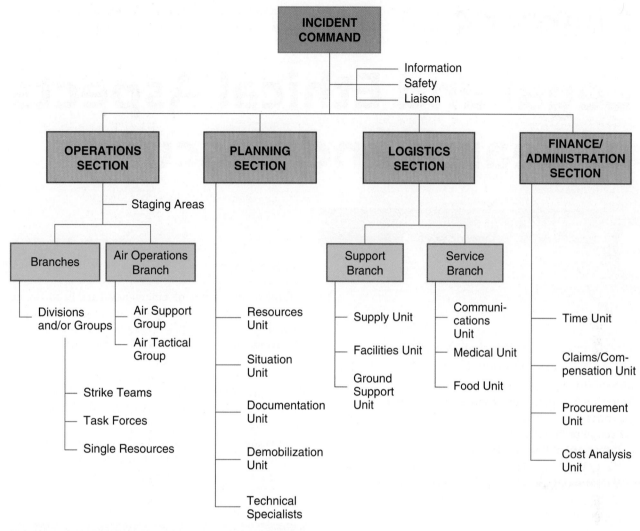

Figure 3–10 The Incident Command System (ICS) organizational model.

7. Organize and brief any subordinates assigned to you.

8. Brief your relief at the end of each operational period and, as necessary, at the time you are demobilized from the incident.

9. Complete required forms and reports and give them to the appropriate person before you leave.

10. Demobilize according to plan.

Incident An occurrence caused by either humans or natural phenomena, that requires action by emergency service personnel to prevent or minimize loss of life or damage to property and/or natural resources.

Incident Action Plan (IAP) Contains objectives reflecting the overall incident strategy and specific tactical ac-

tions and supporting information for the next operational period.

Incident Command System (ICS) A standardized organizational structure used to command, control, and coordinate the use of resources and personnel that have responded to the scene of an emergency.

References

Homeland Security, Department of [DHS]. (2004). National Incident Management System. Washington, D.C.: U.S. Dept. of Homeland Security, March 1, 2004.

National Wildfire Coordinating Group (NWCG). (1994). *The Incident Command System National Training Curriculum*, Modules 1–17. Developed by the Interagency Steering Group. Boise, ID: National Interagency Fire Center, Division of Training.

Chapter 4

Legal and Ethical Aspects of Search and Rescue

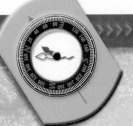

Objectives

Upon completion of this chapter and the related course activities, the student will be able to meet the following objectives:

Describe the relevance of the following legal concepts to SAR:

Scope of Practice. (p. 35)

Standard of Care. (p. 35-36)

Duty to Act. (p. 36)

Engendered Reliance. (p. 36-37)

Negligence. (p. 37)

Abandonment. (p. 37)

Consent. (p. 37-38)

Documentation. (p. 38-39)

Confidentiality. (p. 39)

Define "volunteer" according to the Volunteer Protection Act. (p. 39-40)

Describe the legal philosophy of a searcher entering private property within his or her community. (p. 41)

Do No Harm

A fundamental tenet of emergency care is to do no more harm. SAR personnel who act in good faith and according to an appropriate standard of care can usually avoid legal problems. But laws, regulations, and standards vary across the United States and from country to country, on all issues related to emergency response, including search and rescue (Figure 4–1).

Situations may also arise that require more than just knowledge of the law. Ethical questions can challenge

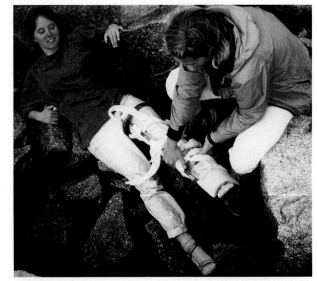

Figure 4–1 A fundamental tenet of emergency care is to do no more harm. SAR personnel who act in good faith and according to an appropriate standard of care can usually avoid legal problems.

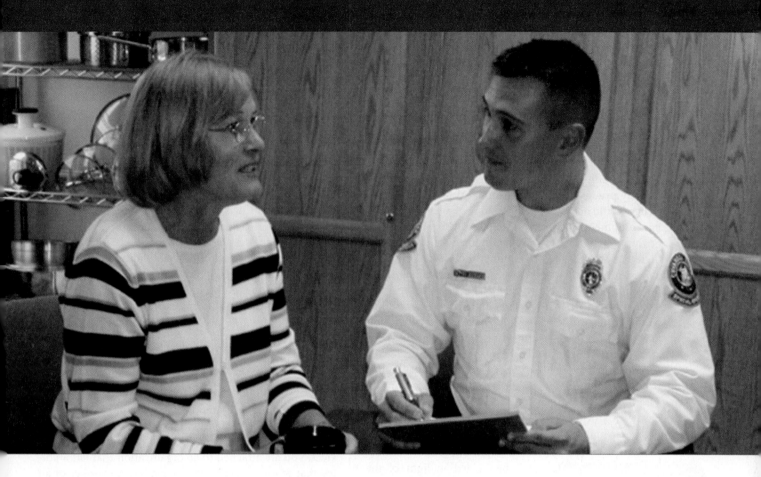

even the most seasoned SAR professional and must be anticipated as well.

This chapter is not meant as a substitute for competent legal council. Rather, it is meant to guide SAR personnel as they consider legal and ethical issues and serve as an aid to help develop questions to ask legal council.

Review of local and state laws cannot be a one-time task. Laws are often revised and technology, standards, news media, and human interests are constantly changing. SAR organizations and personnel should regularly review the relevant and applicable local and state laws and regulations. They should also seek professional legal advice when questions arise. Some states do not have laws related to SAR, and teams located in those states should research their legal position further prior to providing services to the public.

Legal Fundamentals

Some legal issues applicable to the provision of emergency care are so important that they are considered essential knowledge for all SAR personnel. Although a comprehensive overview of legal issues related to SAR cannot be provided here, some of the most important issues related to emergency services personnel will be reviewed in the context of SAR. SAR organizations and personnel have a responsibility to seek competent legal council when questions arise.

Scope of Practice

The scope of practice, or services a SAR organization is able to provide, is usually outlined by state law in the United States. If a SAR organization utilizes the services of medically trained personnel, such as emergency medical technicians, the care they render may be guided by a separate scope of practice. The important point to remember is that all emergency responders, including SAR personnel, have a responsibility to provide proper and consistent care and services that fall within their authorized scope of practice.

Standard of Care

All rescue personnel are required by law to act or behave toward others in a certain way regardless of the activity involved. Depending on the situation, one may have a duty to either act or not act. Generally, it is expected that when one's activities have the potential to cause injury or harm, he or she should be concerned about the safety and welfare of others. How one acts or behaves is called a <u>standard of care</u>.

Several factors influence the standard of care and therefore the appropriateness of one's conduct. Local customs, statutes, ordinances, regulations, and professional and institutional standards all have a bearing on the measure of one's actions.

By definition, the standard of care is, "…how a reasonably prudent person with similar training and experience would act under similar circumstances, with similar equipment, and in the same place" (Browner, Pollak, & Gupton, 2002, p. 67). Generally, medically trained individuals are expected to conduct themselves the same way as other individuals trained to the same level. But, for example, an EMT would not be held to the same standard of care as a physician. Similarly, SAR personnel would be held to the same standard of care as other, similarly trained SAR personnel and teams from the same area. Because these standards are often based on locally accepted practices and protocols, a SAR team in Virginia may be held to the same standard as other SAR teams in Virginia, but would not likely be held to the same standard as a SAR team from California, even if their training were similar.

In addition, one's conduct will be judged in light of the current situation (including all the likely confusion), the needs of those who requested assistance, and the specific equipment available. Local customs and practices help define the standard of care required. However, standards of care may also be imposed by statutes, ordinances, regulations, or case law. In many areas, violation of one of these standards is said to cause a type of negligence.

Professional or institutional standards may also come into play in addition to those imposed by law. Organizations and associations involved in SAR can establish standards of care that may be admitted as evidence in determining the appropriateness of one's actions. Any rules and procedures of a specific SAR team, service, or organization with which one is affiliated may also be considered "institutional standards." The state agency responsible for SAR may have regulations or directives that apply. State or regional SAR teams may have standard practices and procedures that apply. The *National SAR Plan*, the *National SAR Supplement,* the *International Maritime and Aeronautical SAR* (IAMSAR) *Manual,* and similar widely-accepted documents may have proce-

dures, policies, and/or guidance that may be relevant to determining the standard of care in any particular SAR situation.

As a minimum, the standard of care is "ordinary care"—the expectation that anyone who offers assistance will exercise reasonable care and act prudently. Anyone who acts prudently, reasonably, and according to the accepted standard minimizes any threat of civil liability.

To maintain this standard of care within the scope of your state's provisions, certification, and licensing requirements, it becomes necessary for all SAR personnel to acquire sufficient training and, during operations, never exceed the level of training received. Creating, updating, following, and training to accepted group training standards also minimizes exposure to liability.

Duty to Act

An individual's responsibility to provide care or services is called <u>duty to act</u>. This responsibility may come from law or be secondary to the function being performed.

For example, a bystander is under no obligation to assist a stranger in distress. However, there is likely a duty to act if you are charged with providing SAR services, you are attached to an organization that has a policy that requires you to act, or you are a member of an organization that represents itself to the public as providing SAR services. In these situations, an unpaid volunteer is no different than a paid professional in that once a mission has been accepted, arbitrarily refusing to act is no longer an option.

If you or your organization begins to provide services or treatment, you have a legal duty to continue. If you are out of your jurisdiction and come upon an emergency, you may not have a legal obligation to act, but you have a moral and ethical duty to act because of your special training and expertise.

It is also possible for SAR organizations to enter into agreements with local and/or state government agencies that oblige the organization to respond when called (often called a Memorandum of Understanding or MOU). This may constitute a duty to act. The requirements and ramifications of any such agreements must be fully understood by everyone in the organization.

Engendered Reliance

When SAR service "users" assume that a SAR provider will provide a certain level of service, it is called <u>engendered reliance</u>. As long as the expectations of the users match the capabilities of the providers, there is no problem. But if, for example, the capability of the SAR provider is reduced and the need for, and expectation of, the higher level or specific service remains, a discrepancy arises. If a SAR organization fails to provide the service on which the user has become reliant, the organization may be held liable for the discrepancy. For a number of reasons, some SAR organizations have advertised a higher level of service based on only one or two individuals' skills and abilities. The advertising of the increased capability may engender reliance on the organization and a level of capability that does not truly exist. This can be a legal problem.

Does your SAR organization advertise a service that it cannot realistically provide? What happens when your organization's ability to provide a service goes away, but the need for the service still exists? Is your organization obligated to find a way to provide SAR service for your area? These are questions to ask of legal council when you or your organization seeks to offer services for your response area. One way to help avoid these types of problems is to make sure your group has a clear, concise, and updated mission statement giving the public a realistic expectation of what your group can and cannot do.

Negligence

The outcome of even the best run SAR incident is always unpredictable. Unfortunately, the subject of a SAR incident can allege that the care rendered, or the rescue performed, was improper, inadequate, or negligent. Negligence is the failure to provide the same care someone with similar training and in a similar situation would provide. It is a departure from the accepted standard of care that results in the noticeable harm of another. The determination of negligence requires that all four of the following factors be present:

1. **Duty** - The rescuer had a duty to act reasonably within his or her training.
2. **Breach of Duty** - The rescuer failed to perform that duty and did not act within the accepted and reasonable standard of care.
3. **Damages** - The subject was injured or harmed.
4. **Cause** - The rescuer's failure was the cause of the victim's injury or loss.

The heavy burden to prove these four requirements is a strong deterrent against frivolous and unjustified lawsuits.

Abandonment

Abandonment is the "…unilateral termination of care… without the patient's consent and without making any provisions for continuing care…" (Browner et al., 2002,

p. 69). In almost all cases, once started, providers have a duty to continue care until an equally competent person assumes responsibility. Not performing this duty can harm the patient and may provide the basis for negligence. Abandonment can result in both civil and criminal actions against SAR personnel and should be taken very seriously.

Consent

Usually, the initiation of care for conscious, mentally competent adults requires permission or consent. If an adult is in control of his or her actions, he or she has the right to refuse care and cannot be treated against his or her will. Furthermore, treating a patient against his or her will may also be grounds for assault and/or battery.

Consent can be expressed or implied and may involve the care of a minor or a mentally incompetent person. Expressed consent is granted when a person expressly authorizes another— usually verbally—to provide care or transportation. This type of consent must be "informed." That is, the person granting permission must be made aware of the potential risks, benefits, and alternatives before giving his or her consent. To give expressed consent, a person must be of legal age and be mentally competent to make decisions. This consent may also be limited. For example, a person may grant permission for treatment, but not transportation off the mountain or to the hospital.

In a true emergency, when a person is injured and unable to provide expressed consent, or if a life-threatening situation exists, the law assumes the person would grant permission for treatment and transportation anyway. This is called implied consent and applies any time a person is physically unable to give expressed consent. In many situations, the law also allows a spouse or a close relative to give consent for individuals who are unable to give consent for themselves.

In most situations, a parent or legal guardian is required to give consent for the treatment or transportation of a minor. However, depending on the state, a minor may be able to be treated like an adult for the purposes of consenting to medical care if he or she is emancipated, married, or pregnant. Some states also allow minors to give valid consent for medical care depending on their level of maturity and/or age. Implied consent is the same for minors as it is for adults.

> **INFO**
> **Terms Related to Consent**
> Assault – Unlawfully placing a person in fear of immediate bodily harm without the person's consent.
> Battery – Unlawfully touching a person.
>
> SAR Tips

Regardless, consent should be obtained from a minor's parent or guardian whenever possible.

Incidents involving mentally incompetent adults pose problems similar to those involving minors because they cannot give informed consent. Therefore, consent should be obtained from someone legally responsible, such as a legal guardian. Because this is often not easy to obtain, many states have protective custody statutes allowing such a person to be taken to a medical facility under the authority of a law enforcement officer. Of course, if a true emergency exists, implied consent can usually be assumed.

Occasionally, forcible restraint may be required of a mentally disturbed individual before emergency care can be rendered. Often, if you believe that an individual will injure him- or herself, or others, state statutes allow you to legally restrain the subject. However, there will always be specific guidelines and procedures to follow to get this accomplished. For example, some states allow only law enforcement officers to restrain people who are a threat to themselves or others. Regardless of the specific state, SAR personnel must be thoroughly informed about local laws, and SAR organizations must have clearly defined protocols describing exactly how to deal with these issues. The thing to remember is that competent adults have the right to expressly refuse assistance, but this refusal should be thoroughly documented.

Documentation

Most legal experts agree that a complete and accurate record of a SAR incident is an important safeguard against legal complications. The absence of such a record, or if such a record is incomplete, may mean that someone would have to testify regarding the events and activities related to the incident from memory alone. In the face of aggressive cross examination, this could be inadequate or embarrassing, and could raise questions about the appropriateness of other aspects of the incident (Figure 4–2).

Courts in the United States consider an action or procedure that was not recorded as not being performed. They also consider an incomplete, poorly written, or messy report as evidence of incomplete or unprofessional care. To avoid both of these potentially dangerous pitfalls, actions and events should be completely, accurately, and neatly documented on appropriate forms. This type of comprehensive documentation can also be used to evaluate how well SAR personnel operated and managed the incident. This can be invaluable when seeking opportunities for improvement.

The requirement to document fully and properly must also extend to training records (both personal and

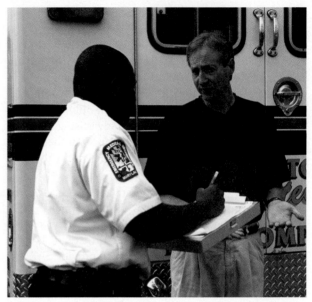

Figure 4–2 A complete and accurate record of a SAR incident is an important safeguard against legal complications.

team), equipment usage and maintenance records, and the documentation of any other requirements of SAR teams and personnel. If they are not fully documented, the assumption is that they did not occur.

The length of time that various records, such as training records, incident records, or equipment maintenance records, must be retained and how they must be disposed of are often addressed in laws or rules called Records Retention Schedules that vary from state to state. These schedules provide a description of the various documents and indicate the length of time each must be maintained as well as its ultimate disposition. Retention periods take into consideration local, state, and federal requirements as well as those of professional bodies such as accrediting and licensing agencies that may apply.

Documentation Tips

Here are some tips on how to record events effectively.

1. Use the correct form and write in ink, not pencil.
2. Write the incident number or name on every page used.
3. Record the complete date and time of each entry.
4. Avoid general and vague terms and expressions. Be specific.
5. Use standard, accepted abbreviations only.
6. Do not use a term if you are unsure of its meaning.

7. Document all actions and observations completely.

8. Document any changes to situations or conditions already noted.

9. Document protective measures used.

10. Document activities and procedures only after they are completed, never before.

11. When using a pre-printed form, write on every line.

12. Sign every entry.

13. Fill in omitted items as new entries with the correct time and date. Do not backdate or add to previously written entries.

14. Draw a single, thin, horizontal line through errors. Never erase them. Document the date and time of every change.

15. Be completely truthful in everything that is written.

Confidentiality

Communications between rescuers and a patient, especially if medical care has been rendered, are considered confidential and generally should not be disclosed without the expressed permission of the subject (patient). As a minimum, information that must be kept confidential includes the patient's medical history, treatment, and examination findings. However, any information pertaining to a subject's condition and situation, and indeed all incident-related information, should also be kept confidential. Even if the law does not require it, professionalism does.

SAR personnel must also be mindful of what they say during SAR operations. News agencies, interested parties, and family members may ask questions directly of field personnel, and these questions must be referred to the individual(s) tasked with responding to such inquires by the Incident Commander. Such inquiries deserve accurate and complete responses, and SAR field personnel are frequently not in the best position to provide the best answers.

Laws that Affect SAR Personnel

The purpose of some of these laws is to encourage individuals who otherwise do not have a duty to act to assist others without the fear of lawsuits. The actual language of these laws varies greatly from state to state, but many apply to anyone who might offer assistance in an emergency. Other laws protect the patient. Laws that protect the responder do not prevent frivolous lawsuits from being filed, but they do make it more difficult for plaintiffs to prevail when care was rendered in good faith, with consent and within the scope of the volunteer's training.

Good Samaritan Laws

Good Samaritan laws have been passed in most states in the United States. They are based on the principle that when one person provides reasonable help to another, the helper should not be liable for errors and omissions that are made when the care is provided in good faith. Some requirements of the application of these laws usually include that the care was given in good faith, it was given without compensation, and the caregiver did not exceed his or her medical training or license. However, these laws do not prevent one from being sued. They just provide an affirmative defense should one get sued for rendering care.

Laws that grant immunity to official providers of emergency care, such as fire fighters and emergency medical technicians, exist in some states but they vary widely from state to state. In all cases, these types of laws do not protect any care provider from the willful or wanton failure to exercise due care that is characterized by gross negligence.

Since these laws vary from state to state, the applicability of these laws to volunteer SAR personnel and organizations should be investigated thoroughly at the local and state levels.

Volunteer Protection Act of 1997

On June 18, 1997, the Volunteer Protection Act (VPA) was enacted into law by the U.S. Congress (111 Stat. 218). The purpose of the act is to limit lawsuits against volunteers serving nonprofit public and private organizations and governmental agencies. The VPA was enacted in response to volunteers withdrawing from service to nonprofit organizations because of concerns about liability. By limiting lawsuits against such volunteers, it was thought that the number of volunteers would increase, thus promoting the ability of nonprofit organizations and governmental entities to provide services at a reasonable cost.

Selected Definitions from the Volunteer Protection Act of 1997

The term "volunteer" means an individual performing services for a nonprofit organization or a governmental entity who does not receive:

a. compensation (other than reasonable reimbursement or allowance for expenses actually incurred); or

b. any other thing of value in lieu of compensation, in excess of $500 per year, and such term includes a volunteer serving as a director, officer, trustee, or direct service volunteer.

The term "nonprofit organization" means:

a. any organization which is described in section 501(c)(3) of the Internal Revenue Code of 1986 and exempt from tax under section 501(a) of such Code and which does not practice any action which constitutes a hate crime referred to in subsection (b)(1) of the first section of the Hate Crime Statistics Act (28 U.S.C. 534 note); or

b. any not-for-profit organization which is organized and conducted for public benefit and operated primarily for charitable, civic, educational, religious, welfare, or health purposes and which does not practice any action which constitutes a hate crime referred to in subsection (b)(1) of the first section of the Hate Crime Statistics Act (28 U.S.C. 534 note).

It is important to note that the VPA does not limit the potential liability of nonprofit organizations. Rather, the VPA was intended to protect the individual volunteer from litigation. In addition, common law will hold nonprofit organizations liable for the negligence of its volunteers, even if that volunteer enjoys immunity under the VPA or similar state law.

To make the most of the protection provided by the VPA, clear direction must be provided to volunteers, including defining the scope of each volunteer's authority. For the VPA to apply, four requirements must be met. Volunteers must:

1. Be acting within their scope of responsibility in their organization.
2. Be properly licensed or certified (i.e., authorized).
3. Not cause harm by gross negligence or any similarly inappropriate type of misconduct.
4. Not cause harm by the operation of a motor vehicle, aircraft, or other vehicle for which an operator's license or insurance is required by the state.

Although the VPA preempts state statute where "such laws are inconsistent with the act," except where state laws provide better or additional coverage, there are ways that states can preempt or restrict parts or all of this law for their area based on certain criteria. SAR volunteers and organizations that use volunteers must research carefully and know how the law applies to them in their respective states.

Health Insurance Portability and Accountability Act of 1996 (HIPAA)

The Health Insurance Portability and Accountability Act (HIPAA) of 1996 took effect in the United States on April 14, 2003. It is the first-ever set of federal privacy standards to protect patients' medical records and other health information provided to health plans, doctors, hospitals, and other health care providers. Developed by the U.S. Department of Health and Human Services (HHS), these new standards provide patients with access to their medical records and more control over how their personal health information is used and disclosed. They represent a uniform, federal floor of privacy protections for consumers across the country. State laws providing additional protections to consumers are not affected by this new rule.

HIPAA included provisions designed to encourage electronic transactions and also required new safeguards to protect the security and confidentiality of health information. The final regulation covers health plans, health care clearinghouses, and those health care providers who conduct certain financial and administrative transactions (e.g., enrollment, billing, and eligibility verification) electronically. Most health insurers, pharmacies, doctors, and other health care providers are now required to comply with these federal standards.

Although SAR personnel and organizations are not specifically mentioned in the law, there is a possibility that the strict requirements of this law could apply to both. It is important that SAR organizations obtain legal council regarding how this might affect their group and operations. On the issue of whether your organization is a "covered entity" (i.e., HIPAA applies), Wirth & Wolfberg (2003) offer some sound advice.

> Even if your service is not a covered entity, it is still important to have strict policies on confidentially of patient information and procedures for release of patient care reports. HIPAA will likely become a "standard of care" when it comes to patient privacy, so even if you aren't covered under the law, [a group should] institute reasonable safeguards that are similar to the HIPAA Privacy rule to ensure that you are following the best practices possible. Establish basic policies and educate all squad [group] members on the importance of following the Golden Rule of HIPAA in your . . . squad: "What You Hear Here, What You See Here, When You Leave Here, Let it Stay Here!"

In addition to federal laws, there are many state and local laws that affect SAR personnel and organizations. Laws and protocols are often very different from state to state or even jurisdiction to jurisdiction, and this can present special challenges for SAR responders responding to those areas. In all cases, SAR groups must do their homework and research the laws for their areas of responsibility to know exactly how they will be affected.

Other Legal Considerations

SAR personnel usually have no more right to trespass than anyone else. But, an understanding of what constitutes trespassing, how to avoid it, and when it is not an issue is important to staying out of legal trouble.

Because everything discovered at a SAR incident should be treated as if it were evidence of a crime, some understanding of the legal responsibilities of SAR personnel at the scene where evidence or a subject is found is also important.

Trespassing

Trespassing is the act of passing beyond a boundary onto one's property (land) without the owner's permission. Property owners usually convey their interest in preventing trespassing by posting a sign that clearly states "No Trespassing." In SAR, a searcher might be trespassing if he or she travels on or across property without proper permission. Generally, SAR personnel have no more right to trespass than anyone else, but there may be some exceptions.

Trespassing falls into three general categories:

1. *Criminal trespass,* where someone willfully enters property that he or she knows has been posted "No Trespassing."
2. *Innocent trespass,* where someone enters the property in such a way that he or she is unaware that the land is posted.
3. *Trespass to save a life,* where someone is able to see a person in distress on the posted property and justify the trespass.

Before traveling onto private property, it is always advisable to obtain permission from the property owner. If permission is denied, entry should not be made, and the refusal must be documented and reported to the Incident Commander. In most cases, a call by the local law enforcement agency is sufficient to convince a landowner to permit SAR personnel to access the property, but a search warrant may occasionally be necessary.

If a landowner asks searchers to leave, even if the property is not "posted," searchers must honor the request. You can minimize problems by including uniformed law enforcement officers on a team that may need to cross posted property.

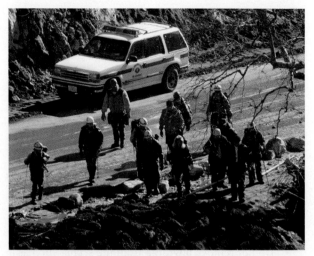

Figure 4–3 SAR personnel arriving first on the scene have a responsibility to secure the area and prevent others from contaminating or modifying evidence.

Incident Site Procedures

Because "what happened?" is a question that will always be asked after an incident, and because a crime could have been committed, everything discovered at a SAR incident should be treated as if it were evidence of a crime. By following a few simple rules, the chances of preserving evidence and maintaining the chain of custody can be maximized.

Secure the Area

SAR personnel arriving first on the scene have a responsibility to secure the area and prevent others from contaminating or modifying evidence. Toward this end, the area should be cordoned off as best as possible and access to the immediate area should be controlled. Of course, care must be provided to injured subjects, but beyond this nothing should be disturbed. In addition, anything that was changed by the treatment of injuries should be noted (**Figure 4–3**).

Document the Scene

After securing the scene and controlling access, someone on site should fully document the scene including anything added, removed, moved, or changed by SAR personnel, even if it was unintentional. This process, however, should not delay summoning the responsible law enforcement agency to the scene (if not already there) to accept responsibility for the scene from SAR personnel. The scene should not be vacated for any purpose after it is secured or it could affect the acceptability of certain evidence. Once established, someone should always retain control over the scene to maintain the chain of custody.

Preserve the Scene

Carter (2002) described a useful set of guidelines for preserving the scene at a SAR incident, which is paraphrased below.

- If the subject(s) appears to be dead when first approached, do the minimum possible to confirm death.
- If the subject is hanging, do not cut down.
- If there is a firearm present, use caution; it may be cocked and have a live round in the chamber. Many weapons chamber a new round after firing and are immediately ready to fire again.
- Do not add anything to the scene, such as cigarette butts, candy wrappers, or scrap paper.
- Do not remove anything from the scene, such as a weapon or the subject's wallet.
- Document the scene exactly with notes, sketches, and photographs. Note any additions, deletions, or alterations (your footprints are additions). Photograph from at least four angles. Investigating authorities will confiscate all notes.
- Note the date and time for all actions and the names and functions of all people present.
- If you are the first on scene, you are responsible for scene security. Do not leave until relieved by a properly identified law enforcement officer. Always get a signed receipt for the scene. It may be necessary to prove later that you were properly relieved.
- Always remember that you may have to testify in court as to what you saw, what you did, and why you did it.

Specific information about handling evidence is in Chapter 14, Search: Background and Related Issues.

General Suggestions

It is impossible to summarize all relevant aspects of the law as it relates to SAR in this text. However, following some simple suggestions can minimize both liability and legal challenges:

1. Do not work in constant fear of being sued. Knowing your job and doing it well go a long way toward minimizing liability.
2. Always act in good faith and according to an appropriate standard of care. Do what you know you should.
3. Seek professional legal advice when specific legal questions arise.
4. Provide proper and consistent care at all times. Treat everyone with the same high level of care.
5. Become familiar with the standard of care in your area. At a minimum, act prudently, reasonably, and according to the accepted standard.
6. Acquire sufficient and appropriate training and, during operations, never exceed the level of training received.
7. Keep training up to date.
8. Become and stay familiar with any local and state agreements entered into by your organization.
9. Do not advertise or suggest a higher level of capability than you or your organization can realistically provide.
10. Once started, continue care until properly relieved.
11. Become familiar with the various types of consent and receive consent before providing care and/or transportation.

12. Maintain and become familiar with the local protocol that describes how to deal with situations that may require forcible restraint.

13. Fully and properly document the following: all activities and observations at a SAR incident, all training (both personal and team), and all equipment usage and maintenance.

14. Treat all information related to a SAR incident as confidential.

15. Become familiar with, and abide by, Good Samaritan laws, the Volunteer Protection Act, HIPAA, and other local, state, and federal laws that affect SAR personnel in your area.

16. Become and stay familiar with the procedures used locally in handling evidence at a SAR incident site.

SAR Terms

Abandonment The unilateral termination of care without the patient's consent and without making any provisions for continuing care.

Duty to Act An individual's responsibility to provide care or services. This responsibility may come from law or be secondary to the function being performed.

Engendered reliance The assumption by SAR service "users" that a SAR provider will provide a certain level of service.

Expressed consent Granted when a person expressly authorizes another—usually verbally—to provide care or transportation.

Good Samaritan Laws Laws that limit liability when one person provides reasonable help to another in good faith.

Implied consent When a person is injured and unable to provide expressed consent, the law assumes the person would grant permission for treatment and transportation anyway.

Negligence The failure to provide the same care someone with similar training and in a similar situation would provide.

Standard of care How a reasonably prudent person with similar training and experience would act under similar circumstances, with similar equipment, and in the same place.

Trespassing The act of passing beyond a boundary onto one's property without the owner's permission.

References

Browner, B., Pollak, A., & Gupton, C., Eds. (2002). *Emergency Care of the Sick and Injured*. American Academy of Orthopaedic Surgeons. Sudbury, MA: Jones and Bartlett Publishers.

California Department of Forestry. (1983). *Field Operations Guide ICS 420-1*. Stillwater, OK: Fire Protections Publications, Oklahoma State University.

Carter, D. (2002). *Field Team Member Manual*, 4th Ed. W. White, M. Pennington, & R. Glen, Eds. Ruthers Glen, Virginia: Search and Rescue Training Associates, Inc.

United State Congress. (1997). *Volunteer Protection Act of 1997*. Text, 105th Congress, 1st Session. Public Law 105-19. Washington, D.C. Retrieved on 15 August 2003 from http://www.explorium.org/PL_105-19.htm.

Wirth, S. & Wolfberg, D. (2003). *Law bytes: Are you really covered under the new HIPAA privacy rule?* Retrieved on 19 June 2003 from www.merginet.com/scripts/emsnews/print/503_17.shtml.

Chapter 5

Physiology and Fitness

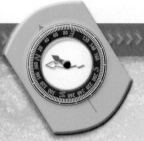

Objectives

Upon completion of this chapter and the related course activities, the student will be able to meet the following objectives:

Demonstrate awareness of and need for identifying your personal limitations and strengths as a member of a search crew. (p. 55)

Describe how, in each of the following processes, the human body loses heat:
Radiation. (p. 47)
Conduction. (p. 47)
Convection. (p. 48)
Evaporation. (p. 48)
Respiration. (p. 49)

Describe the heat production and heat loss balance equation of the human body. (p. 46)

Describe the basic water and chemical needs of the human body. (p. 45-46)

List the average daily food and water requirements of the human body in average, cold, and hot environments. (p. 44-46)

Physiology

The foundation for comfortably living and working in the outdoors is an understanding of the human body. This understanding need not be on the level of a physician, but one should have some comprehension of how the body reacts to or is affected by the environment. In short, SAR personnel must have a working knowledge of human biological survival (the necessities and priorities of life), including a fundamental understanding of issues related to nutrition, hydration, and thermoregulation.

Food and Nutrition

It takes several hours for most foods to become available to the body as energy. The old saying, "You are what you eat," is an accurate statement. But, more accurate is the statement, "What you eat today is what you run on tomorrow." So, in order to be optimally prepared, SAR personnel must eat a well-balanced diet every day so that they are best prepared for peak performance when they are called.

Because excellent references are readily available on this topic, proper nutrition and diet will not be addressed here in any detail. However, this does not mean that these subjects are not important to SAR personnel. They are critically important; so much so that they should receive comprehensive examination beyond what is possible here. The U.S. Department of Health publishes dietary guidelines with which all SAR personnel should be familiar. Nutritional planning and discipline are essential if one expects to be able to work today at a SAR incident on the fuel he or she ingested yesterday.

Humans in arctic or cold environments consume more calories than those in warm climates. It has been estimated that this increase could be as great as 2000 extra calories per day. For this reason, long-lasting, high-energy

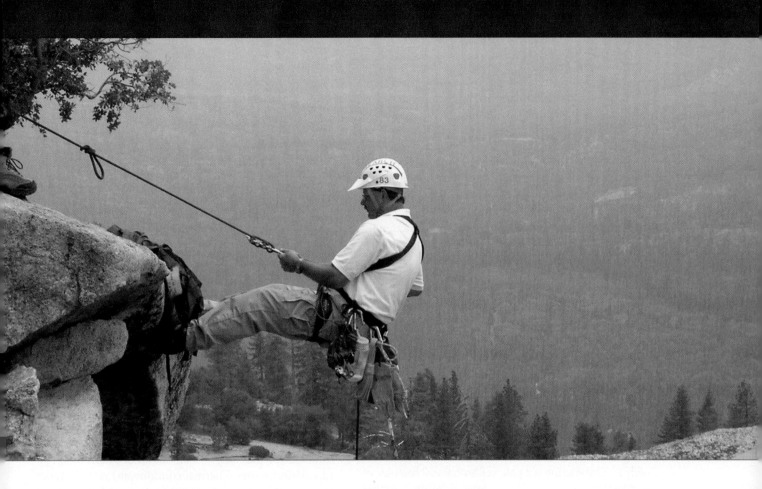

foods become more of a critical factor in cold weather than in other climates. As a point of reference, the basic metabolic rate measured under standard conditions is about 1400 to 1800 calories per day, just to maintain the body at its least active waking level (obviously this varies from individual to individual). **Table 5–1** shows estimated caloric needs of individuals by level of activity. Using this table, it can be shown that a 165-pound (75-kilogram) male participating in heavy activity (like field SAR operations) would require just over 3700 calories per day.

Table 5–1	Estimated daily calorie needs of athletes by activity level	
Activity Level	Male Calories per lb	Female Calories per lb
Light	17	16
Moderate	19	17
Heavy	23	20

Source: Data are adapted from Baechle & Earle, 2000, p. 253.

Water and Hydration

Water is essential for proper body function. The human body may be able to survive for as long as a month without food but only a matter of days without water. Approximately two thirds of one's body weight is water. Two thirds of this water is inside body cells (intercellular), and the other one third is in the veins, body cavities, and other spaces. Maintaining adequate fluid balance is vitally important to survival, let alone being able to work under stress. No other nutrient affects athletic or work performance more than water, so consuming an adequate amount of water is vital to being able to perform any sort of activity including SAR.

Water is so essential that a 1% decrease in normal levels makes us thirsty. When body water levels fall below a certain level, saliva decreases, the throat gets dry, and the urge to drink follows. As the body continues to lose water, the viscosity of the blood increases, performance decreases, early fatigue sets in, and muscle cramping may occur. Headache, dizziness, nausea, irritability, and vomiting are also signs and symptoms of dehydration. A 10% water level drop (6% of body weight) impairs thinking and judgment. Twenty percent loss is usually fatal. The time required for such a large fluid loss depends on environmental circumstances and what types of conservation methods are used.

During hard work, the muscles produce an excess of heat, which must be dissipated or the body will overheat. This is why you sweat. For every 600 calories of heat the body generates, you can lose about 1 liter of fluid in the form of sweat. Clothes that do not allow the evaporation of sweat, or a humidity level that does the same, will cause overheating in a hot environment. It is the actual evaporation of moisture from the skin that cools the body, not just the sweating.

An inactive person requires a minimum of 1.2 liters of water a day to keep all body systems functioning properly. Small levels of activity (walking, normal daily actions) can easily double this requirement. High humidity can again double the needed amount, as can physical exertion. It is not unusual to require 8 to 10 liters of water per day under extreme conditions.

In moderate temperatures, people have survived 17 days without water. Conversely, in a hot desert environment one might last only a few hours, since physical exertion under these conditions can cause the loss of 2 to 3 liters of water per hour to sweat. Beyond normal methods of water loss, vomiting, sickness, excessive urination, and diarrhea can all contribute to rapid dehydration.

Proper re-hydration requires one to drink water slowly until the urine is a pale yellow color. The color of the urine is a good test for dehydration: deep amber urine (usually in small quantities) signifies dehydration; pale yellow (usually in great quantities) signifies adequate hydration. Re-hydrating with water is just fine, but a sports drink like Gatorade® or an equivalent will also help replace electrolytes lost through sweating and the taste may encourage one to drink more. This may be important because most people stop drinking fluids before they are adequately re-hydrated. Research shows that people will drink more of a flavored beverage than plain water (Passe, et al., 2000; Wilk & Bar-Or, 1996) and so it is recommended that a dry, flavored sports drink mix (Gatorade®, G-Push®, Ultima®, Cytomax®, etc.) be carried with water. Treated water also can be made more palatable by adding a flavored mix.

It is possible to drink large amounts of water and have little fluid increase due to salt or electrolyte deficiency. Salt deficiency is often underestimated when a person is not acclimated to the heat and sun. Typical hot weather appetite loss adds to possible imbalance. Salt in pill form or directly dissolved in fluid is recommended for persons perspiring heavily in hot weather. However, salt or salt pills should be taken cautiously. Without adequate water, they can do more harm than salt deficiency. Never take salt if water supplies are short. In addition, many commercial salt pills tend to nauseate some people to the point of vomiting, worsening the problem, while others pass the pills straight through the digestive system in the same form. Buffered salt tablets seem less troublesome to most people.

Key Points

- Water is more essential than food and lack of it will kill you quicker than lack of food.
- It is impossible to perform at any reasonable level without the proper intake of fluids.
- Food should be eaten only when there is enough water to drink. Do not eat if water is scarce.
- Consider the use of flavored sports drink mixes to encourage fluid intake and to cover the taste of treated water.
- Use salt tablets with caution, only when excessive sweating has occurred in a short period of time, and only when there is plenty of water to drink.

Body Temperature Regulation

As warm-blooded animals (homeotherms), humans possess a thermal regulatory system that maintains the body temperature at about 99°F (37°C), regardless of environmental fluctuations. Since the body constantly produces heat, heat must be transferred to the environment for the body to maintain a constant temperature. Heat balance (thermal equilibrium) is the balance between the rate of heat production and the rate of heat loss.

The Heat Balance Equation

Those interested in maintaining a normal body temperature must do two things: maintain a healthy, well-nourished body (control of heat production), and adjust the clothing system as required (control of heat loss). Nutrition is discussed in the previous section and clothing systems are addressed in Chapter 7.

The body's primary method of regulating its temperature involves finely adjusting the flow of heated blood between its core (brain, heart, lungs) and periphery (skin, arms and legs). Generally, blood is pushed to the skin and extremities for cooling, and shunted to the core to preserve heat.

The human body is constantly producing heat through metabolism and muscle movement. The body may also absorb heat from its environment. Much of this heat must be dissipated to our clothing and the environment if a constant inner body core temperature is to be maintained. For brief periods the body can even store a little excess heat in its outer tissues. If heat loss exceeds production, the body will draw on this stored heat. In the end, heat loss must equal heat production and absorption if a thermal equilibrium is to be maintained.

Heat is produced in the body in two ways: as a natural by-product of certain chemical reactions (exothermic metabolism), and as a by-product of muscle movement (work). However, the body can also derive heat through absorption of radiant energy from the sun or other heat source.

An individual's metabolic rate (or calorie production) is highly variable and differs from person to person. For the average male, it can range from 70 calories per hour while sleeping to 524 calories per hour during strenuous work.

On a clear day, the unclothed body can absorb as much as 230 calories per hour of the sun's heat energy. In very hot environments, radiated heat gain can cause overheating problems, so the body must be protected from it. In cold environments, layers of clothing and/or shelter can reduce radiated heat loss. The color of clothing can also make a difference. The darker the clothing, the more radiant heat energy will be absorbed. The lighter the clothing color, the more radiant heat energy is reflected. So, wear dark-colored clothing in cold environments and light-colored clothing in hot environments.

As the body's core temperature begins to rise, two things happen: blood vessels in and near the surface of the skin dilate (enlarge) to help release the blood's latent heat to the environment, and sweating begins. The subsequent evaporation of perspiration from the skin releases a tremendous amount of heat energy. The hot blood being pumped from the body's core to the skin is also cooled by convection, conduction, and radiation.

The reverse takes place when the body is exposed to a cold environment or its core temperature drops (**Figure 5–1**). Blood vessels constrict and circulation to the surface of the skin and periphery is limited to reduce heat loss. Less blood going to the surface of the skin means less heat lost to the environment. Shivering also begins. In extreme circumstances, circulation may be cut off almost entirely to the most distant appendages (fingers, toes, ears, and nose), thus predisposing them to local cold injuries like frostbite.

Since the brain is a critical "core" organ, the head and neck continue to receive full blood flow even under cold stress. Because these areas of the body are very vascular (contain many blood vessels, some quite large), the blood flowing to these areas can release a great deal of heat to the environment if they are not protected. This is why it is critically important to cover and protect the head and neck in cold environments.

Muscular activity can increase one's metabolic rate for short periods by as much as 750%. However, different types of muscular activity produce different results.

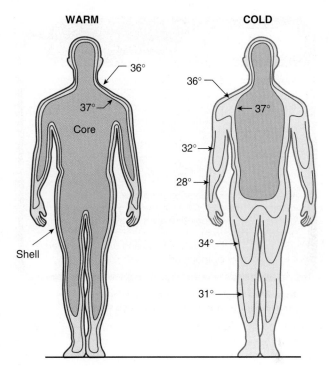

Figure 5–1 Reaction of the body to cold (C°).

Shivering and isometric exercises (working one muscle group against another without movement) will make heat immediately available to the body without heavy perspiration. Thus, these methods are preferred over running or strenuous activity. In addition, isometrics can be done in a sleeping bag or sitting in a chair. At least 10 minutes of exercise may be needed for the desired effect.

Methods of Heat Transfer

Heat transfer is the loss of heat to the environment. There are several methods by which this occurs, including: radiation, conduction, convection, and evaporation. Perspiration and respiration cause evaporative heat loss (**Tables 5–2** and **5–5**).

Radiation during a cold day will amount to about 5% of the total heat loss from a clothed body. The only heat that can be lost by radiation is that which escapes from bare skin or reaches the outer layer of clothing. The higher the temperature of the radiating surface, the faster heat will be lost through this method. The harder one works, the hotter the skin becomes and the greater the heat that will be released by radiation. This is why in an emergency situation in the cold, one should only perform the activities that are absolutely necessary for survival.

Conduction normally plays a very small part in total heat loss during everyday activities. However, this method

| Table 5-2 | Heat loss breakdown |

Percent	Cause
60	Radiation (from nude body at rest in a thermoneutral environment)
18	Convection (at rest)
3	Conduction
15	Evaporation from skin
7	Evaporation from lungs (respiration)
3	Excretion of feces and urine (considered evaporation)

Note: Percentages are averages and may not sum to 100%
Source: Cornell University Ergonomics web site

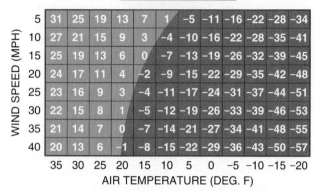

Wind Chill Chart

Figure 5-2 More information on wind chill is available on the National Oceanic and Atmospheric Administration (NOAA) web site.

of heat loss can be a major source of discomfort and cause serious problems in severe climates and hostile environments. For example, sitting or lying directly on snow, ice, the cold ground, metal, or any good conductor of heat will result in continual loss of valuable calories. Since heat flows from hot objects to cold objects and flows fastest when there is a great temperature differential, the only effective way to prevent conductive heat loss is to separate your body from any cold surface with an insulating layer. Moisture imbedded in clothing reduces the amount of trapped air and thus increases conductive heat loss through the material.

A nonconductive material is one that when heated on one side will stay cool on the other. The most efficient insulator "material" is air, and clothing systems take advantage of this fact. The problem with air that is not trapped is that it circulates. As free moving air next to the body absorbs heat, it expands and rises. Immediately, new cooler air moves in and replaces this moving warm air. This is natural convection, and it takes place as a result of both wind and the bellows action of clothing as the wearer moves. Even though air is a poor conductor, it can facilitate the transfer of heat because of its mobility within a clothing system. To properly utilize air's insulation qualities, it must be trapped and prevented from moving.

To prevent *convective* heat loss, air movement (wind) around the body must be either eliminated or significantly reduced. Under emergency cold conditions, just getting out of the wind can be a life saver. Convection is the reason for the Wind Chill Index (**Figure 5-2**), which

accounts for wind when it illustrates how cold people feel when outside. Wind chill is based on the rate of heat loss from exposed skin caused by wind and cold. As the wind increases, it draws heat from the body, driving down skin temperature and eventually the core temperature. Therefore, the wind makes the body FEEL much colder. If the air temperature is 0°F and the wind is blowing at 15 mph, the wind chill is −19°F. At this wind chill temperature, exposed skin can freeze in minutes. The only effect wind chill has on inanimate objects, such as car radiators and water pipes, is to shorten the amount of time for the object to cool. The inanimate object will not cool below the actual air temperature.

When heat and humidity combine to reduce the amount of evaporation of sweat from the body, outdoor physical activities becomes dangerous even for those in good shape. Similar to the wind chill index, the heat index is used to measure the amount of discomfort during the summer months when heat and humidity often combine to make it feel hotter than it actually is (**Table 5-3**).

Convective heat loss can also occur in water. In water, body heat is lost 25 times faster than in air (**Table 5-4**). Swimming in cold water uses more body heat and significantly reduces survival time. The reason: Cold water absorbs more heat than cold air as it moves past the body.

The last form of heat loss is *evaporation*. Respiration and perspiration both involve evaporative heat loss and are often overlooked as significant heat loss methods. Evaporation of one ounce of water releases about 17 kilocalories. A <u>kilocalorie</u> is the amount of heat required to raise the temperature of one kilogram of water one degree centigrade or about 1000 calories.

Table 5-3 — Heat index table

Apparent Temperature*

Relative Humidity	Air Temperature										
	70	**75**	**80**	**85**	**90**	**95**	**100**	**105**	**110**	**115**	**120**
30	67	73	78	84	90	96	104	113	123	135	148
35	67	73	79	85	91	98	107	118	130	143	
40	68	74	79	86	93	101	110	123	137	151	
45	68	74	80	87	95	104	115	129	143		
50	69	75	81	88	96	107	120	135	150		
55	69	75	81	89	98	110	126	142			
60	70	76	82	90	100	114	132	149			
65	70	76	83	91	102	119	138				
70	70	77	85	93	106	124	144				
75	70	77	86	95	109	130					
80	71	78	86	97	113	136					
85	71	78	87	99	117						
90	71	79	88	102	122						
95	71	79	89	105							
100	72	80	91	108							

*The Effects on the Human Body

>130	Serious heat injury highly likely with continued exposure
105–130	Serious heat injury likely with prolonged exposure
90–105	Heat injury possible with prolonged exposure
80–90	Exercise more fatiguing than usual; watch for heat cramps and heat exhaustion

Source: National Oceanic and Atmospheric Administration

The majority of evaporative heat loss is through sweating. Even without heavy sweating, this loss amounts to about 20% of the total and is referred to as insensible perspiration. Insensible perspiration is the continuous, imperceptible drying out of the skin. It is estimated that one loses about 1-1/2 pints of moisture per day through this process. Although perspiration in the form of sweat can be controlled, insensible perspiration cannot.

In most cold circumstances, respiratory heat loss is not considered significant. However, in an extremely cold environment where any calorie loss is important, the respiratory system is converting subzero temperature air to 98.6°F in less than 18 inches of space (the length of your airway and lungs). This requires a substantial investment of calories by the body. With the addition of a simple rebreather (an improvised thickness of clothing, material or structure that preheats inhaled air, e.g., a scarf, piece of clothing, sock or tube-shaped hood), one can significantly reduce respiratory heat loss.

Fitness

The importance of <u>physical fitness</u> in SAR or why being fit contributes to field SAR operations should be obvious. What may need to be stated, though, is that a lack of conditioning and fitness has been repeatedly identified as one of the most common problems faced in the field by SAR personnel and managers. This has undoubtedly resulted in reduced effectiveness and increased safety risk.

Maintaining a regular program of physical conditioning provides a head start toward coping with stressful emergencies in hostile environments. Not everyone must be a flawless physical specimen, but a reasonable fitness level is necessary for optimal performance, especially in the field. However, running and other serious exercise is understandably not for everyone. Fortunately, there can be a place in SAR for virtually anyone who wants to participate, as long as every individual recognizes and shares his or her limitations.

Because fitness has been recognized as such a widespread problem in SAR—much like it has been recognized as a problem in modern society in general—it seems prudent to review some of the very basic issues related to this important topic.

Making a Commitment

The first important step on the path to physical fitness is to seek information, and the second is to decide that you are going to be physically fit. The information provided here is designed to help you reach that decision and your goal.

The decision to carry out a physical fitness program to prepare for SAR cannot be taken lightly. It requires a lifelong commitment of time and effort. Exercise must

Table 5–4	Cooling rate of body in water	
Water Temperature		Core Body Cooling Rate
°F	°C	°C/Hour
68	20	0.5
59	15	1.5
50	10	2.5
41	5	4.0
32	0	6.0

Note: In cold water, body heat is lost 25 times faster than in cold air due to convective heat loss.
Source: Professor Alan Hedge, Cornell University, 1/2002.

Table 5–5	The effect of various surface (skin) and core temperatures					
Skin (Shell) Temperature				Core Temperature		
°C	°F	Condition	°C	°F	Condition
>45	>113	Burns	>42	>108	Fatal
42	108	Pain	41	106	Coma, convulsions
40	104	Uncomfortably hot	39.5	103	Upper acceptable limit, drowsiness
25	77	Uncomfortably cold	37	98.6	Normal
5	41	Numbness	35.5	96	Lower acceptable limit, mental dullness
0	32	Frostbite	34.5	94	Shivering diminishes, extreme mental slowness
<−0.6	<31	Skin freezes	33	91	Coma
			<33	<91	Deep coma, death
			27	81	Heart stops, death

Source: Professor Alan Hedge, Cornell University, 1/2002.

become one of those things that you do without question, like bathing and brushing your teeth. Unless you are convinced of the benefits of fitness and the risks of unfitness, you will not succeed.

Patience is essential. Don't try to do too much too soon and don't quit before you have a chance to experience the rewards of improved fitness. You can't regain in a few days or weeks what you have lost in years of sedentary living, but you can get it back if you persevere. The prize is worth the price.

The following paragraphs contain the basic information you need to begin and maintain a personal physical fitness program. These guidelines are intended for the average healthy adult, and explain what your goals should be, and how often, how long, and how hard you must exercise to achieve them. Information is also provided that will make your workouts easier, safer, and more satisfying. The rest is up to you.

Checking Your Health

If you are under 35 and in good health, you probably do not need to see a doctor before beginning an exercise program. But if you are over 35 and have been inactive for several years, you should consult your physician, who may or may not recommend a graded exercise test. Other conditions that indicate a need for medical clearance are:

- High blood pressure
- Heart trouble
- Family history of early stroke or heart attack deaths
- Frequent dizzy spells
- Extreme breathlessness after mild exertion
- Arthritis or other bone problems
- Severe muscular, ligament, or tendon problems
- Other known or suspected disease

Vigorous exercise involves minimal health risks for persons in good health or those following a doctor's advice. Far greater risks are presented by habitual inactivity and obesity.

Defining Fitness

Physical fitness is to the human body what fine-tuning is to an engine. It enables us to perform up to our potential. Fitness can be described as a condition that helps us look, feel, and do our best. According to the President's Council on Physical Fitness and Sports, physical fitness is:

The ability to perform daily tasks vigorously and alertly, with energy left over for enjoying leisure-time activities and meeting emergency demands. It is the ability to endure, to bear up, to withstand stress, to carry on in circumstances where an unfit person could not continue, and is a major basis for good health and well-being.

Physical fitness involves the performance of the heart and lungs, and the muscles of the body. And, since what we do with our bodies also affects what we can do with our minds, fitness influences to some degree qualities such as mental alertness and emotional stability.

As you undertake your fitness program, it's important to remember that fitness is an individual quality that varies from person to person. It is influenced by age, sex, heredity, personal habits, exercise, and eating practices. You can't do anything about the first three factors. However, it is within your power to change and improve the others where needed.

Knowing the Basics

Physical fitness is most easily understood by examining its components, or "parts." There is widespread agreement that these four components are basic:

- *Cardiorespiratory Endurance* – The ability to deliver oxygen and nutrients to tissues and to remove wastes, over sustained periods of time. Long runs and swims are among the methods employed in measuring this component.
- *Muscular Strength* – The ability of a muscle to exert force for a brief period of time. Upper-body strength, for example, can be measured by various weight-lifting exercises.
- *Muscular Endurance* – The ability of a muscle, or a group of muscles, to sustain repeated contractions or to continue applying force against a fixed object. Pushups are often used to test endurance of arm and shoulder muscles.

- *Flexibility* – The ability to move joints and use muscles through their full range of motion. The sit-and-reach test is a good measure of flexibility of the lower back and backs of the upper legs.

"Body Composition" is often considered a component of fitness. It refers to the makeup of the body in terms of lean mass (muscle, bone, vital tissue, and organs) and fat mass. An optimal ratio of fat to lean mass is an indication of fitness, and the right types of exercises will help you decrease body fat and increase or maintain muscle mass.

A Workout Schedule

How often, how long, and how hard you exercise, and what types of exercises you do should be determined by what you are trying to accomplish (**Figure 5–3**).

Your goals, your present fitness level, age, health, skills, interests, and convenience are among the factors you should consider. For example, an athlete training for high-level competition would follow a different program than a person whose goals are good health and the ability to meet work and recreational needs.

Any exercise program should include something from each of the four basic fitness components described previously. Each workout should begin with a warm up and end with a cool down. As a general rule, space your workouts throughout the week and avoid consecutive days of hard exercise.

Here are the amounts of activity necessary for the average healthy person to maintain a minimum level of overall fitness. Included are some of the popular exercises for each category.

- *Warm Up* – Five to ten minutes of exercise such as walking, slow jogging, knee lifts, arm circles or trunk rotations. Low intensity movements that simulate movements to be used in the activity can also be included in the warm up.

- *Muscular Strength* – A minimum of two 20-minute sessions per week that include exercises for all the major muscle groups. Lifting weights is the most effective way to increase strength.

- *Muscular Endurance* – At least three 30-minute sessions each week that include exercises such as calisthenics, push-ups, sit-ups, pull-ups, and weight training for all the major muscle groups.

- *Cardiorespiratory Endurance* – At least three 20-minute bouts of continuous aerobic (activity requiring oxygen) rhythmic exercise each week. Popular aerobic conditioning activities include brisk walking, jogging, swimming, cycling, rope jumping, rowing, cross-country skiing, and some continuous action games like racquetball and handball.

- *Flexibility* – Ten to 12 minutes of daily stretching exercises performed slowly, without a bouncing motion. This can be included after a warm-up or during a cool down.

- *Cool Down* – A minimum of 5 to 10 minutes of slow walking, low-level exercise, combined with stretching.

A Matter of Principle

The keys to selecting the right kinds of exercises for developing and maintaining each of the basic components of fitness are found in these principles:

- *Specificity* – Pick the right kind of activities to affect each component. Strength training results in specific strength changes. Also, train for the specific activity you are interested in. For example, optimal hiking performance is best achieved when the muscles involved in walking are trained for the movements required. It does not necessarily follow that a good runner is a good swimmer.

- *Overload* – Work hard enough, at levels that are vigorous and long enough to overload your body above its current level, to bring about improvement.

- *Regularity* – You can't hoard physical fitness. At least three balanced workouts a week are necessary to maintain a desirable level of fitness.

- *Progression* – Increase the intensity, frequency, and/or duration of activity over periods of time in order to improve.

Some activities can be used to fulfill more than one of your basic exercise requirements. For example, in addition to increasing cardiorespiratory endurance, running builds muscular endurance in the legs, and swimming develops the arm, shoulder, and chest muscles. If you select the proper activities, it is possible to fit parts of your muscular endurance workout into your cardiorespiratory workout and save time.

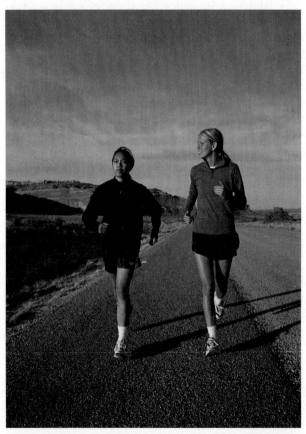

Figure 5–3 How often, how long, and how hard you exercise, and what types of exercises you do should be determined by what you are trying to accomplish. Field SAR work is physically demanding and requires a moderate to high level of fitness.

What Kind of Exercise?

Although any kind of physical movement requires energy (calories), the type of exercise that uses the most energy is **aerobic exercise**. The term "aerobic" is derived from the Greek word meaning "with oxygen." Jogging, brisk walking, swimming, biking, cross-country skiing, and aerobic dancing are some popular forms of aerobic exercise. Aerobic exercises use the body's large muscle groups in continuous, rhythmic, sustained movement, and require oxygen for the production of energy. When oxygen is combined with food (which can come from stored fat) energy is produced to power the body's musculature. The longer you move aerobically, the more energy needed and the more calories used. Regular aerobic exercise will improve your cardiorespiratory endurance, which is the ability of your heart, lungs, blood vessels, and associated tissues to use oxygen to produce energy needed for activity. You will build a healthier body while getting rid of excess body fat.

In addition to the aerobic exercise, supplement your program with muscle strengthening and stretching exercises. The stronger your muscles, the longer you will be able to keep going during aerobic activity, and the less chance of injury.

How Much, How Often?

Experts recommend that you do some form of aerobic exercise at least three times a week for a minimum of 20 continuous minutes. Of course, if that is too much, start with a shorter time span and gradually build up to the minimum. Then gradually progress until you are able to work aerobically for 20 to 40 minutes. If you need to lose a large amount of weight, you may want to do your aerobic workout five times a week.

It is important to exercise at an intensity vigorous enough to cause your heart rate and breathing to increase. How hard you should exercise depends to a certain degree on your age, and is determined by measuring your heart rate in beats per minute.

The heart rate you should maintain during exercise is called your **target heart rate**, and there are several ways you can arrive at this number. The simplest is to subtract your age from 220 and then calculate 60% to 80% of that figure. Beginners should maintain the 60% level; more advanced can work up to the 80% level. This is just a guide, however, and people with any medical limitations should discuss this formula with their physician.

You can do various types of aerobic activities, such as walking one day and riding a bike the next. Make sure you choose an activity that can be done regularly, and is enjoyable for you. The important thing to remember is not to skip too many days between workouts or fitness benefits will be lost. If you must lose a few days, gradually work back into your routine.

Controlling Your Weight

Just about everybody seems to be interested in weight control. Some of us weigh just the right amount; others need to gain a few pounds. Most of us "battle the bulge" at some time in our life. Whatever our goals, we should understand and take advantage of the important role of exercise in keeping our weight under control.

Carrying around too much body fat is a major nuisance. Yet excess body fat is common in modern-day living. Few of today's occupations require vigorous physical activity, and much of our leisure time is spent in sedentary pursuits.

Recent estimates indicate that 34 million American adults are considered obese (20% above desirable weight). Also, there has been an increase in body fat levels in children and youth over the past 20 years. After infancy and early childhood, the earlier the onset of obesity, the greater the likelihood of remaining obese. Excess body fat has been linked to such health problems as coronary heart disease, high blood pressure, osteoporosis, diabetes, arthritis, and certain forms of cancer. Some evidence now exists showing that obesity has a negative effect on both health and long life.

Exercise is associated with the loss of body fat in both obese and normal weight persons. A regular program of exercise is an important component of any plan to help individuals lose, gain, or maintain their weight.

The key to weight control is keeping energy intake (food) and energy output (physical activity) in balance. When you consume only the necessary calories your body needs, your weight will usually remain constant. If you take in more calories than your body needs, you will put on excess fat. If you expend more energy than you take in you will burn excess fat.

Exercise plays an important role in weight control by increasing energy output, calling on stored calories for extra fuel. Recent studies show that not only does exercise increase metabolism during a workout, but it causes your metabolism to stay increased for a period of time after exercising, allowing you to burn more calories.

How much exercise is needed to make a difference in your weight depends on the amount and type of activity, and the amount you eat. Aerobic exercise burns body fat. A medium-sized adult would have to walk more than 30 miles to burn up 3,500 calories, the equivalent of one pound of fat. Although that may seem like a lot, you don't have to walk the 30 miles all at once. Walking a mile a day for 30 days will achieve the same result, providing you don't increase your food intake to negate the effects of walking.

If you consume 100 calories a day more than your body needs, you will gain approximately 10 pounds in a year. You could take that weight off, or keep it off, by doing 30 minutes of moderate exercise daily. The combination of exercise and diet offers the most flexible and effective approach to weight control.

Since muscle tissue weighs more than fat tissue, and exercise develops muscle to a certain degree, your bathroom scale won't necessarily tell you whether or not you are "fat." Well-muscled individuals, with relatively little body fat, invariably are "overweight" according to standard weight charts. If you are participating in a regular program of strength training, your muscles will increase in weight, resulting in an overall body weight increase. Body composition is a better indicator of your condition than body weight.

Lack of physical activity causes muscles to become soft, and if food intake is not decreased, added body weight is almost always fat. Once-active people, who continue to eat as they always have after settling into sedentary lifestyles, tend to suffer from "creeping obesity."

Benefits of Exercise in a Weight Control Program

The benefits of exercise are many, from producing physically fit bodies for SAR to providing an outlet for fun and socialization. When added to a weight control program these benefits take on increased significance.

It has already been noted that proper exercise can help control weight by burning excess body fat. It also has two other body-trimming advantages: (a) exercise builds muscle tissue and muscle uses calories up at a faster rate than body fat; and (b) exercise helps reduce inches and a firm, lean body looks slimmer even if your weight remains the same.

Remember, fat does not "turn into" muscle, as is often believed. Fat and muscle are two entirely different substances and one cannot become the other. However, muscle does use calories at a faster rate than fat, which directly affects your body's metabolic rate or energy requirement. Your basal metabolic rate (BMR) is the amount of energy required to sustain the body's functions at rest and it depends on your age, sex, body size, genes, and body composition. People with high levels of muscle tend to have higher BMRs and use more calories in the resting stage.

Some studies have even shown that your metabolic rate stays elevated for some time after vigorous exercise, causing you to burn more calories throughout your day. Additional benefits may be seen in how exercise affects appetite. A lean person in good shape may eat more following increased activity, but the regular exercise will burn up the extra calories consumed. On the other hand, vigorous exercise has been reported to suppress appetite. Physical activity can be used as a positive substitute for between meal snacking.

Better Mental Health

The psychological benefits of exercise are equally important to the weight conscious person. Exercise can decrease stress and relieve tensions that might otherwise lead to overeating. Exercise builds physical fitness, which in turn builds self-confidence, enhanced self-image, and a positive outlook. When you start to feel good about yourself, you are more likely to want to make other positive changes in your lifestyle that will help keep your weight under control.

In addition, exercise can be fun, provide recreation, and offer opportunities for companionship. The exhilaration and emotional release of participating in sports or other activities are a boost to mental and physical health. Pent-up anxieties and frustrations seem to disappear when you are concentrating on returning a serve, sinking a putt, or hiking that extra mile.

Tips to Get Started

Hopefully, you are now convinced that in order to successfully manage your weight you must include exercise in your daily routine. Here are some tips to get you started:

1. Check with your doctor first. Since you are carrying around some extra "baggage," it is wise to get your doctor's "OK" before embarking on an exercise program.

2. Choose activities that you think you'll enjoy. Most people will stick to their exercise program if they are having fun, even though they are working hard.

3. Set aside a regular exercise time. Whether this means joining an exercise class or getting up a little earlier every day, make time for this addition to your routine, and don't let anything get in your way. Planning ahead will help you get around interruptions in your workout schedule, such as bad weather and vacations.

4. Set short-term goals. Don't expect to lose 20 pounds in two weeks. It has taken awhile for you to gain the weight; it will take time to lose it. Keep a record of your progress and tell your friends and family about your achievements.

5. Vary your exercise program. Change exercises or invite friends to join you to make your workout more enjoyable. There is no "best" exercise—just the one that works best for you. It won't be easy, especially at the start. However, as you begin to feel better, look better, and enjoy a new zest for life, you will be rewarded many times over for your efforts.

Tips to Keep Going

- Adopt a specific plan and write it down.
- Keep setting realistic goals as you go along, and remind yourself of them often.
- Keep a log to record your progress and make sure to keep it up-to-date.
- Include weight and/or percent body fat measures in your log. Extra pounds can easily creep back.

- Upgrade your fitness program as you progress.
- Enlist the support and company of your family and friends.
- Update others on your successes.
- Avoid injuries by pacing yourself and including a warm-up and cool down period as part of every workout.
- Reward yourself periodically for a job well done!

Admitting Limitations

You must make a realistic assessment of your physical abilities without being nostalgic and recalling earlier athletic achievements. Males reach their physiological prime in their late teens and females in their early teens. This does not rule out fitness at a later time in your life, however. If you are to maintain optimum performance, you must not try to do more than you are capable of achieving. Assess your physical limitations realistically and restrict your activities accordingly. There is as much to do for those who are not up to arduous field work, as there is for the marathon runner. Do not compare yourself with others since we all set our own limits. Everyone is different.

In general, when you are prepared physically, you will know the limits of that condition. Being prepared is preferred to finding out about your lack of conditioning after a futile and dangerous attempt at working in the field. Remember that when search and rescue personnel become disabled, injured, or ill, focus is drawn away from the victim. Knowing when to stay out of the field is a prime example of when your brain becomes your primary survival tool.

Mental Fitness

Keeping your body in condition virtually assures your ability to think clearly and concentrate for long periods of time. Both mental and physical conditioning are required for searching and surviving. The time will come when alertness, resourcefulness, and mental toughness will get you through a tight spot. You must be prepared for that eventuality.

In everything you do—work, play, school, relationships, etc.—mental preparedness can be accomplished by following some simple "self" guidelines. The following tips also help in maintaining a proper attitude of safety, in life as well as SAR.

- **Be thorough.** When you begin something, finish it and do it right. Perseverance is an essential survival tool.
- **Be confident and willing to learn.** Confidence comes through training and experience. Learn essential skills and practice what you learn. If you do something right, remember what and how you did it and do it that way the next time. If you do something wrong, remember what and how you did it and do it differently the next time. Learn something from every experience.
- **Be conscientious.** There is a good chance that no one will be around to watch what you are doing. Your activities must be guided by your own standards—set them high. Your peace of mind is your greatest, and sometimes only, reward.
- **Be assertive.** Take advantage of new experiences. Push yourself beyond what you have done in the past without being foolish. Take the lead to get things accomplished. Don't be afraid to take a safer route or to recheck your bearings.

SAR Terms

Aerobic exercise Exercise that combines food (often fat) with oxygen to produce energy for the body and that leads to cardiorespiratory endurance.

Basal metabolic rate The amount of energy required to sustain the body's functions at rest.

Heat transfer The loss of heat to or from the environment through radiation, conduction, convection, or evaporation.

Kilocalorie The amount of heat required to raise the temperature of one kilogram of water one degree centigrade or about 1000 calories.

Physical fitness According to the President's Council on Physical Fitness and Sports, physical fitness is the ability to perform daily tasks vigorously and alertly, with energy left over for enjoying leisure-time activities and meeting emergency demands.

Target heart rate The heart rate you should maintain during exercise.

References

Armsey, T.D., & Green, G.A. (1997). Nutrition supplements: Science vs hype. *The Physician and Sports Medicine*, 25(6), 76–84.

Baechle, T.R., & Earle, R.W. (2000). *Essentials of Strength and Conditioning* (2nd ed.). Champaign, IL: Human Kinetics.

Chapter 6

Survival and Improvisation

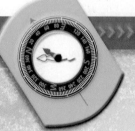

Objectives

Upon completion of this chapter and any course activities, the student will be able to meet the following objectives:

List and prioritize the necessities of life. (p. 58)

Describe the four parts of the initial response to a life-threatening situation. (p. 60-61)

Demonstrate awareness of the term "comfort zone" and describe how it relates to SAR. (p. 61)

List at least five ways to control fear. (p. 61-62)

Explain the survival situation plan, STOP (stay, think, observe, plan). (p. 62-63)

Define positive mental attitude. (p. 58)

Differentiate between the requirements for short-term versus long-term survival. (p. 56-84)

List at least three basic considerations for shelters. (p. 67-69)

List at least three methods of water purification. (p. 82)

Describe methods used to construct a fire. (p. 69-74)

List at least three basic considerations for signals. (p. 74-76)

Describe some considerations in personal waste disposal. (p. 82)

Describe three methods used for personal cleanliness in the outdoors. (p. 82-83)

What Is Survival?

Traditional definitions of survival imply primitive conditions, living off the land, or battling the elements to live through some precarious predicament in the wilderness. Depending on one's perspective, survival means different things to different people.

A survival situation is one in which an individual's very existence is threatened. Some kind of action is necessary to alleviate a threat to life. To survive is to continue existing, to live despite some event or adverse set of circumstances. Survival is simply living a minute longer by any means possible.

The ability to survive is infinitely more complex than merely being able to "live off the land." Statistics show that nearly all survival situations today are short term (72 hours or less), as the more publicized long-term survival experiences comprise fewer than 5% of all incidents. To establish an effective, rational response to any survival situation, it is imperative to realize that actions and needs must be prioritized. Preconceived ideas about survival can precipitate actions when stressed, and the results can be fatal. First-hand accounts and interviews of survivors substantiate the fact that the decisions made in the first hours or minutes of an emergency have a great bearing on the ultimate outcome (Figure 6–1).

It is essential to understand the human body, not as thoroughly as a physician understands it, but how it reacts to or is affected by environmental stress. A working knowledge of how to manage your body properly in an emergency is the key to survival. Proper body management is defined as the maintenance and control of your essential (limited) body resources and problem-solving capabilities. If mismanaged, body upsets will result and directly affect one's ability to survive in any environment for any period of time.

The greatest obstacle an individual will have to overcome is an inappropriate mental attitude. Since so much of survival is dealing with psychological challenge, the brain

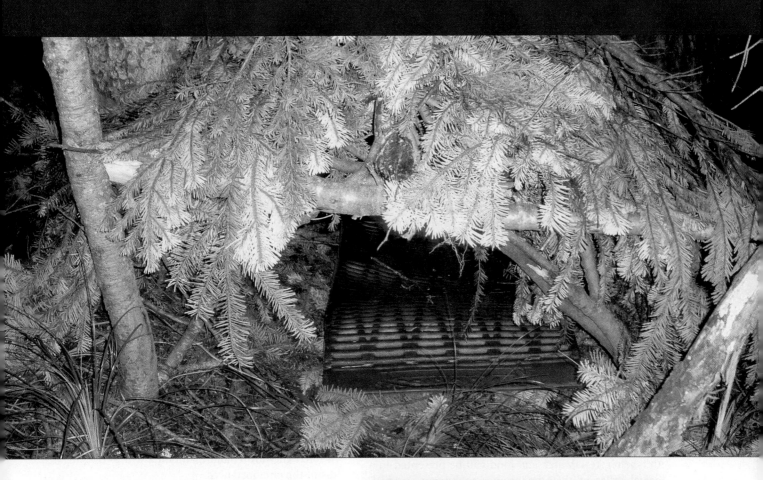

becomes the individual's most important survival tool. Recognizing and acquiring the body's physical needs will always require the capacity for analytical thought that is based in previous experience and training. Thus, the body and mind are inseparable when it comes to survival.

People live, work, and play in a comfort zone. Just as people differ in their abilities, comfort zones and their limits also differ from person to person. Since people are creatures of habit, and the technology they have created takes much of the unexpected out of their lives, most rarely venture outside of their comfort zones. Studies of those who perform high-risk and challenging activities show that those who operate on the outskirts of their comfort zones and continually push their limits react better in an emergency. Under repeated stress situations, people learn to make more and more effective adjustments. However, most people rarely experience an emergency, so their typical response is to display disorganized and shock-like behavior. Rational, coherent thinking that calls upon similar situations from past training and experience will, in most cases, be the most effective method for gaining control of the situation.

Modern technology has accustomed people to light-switch conveniences that eliminate thirst, hunger, cold, heat and, in most cases, fear. In an unexpected survival situation, confidence and self-reliance will play a key role in determining the ultimate outcome of

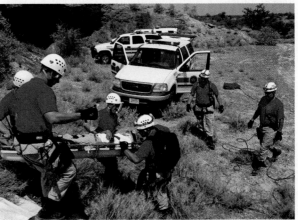

Figure 6–1 Decisions made in the first hours or minutes of an emergency have a great bearing on the ultimate outcome of the situation.

that experience. Unfortunately, people are not only dependent upon their technology but are products of a culture that has little need for individuals to be self-reliant on a daily basis. Self-reliance is developed through actual experience and dependence on one's self for everyday needs. There is no substitute for actually having performed a task that is designed to save lives.

The Necessities of Life

What does it actually take for a human being to stay alive for an indefinite period of time? Typical answers might include clothes, a house, a car, and three meals a day. However, several thousand years ago humans did not have these conveniences, yet they still survived. By listing the necessities of life and asking the question, "how long can a human live without each item," it is possible to prioritize these necessities. The time factors involved with this type of analysis should be in terms of minutes, hours, days, and weeks. Although this approach may seem elementary, it will provide a foundation for good judgment when dealing with all life-threatening emergencies (**Table 6-1**).

SARTips

INFO
The Necessities of Life
1. Will to Live/Positive Mental Attitude (PMA)
2. Air/Oxygen
3. Shelter/Clothing, Warmth
4. Rest
5. Signals (if you expect to be found)
6. Water
7. Food

Priority 1: Positive Mental Attitude

Air, shelter, rest, water, and food will be presented in a logical order of their importance to human survival. However, an often overlooked but vital priority is a mental attitude that is positive in nature and appropriate in its perspective for a given situation. This is usually the result of a thorough background in the knowledge and skills necessary to preserve human life in a hostile environment.

An extremely important part of emergency response from an individual's standpoint is the "whole person concept." An understanding of this basic theorem enables a person to better put into perspective the priorities of any emergency environment. The "whole person concept" as it applies to response is a term that ties together both mental and physical body processes. Simply put, what affects a person physically also affects a person mentally, and whatever affects a person mentally will ultimately affect a person physically. Realization of this fact alone can have a tremendous impact on anyone's ability to cope with stressful environments.

If all other priorities have been maintained or procured, but an individual lacks the will to live or the ability to cope with the situation mentally because of physical condition, then all is lost. People are at the mercy of the elements and whatever luck might be thrown their way. The power of the mind must never be underestimated.

It is worth a note of caution here to emphasize that although a positive mental attitude (PMA) should be number one on the list of priorities, it is possible to take negative action even though your attitude is positive. Mental attitude must not be misconstrued as a cure-all for survival situations. PMA does very little to analyze the body's enemies, recognize a threat to life, or understand the counteractions necessary in an emergency situation. In the majority of cases it must be coupled with proper education, training, and experience.

Will to Live

To further clarify PMA, it is helpful to break the concept down into two areas. The first is the "will to live." The will to live can be described as an overwhelming urge to survive no matter what the odds or circumstances. It has been debated extensively as to whether humans have a natural instinct for preservation. Numerous war accounts over the last century suggest that death often seems to be the easiest way out during periods of extreme physical and mental stress. People have the power to will themselves to death. Similarly, they also have the power to will themselves to live. To survive in a challenging situation, one must be able to focus on survival, visualize the future, and maintain a will to live, regardless of the circumstances.

Whole Person Concept

The second area of a PMA deals specifically with the "whole person concept" and a person's problem-solving ability. It is possible to be thoroughly knowledgeable, experienced, have a PMA commensurate with the situation, and still not operate at 100 percent of your capability.

Those with a PMA that is appropriate in its perspective for a given situation coupled with a strong will to live ultimately are in the best position to assess the situation realistically and prioritize what needs to be accomplished during any survival situation.

Priority 2: Air

Breathing is essential to maintain life on a minute-by-minute basis. Air, specifically its life-sustaining component, oxygen, must be the second priority. The average survival time without air is measured in minutes.

Priority 3: Shelter

Inherent to most survival situations is coping with inclement weather. Since human beings are designed to live naked only in areas where temperatures are very close to that of the body, environments outside this realm pose a variety of body protection problems. Anything that protects the body can be called shelter. Clothing is shelter in close proximity to the body.

How to provide adequate shelter for a specific environmental situation is the dilemma. There are temperature extremes in the United States where inadequate shelter could cut survival time to a few hours and in some cases it could be reduced to one hour or less. Fire and warmth also can be considered under shelter because, by definition, they help maintain the body's temperature in a cold environment.

Priority 4: Rest

As mentioned earlier, energy levels within the body are vitally important and significantly impact the ability to cope with any given situation. There is a good possibility that it may not be possible to renew or increase energy levels during an emergency. In survival situations it is imperative to conserve what is already present in the body. One of the most efficient ways of doing this is through adequate rest. The human body is a wonderful machine that is capable of doing amazing things when provided with proper care and maintenance. Timely periods of rest in stressful situations conserve energy for future use, and rest rids the body's tissues of carbon dioxide, lactic acid, and other body wastes. Taking a short time for rest will also provide time for reflection and analysis of the situation. Mental rest is just as important as physical rest, if not more so. Extreme stress periods (both physical and mental) with no rest can significantly decrease survival time.

Priority 5: Signals

If you are lost or immobilized and become the subject of a search, it is important for searchers to be able to find you. In this situation, deploying some type of signal(s) could be helpful. Details on signaling are presented later in this chapter.

Priority 6: Water

It is generally accepted that water and its associated problems, such as dehydration and whether it is potable or not, are among the most pressing in any survival situation. The body is comprised of approximately two thirds water that is stored within its tissues, circulatory system, and internal organs. Water is essential for body temperature regulation, waste elimination, and digestion of food. While at rest with no activities, the body utilizes approximately two quarts of water a day merely to carry on normal body functions. Consumption of any amounts

less than this will result in dehydration. Activity of any kind drastically increases the body's requirements for water. Therefore, it is not the water that should be rationed, but one's sweat and activity. A 2.5% water deficit can occur in as little as a few hours, and this can result in a 25% loss of efficiency. Extreme conditions without water could cut survival time to a matter of only a few days, even if methods of water conservation are used. Water is high on the list of priorities for maintaining life.

Priority 7: Food

Contrary to popular belief, the human body does not require three meals a day to remain alive. Countless people across the world today live on far less. Many have only one meal a day and some not even that. Records and statistics from survival experiences show numerous accounts of 40- to 70-day periods with no caloric intake. This fact coupled with current records showing that most survival situations last 72 hours or less emphasizes that procurement of food in a survival situation should be *last* on the list of priorities.

Energy levels within the body play an important role in warmth and performance. It is a common fact that high-energy snacks provide additional calories for heat production as well as movement. Although food would play a minor role under most circumstances, cold environments require many calories to maintain normal body temperature. As mentioned earlier, conservation of existing energy levels is the best strategy when survival is an issue.

Table 6–1	Necessities of life and survival time	
Necessities of Life in Priority Order	**Survival Time if Requirement Not Fulfilled**
Positive mental attitude and will to live	Depends entirely upon you
Oxygen in air	3 to 5 minutes
Body shelter from extreme temperatures	3 to 4 hours, depends upon the environment
Rest (mental as well as physical)	30 hours in extremes
Water	3 days in extremes
Food	3 weeks or more

Surviving SAR: Selected Thoughts

- The same environment that caused another person(s) problems can also cause difficulty for you.
- You can find yourself doing SAR work in unfamiliar terrain where all the potential hazards are unknown.
- You can become lost or disoriented in unfamiliar areas, especially if you are unprepared in the first place.
- Hazardous areas are some of the first areas to be searched. In your zeal to help others, you can also become a victim if you aren't careful.
- "First Notice" information is often vague. The severity/magnitude of a SAR incident is often misrepresented or misjudged. SAR personnel are quick to venture into situations with less information than is necessary for safe operations.
- The incidence of injury in SAR operations is high. This may be due to poor preparation, adrenaline "poisoning," misdirection by incident managers, or a number of intrinsic problems related to SAR operations.

Mental Aspects of Emergency Response and Survival

A positive mental attitude (PMA), appropriate in its perspective for a given situation, ultimately assumes the highest of all priorities during any survival situation.

SARTips

INFO
Staying out of trouble is the name of the game in SAR operations. When SAR personnel become lost or injured, work efforts are often directed away from the original subject(s).

There is really no way to accurately predict any person's behavior or thought processes during sudden mental and physical stresses. Reactions to every situation will vary greatly with every circumstance and every individual. In general, there are two aspects of emergency response that should be considered by SAR personnel: (1) mental preparation for SAR operations, and (2) immediate response to an emergency situation.

Mental Preparation

Mental preparation is vitally important to safe SAR operations. Anger, fear, frustration, depression, worry, and anxiety all affect a person's ability to concentrate. Anyone who brings their problems into SAR operations is easily distracted and less able to adjust to any kind of stress. The relationship between mental functions and physical capability has already been discussed.

An accurate prediction on how any one person may react in a life-threatening situation is nearly impossible. What is known is that under repeated stress situations, people will make more and more effective adjustments. There are many things present in everyday life to provide indications of stress performance, but earlier reactions may be the most telling. We must learn to read these indicators and make necessary adjustments.

Response to Life-Threatening Situations

One of the few areas that survival instructors universally agree is the need for controlling the mind, and thus one's actions, in an emergency situation. There are four phases that outline one's response to an emergency. These phases and their characteristics may enable SAR personnel to better understand how to effectively deal with, and mentally manage, any emergency situation. The four phases of initial response to a perceived emergency are: alarm, reaction, response/options, and rest.

Stage I: Alarm
One definition of alarm is a state of alertness as a result of some stimulus. Anxiety appears as a natural reaction to an event as one considers what could happen.

Stage II: Reaction
In the reaction stage, the physical body gears up for action. Anxiety increases as the entire body, both physical and mental, believes that there is a possibility that something is going to happen that will impact it.

- Muscles tighten
- Sweat glands close down
- Sugar is released for energy
- Adrenaline starts to flow
- Heart rate increases

If allowed to progress unregulated, anxiety turns to overt fear. This is the point at which training and/or experience can most impact subsequent events. If SAR personnel have practiced both standard procedures and a methodical approach to attacking the problem, then it is likely that the response will be natural and positive. If the response requires involved thought or lengthy decision-making, chances are that anxiety and fear will increase and influence one's actions. When appropriate action is required in an emergency, there is no substitute for practice and experience.

Stage III: Response and Options

Also known as the "fight or flight" syndrome; adrenaline is released into the system as a response to a stimulus. This phase is often characterized by "scatterbrained" thinking, with no definite plan, and a refusal to believe the situation is really as bad as it is or that it is happening at all. This may quickly progress to complete panic, typified by frozen limbs and mind (including physical weakness, crying, trembling, nausea, or vomiting). An individual might turn and run, stand and do something positive, or merely turn into a shaking blob. It must be understood that anxiety and fear are perfectly natural feelings that can and must be controlled.

The best approach to managing this phase is to apply a methodical approach to the problem, using precise actions and sequential procedures learned through training and practice.

Stage IV: Rest

This stage involves a sharp emotional letdown after high-energy output.

- Eventually, this will come whether wanted or not.
- In many cases, this will be a complete physical and emotional drain.
- Shock will likely occur, so be prepared for it.

Comfort Zones

Humans are basically creatures of habit and are dependent on routine, organization, and some degree of discipline. Once these habits are established, people become comfortable with their behavior and surroundings. People generally become skilled and proficient only after a period of slow, deliberate actions while learning what is expected of them. Everyone establishes these "comfort zones" both physically and mentally. It follows then that whenever a person is placed in a situation that forces use of the outer limits of his/her comfort zone, anxiety and stress are created.

Comfort zone limits vary with each individual in accordance with experience and knowledge. Everyone is unique in abilities, and since a human being is basically a creature of habit, most will go outside of their comfort zones only rarely. Herein is the difficulty of functioning in any emergency environment. Very often, every decision is important and there is little room for mistakes.

At best, decision-making is always difficult and this is even more true in times of emotional upset. The best way to prepare mentally is through self-discipline and practice during everyday routine. Look for opportunities to expand your comfort zone into areas that you may be unsure of now.

Are you a person who continually takes the easy way out or do you tackle everyday problems with a positive attitude and direct approach? These questions can be applied to personal relationships and situations that develop. The answers may give you a good indication of your ability to react under stress.

Good habits in training and everyday life pay off in an emergency.

SAFETY
In order to make sound decisions in stressful situations, establish self-discipline and good habits in your daily training.

Controlling Fear

As any individual approaches comfort zone limits, an unconscious level of fear known as anxiety will be experienced. This is characterized by feelings of uneasiness, general discomfort, worry, and/or depression. These feelings can vary in intensity, duration, and recurrence. If this anxiety is allowed to progress, it may become overt fear. Fear that is unchecked and reinforced by other thoughts or stimuli can quickly turn to panic with complete loss of reasoning. Fearfulness turned to blind panic can cause an experienced person to injure or kill him- or herself—and perhaps others—in the intensity of terror.

INFO
No passion so effectively robs the mind of all its powers of acting and reasoning as fear.
Edmund Burke, 1729–1797
British statesman and political theorist

Training, including knowledge and experience gained in simulated emergencies, reduces the unknown and helps to control fear. When fantasy distorts a moderate danger into a major catastrophe, behavior can become abnormal. If this happens, people may be reacting to feelings and imagination or past traumatic events rather than the actual problem at hand. In such cases people tend to underestimate (rather than overestimate) the danger, which readily leads to reckless, even foolhardy, behavior.

There are many ways to fight fear, but one of the best is to meet it head on. Recognize fear as a natural phenomenon. Try to establish just why it is that you are afraid and accept it as the defense mechanism that it is. Some professionals in the behavior field believe it is beneficial to get mad at your own fears. At least it is a positive action that puts the fear into proper prospective.

To best manage fear in an emergency, make sure you have the following:

- As much knowledge about the situation as possible
- The proper tools and/or equipment for the response
- A positive mental attitude (will to live).

Tell yourself that others have conquered the same situation. There are no clear-cut lines between recklessness and bravery, or caution and panic. That is why it is essential to maintain proper mental control in an emergency.

Symptoms of Fear

Physical Symptoms

- Quickening of pulse, breathlessness
- Dilation of pupils
- Increased muscular tension and fatigue
- Perspiration of hands, feet, and armpits
- Frequent urination
- Dry mouth and throat, high-pitched voice with stammering
- "Butterflies" and faintness caused by empty stomach
- Nausea and vomiting

Mental Symptoms

- Irritability, increased hostility
- Talkative at early stages, later speechless
- Laugh or cry hysterically
- Confusion, forgetfulness, inability to concentrate
- Feeling of unreality, flight, panic, and sometimes stupor

Controlling Your Fear

- Do not try to physically or mentally run away from the situation. Recognize fear for what it is and accept it. Try to learn what your reactions are likely to be by looking at your daily habits.
- Learn how to make decisions quickly and logically by establishing good habits. Take positive action to take control of the situation instead of letting it control you.
- Develop self-confidence by continually expanding your comfort zone to encompass experiences that are unfamiliar. Define your fears and recognize them.
- Realize that "it can happen to me" and be prepared. Be properly equipped and prepared at all times. Always have a number of options in your plan. Prepare for the worst and hope for the best.
- Keep informed and increase your knowledge to reduce the unknown.

- Have procedures mapped out so that you will be busy, if not physically then mentally.
- Set realistic goals.
- Realize that teamwork always accomplishes more than a one-person show.
- Use affirmative self-talk. Talk positively about your actions and your future.
- Do not be afraid of spiritual faith.
- Gather as much information about your situation as possible.
- Cultivate good survival-oriented attitudes. The main goal is survival with everything kept in perspective. The discomforts of the moment are only temporary.

Controlling Fear in Others

- Cultivate mutual support.
- Use good leadership practices.
- Practice and demonstrate discipline as a model for others.
- Demonstrate a positive attitude.
- Do not indicate resentment of others' reactions. Accept a person's right to individual feelings.
- Do not scold others. Accept a person's limitations.
- Comfort others without encouraging them to feel sorry for themselves.
- Involve them in simple tasks; occupy their minds and bodies.

Mental Steps of Managing an Emergency

One way to find answers in a survival situation is to use the mnemonic, STOP:

S – Stay/Stop
T – Think
O – Observe
P – Plan

Stay/Stop at the first sign of trouble. Rushing around will only cause confusion. Stopping helps fight the emotions of anxiety and panic, and greatly improves your chances of surviving. You got yourself into this situation and you can get yourself out. Stop for a moment and be patient. If anyone needs medical assistance, administer first aid.

Think about immediate and future dangers. Analyze the weather terrain and available resources to sustain life. Look for recognizable landmarks or study a map for clues. If you are lost, how long ago did you know where you were? Can you return to that spot? Are there footprints or signs to guide you? Can you hear signs of civilization? Move slowly, and do not make hasty judgments. Think about what the correct future actions should be.

Observe and size up the situation. Look around for immediate hazards that may threaten you. How long until darkness? What is available to work with? Look for the best possible course of action.

Plan the best course of action before implementing any action. Be deliberate and practical. Your plan should be a blueprint based upon the necessities and priorities of life.

Individual Beliefs

Many adult fears and related misconceptions are based upon stories and statements originating during early years of life from unenlightened sources. These thoughts, statements, and stories are stored in the subconscious. Survival and emergency preparedness trainings are important to balance reality and experience against illusion and raw instinct.

Negative feedback inadvertently given during childhood or during any learning process may have a profound effect on behavior and reaction. Negative reaction to fledgling attempts at independence and self-reliance are good examples of how to program them for poor performance in the future. The same principle holds true after a person reaches maturity and receives negative feedback for some type of performance. Negative self-talk has a dramatic negative effect on performance. All people must learn to program themselves and others more positively, remembering that individuals act or react in accordance with what each believes to be true.

The mind is constantly at work picking up information and skills, and the subconscious will never erase whatever is intentionally or unintentionally placed there. In any situation, actions are a reflection of how an individual perceives the environment and the individual in it. In short, the subconscious mind mirrors self-image. If the self-image is strong, the individual will be strong. If the picture is of a weakling, the individual will be weak. More importantly, individuals who think they cannot survive probably will not even try.

Every Survivor Sets a Goal

Hundreds of accounts and personal interviews with those who have undergone trying mental and physical experiences reveal that nearly every survivor has set some type of goal. The goal may have been simply to live or it may have been a combination of staying alive and accomplishing something else. Philosophically, life is comprised of setting one goal after another and taking the trip in between. Many prisoners of war (POWs) who were released after the Vietnam conflict related numer-

ous self-set goals that gave meaning and purpose to staying alive.

The goal-setting process is vital and has been used extensively, but many cheat themselves of its full effect. It has been said that life is truly not the setting of personal goals, but the journeys to reach those goals that makes living worthwhile. If this is true, then constantly learning to readjust goals provides incentive, not only to live, but to give purpose to existence. Likewise, a survivor must readjust goals to suit the situation. Many people have survived tremendously difficult ordeals after crashing a vehicle only to die just after being rescued. Their main goal could have been to be rescued. Perhaps they failed to look beyond that goal and establish new goals. They simply let down and gave up too soon.

We Choose Our Path

We as individuals have the ability to evaluate performance potential during a time of emergency or stress. We are creatures of habit, and do things regularly that will give good indications of how we will react to emergencies.

Nearly always, we choose the path to follow after the onset of an emergency. All of us have the ability to use our mind as a valuable tool or have it work against us as a feared enemy. It is never too late for changing our habits, values, and attitudes to ones that will produce positive mental actions during emergencies.

Maintaining a PMA is the key to successful emergency response and better everyday living. A "can do" attitude is necessary for both survival and SAR work. Solve the problems as they arise, one at a time, and you can stay alive with comfort and safety. Problem solving in itself is a test of your ability to analyze and act in an appropriate way. You must improvise with what you know and with what you have.

As an individual involved in SAR, be prepared. The physical answer to being prepared lies in the clothing and equipment that you will carry. The mental answer of preparedness will be the training, education, and variety of knowledge that you have filed away in your brain.

Defensive Living: A Preparedness Ethic

The emergency preparedness education philosophy of defensive living is best defined as the constant conscious thought process and behavior of an individual to identify or predict situations that will affect his/her comfort or existence. This philosophy is not meant to be an obsession or extreme preoccupation, but rather a conscious development of an individual preparedness attitude to avoid unnecessary emergency situations. Defensive living is the knowledge to recognize dangers, make the proper choices, and have the necessary skills, equipment, and knowledge to cope with adversity.

Defensive living develops self-responsibility to always:

- Reduce the risk factor
- Maintain optimum body efficiency
- Solve the immediate threat problem
- Maintain positive action
- Guard personal comfort

The goal of defensive living is to create in each of us the habits of forethought, awareness, preparedness, and alertness to cope with changing situations that threaten or affect our lives.

Improvisation

Solving the problem of staying alive in any life-threatening situation requires a basic understanding of several concepts. Survival is based on resilience, that is, the ability to overcome difficulties and disappointments. It also requires talent (skills), desire, and the optimism to overcome those difficulties and disappointments. It is essential to understand the nature of threats posed by the natural environment and the corresponding physiological effects on the body. With this knowledge should come an ability to assess the level of threat and establish a set of priorities. While there is no substitute for preparedness, there will always be situations where the right resource to do a job is simply not available. What is available must be adapted to meet the needs at hand. This adapting of one's surroundings to solve problems is called improvisation. Occasionally, procuring the necessities of life is not easily accomplished and one must improvise to accomplish a goal or solve a problem. Being adaptable, that is, capable of improvising, is an important survival skill.

Survivors have used chunks of rotten log for building blocks and bark stripped from fallen trees for floors, walls, and roofs. There are stories of stormbound pioneers who wore bark slab clothing. Nothing is useless when survival is the issue. A car, a downed airplane, or any man-made object contains a potential source of needed materials.

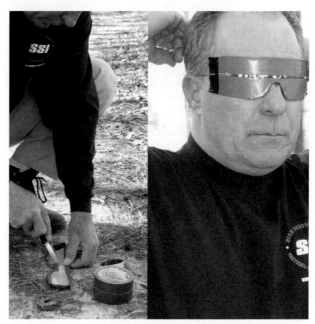

Figure 6–2 Improvising means a person must reason, compare, analyze, and solve problems to accomplish an objective. Shown is a pair of "pinhole" goggles used to enhance or protect vision in the absence of eyeglasses or sunglasses. A knife is used to punch two rows of small holes in a piece of aluminum cut from a soda can (left). Photo courtesy of F. Wysocki, Survival Strategies, Inc.

Improvising means a person must reason, compare, analyze, and solve problems to accomplish an objective (**Figure 6–2**). It involves a basic knowledge of physics, chemistry, mechanics, and common sense to utilize what is available to accomplish the task. It may not be perfect, but adequate for short-time emergency use. As soon as a problem is recognized, decide what is required, and then decide how to do it. Be positive, look around, and try to make what is needed from materials at hand. Prioritize needs using the necessities of life and the following rules and principles of improvising.

Six Simple Steps in the Improvising Process

1. Size up the situation.
   - Determine your needs.
   - What is your priority? Shelter? Fire? Medical?
   - Is there a need that you must take care of first?
   - How was it done in early or primitive times?
2. Identify contingencies.
   - Could the situation get worse if I don't improvise something? If so, how bad could it get?
3. Determine your goal.
   - Exactly what do I need and what is the time frame?

4. Inventory your resources.
   - Available materials and tools.
5. Build a plan.
   - Consider the alternatives: What can I use instead?
   - Keep it simple, and think about simple machines.
   - Select the alternative providing the most efficient use of your materials, time, and energy.
6. Take action.
   - Make your product durable and safe.
   - Remember the real priorities and necessities of life.

Look at resources and materials as a primitive society would look at them: How can I use this piece of material to provide a basic need, or how can this resource be useful to accomplish what task? Think of an object that normally does the job. How is it constructed, what materials is it made of, and what principles does it incorporate? Now, look around and see what is available. Can you construct it from what you have? Try it. Use failures as incentives to try again. Never quit trying.

Useful articles for improvising include:

- Your clothing
- Contents of your pockets
- Other personal equipment
- Items in the natural environment
- Garbage and rubbish
- Stalled transportation

High Priority Needs

Improvised first aid materials include:

- Bandages: clothing, belts or seat belts, sleeping bags, tents
- Splints: sticks and limbs, molding, seat foam, carpet.
- Crutches: limbs and branches, ski poles, tent poles, skis, ice axe
- Neck support: foam rubber in seats, magazines, maps, sleeping pad.

Improvised clothing and shelter materials include:

- Protection: carpet, tent material, garbage bag, stuff sac, and plastic tarp
- Cordage: wire, seat belts, belt, strips from plastic bag or clothes twisted together
- Insulation: upholstery padding, maps, newspaper, carpet, dry grass, and pine needles
- Eye protection: side of soda can with pinholes, paper with pinholes, bark, T-shirt.

Improvised fire starting materials include:

- Spark: battery and wire, lighter striker
- Stove construction: Fill a container with fuel and oil mixed with sand, loamy soil or dirt. As the fire dies down, stir the sand or soil and the flame will flare back up.

Signaling materials include:

- Lights: Battery, a light and some wire (stalled transportation), chemical lights, headlamps, etc.
- Fire: Oil, tires, foam rubber, and hoses all burn with black smoke. Also, upholstery in vehicle.
- Ground signal: Part of an aircraft, boughs, clothing, rocks, logs, shadow from trench.
- Signal mirror: Reflectors, light lens, mirrors, glass, polished metal.

Improvised water procurement materials include:

- Collectors: Black plastic in winter, clear plastic in summer (transpiration bag); condensation on metal surfaces, deep hole in the right location.
- Storage: Zip lock bags, sheet of plastic with tied opening, vehicle parts, rubber gloves, section of tarp, in clothing or shoe (boot).

Shelter

Shelter is anything that protects the body from temperature, weather, insects, or any other life-threatening force or element. In fact, our clothing is the shelter we wear and it constitutes the first line of defense in any environment. Without shelter (adequate protection from the elements and environment) in most places on Earth, humans can only survive for a short time. Without adequate clothing, a shelter is essential. Without adequate clothing and shelter on most of the Earth, a fire is essential. The ability to maintain the body's optimum temperature (98.6°F) and knowledge of how to apply body shelter concepts are essential for comfort and survival in the outdoors. In its simplest form, a shelter may or may not have a heat source, though in colder climates, some form of heat is desirable for additional comfort. In an emergency, (severe weather, inadequate clothing, injured companion), it is important to find protection from the elements as soon as possible.

There are three basic types of shelters that can be utilized in an emergency (Figure 6–3). The first is called

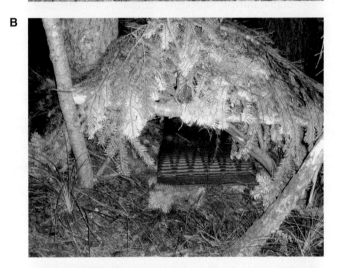

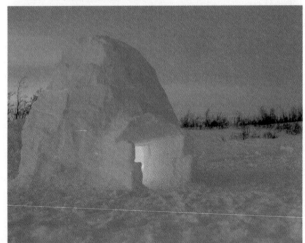

Figure 6–3 Three basic types of shelters can be utilized in an emergency: (A) immediate action, (B) temporary, and (C) long-term.

"immediate action" and can serve to protect an individual within minutes. This type of shelter normally consists of something carried by an individual that can be accessed and put into use very quickly. It serves as an immediate body protection mechanism and is generally small, compact, and lightweight. This type of shelter is commonly usable in water or on land, and can be as simple as a 7-bushel leaf bag or a heavy-duty 55-gallon barrel liner. Many outdoorsman prefer the heavy-duty trash bags utilized by highway departments to pick up trash and other litter.

Temporary shelter can be accessed and utilized in somewhere between 30 and 60 minutes. Minimal energy is expended to construct or access this survival-type shelter. It generally requires improvisation, some basic tools, and knowledge of shelter construction and design. Temporary shelters utilize existing resources from the environment, stalled transportation, or items from a personal preparedness inventory. In many cases this can be a transition to the last type shelter, which is more long term in nature.

The third type of shelter, commonly called long term, is a structure designed to accommodate someone for 72 hours or more. This type of shelter requires substantially more resources and energy to build and incorporates more of what we would like to think of as "creature comforts." It is normally only built when an extended stay is anticipated, but in most cases it would not be necessary.

Three Types of Shelter

1. Immediate action shelter: Can protect you within minutes.
2. Temporary shelter: Can be accessed and utilized in 30 to 60 minutes.
3. Long-term shelter: Designed and built to accommodate someone for 72 hours or more.

While some say, "do like the animals do" and seek shelter by burrowing under foliage or in a protected area, this advice must be qualified. It is virtually impossible to build a waterproof and windproof shelter from natural materials. You must be prepared! There is no substitute for good rain gear, tarps, tents, a good rain fly, and/or adequate clothing. Don't waste reserves of energy and body heat with futile unproductive efforts. Fire and light are pleasant, but starting a fire in rain or snow and/or high wind may be impossible and only serve to waste calories and get clothing wet.

Whenever a situation requires immediate body protection, a shelter can be improvised from what you have with you or around you. Your preparation and the materials at hand will determine a shelter's efficiency. Efficient shelters need little or no external headroom to maintain body warmth. Adequate body shelter can be improvised with the right materials and preparation.

Shelter is a supplement to clothing, and a properly built shelter should protect the body from wind, wet, cold, and insects. Through a lack of adequate body shelter or clothing, the already limited supplies of body heat, energy, and water are quickly lost. Remember, a sleeping bag is a shelter composed of two layers of relatively weatherproof fabric separated by insulating material. Heat produced by the body is retained inside the bag even when outside temperatures drop below freezing.

The efficiency of a sleeping bag is improved by added ground insulation (more trapped dead air space or thickness of material), extra insulating material fabricated in the bag itself, and overhead protection (tent or tarp) from wind and rain. Keep this sleeping bag principle in mind when building emergency shelters.

Build a shelter:

- Simple and small, no bigger than what is absolutely needed for body protection.
- With minimal expenditure of time, energy, and body water.
- To minimize body heat loss or gain through the primary mechanisms of temperature transfer in the body (conduction, convection, radiation, evaporation).

Considerations for Shelter Building

The usefulness and efficiency of a shelter is dependent on many factors, such as where it is built, what it is made from, and the environment in which it is built.

Shelter Location

It would be nice if there were always choices for ideal shelter locations. Sometimes circumstances dictate that we must "hole up" at whatever location or set of circumstances where the need exists. Stalled transportation provides the best source of immediate shelter needs, but many times a vehicle is not available. If caught outside unexpectedly, a good first step is to check the area for possible dangers. Areas to avoid include the following: dry streambeds in desert regions, avalanche chutes in steep rocky high country, rock fall areas, dead trees (snags) with large limbs, exposed mountain saddles or valley openings where strong winds tend to blow, low valley areas in winter or autumn where cold air pockets and/or frost may accumulate, and thick dense woods where moisture tends to accumulate and not dry out. Also, pay attention to insect or animal signs in the area. Slow-flowing river edges with swampy areas tend to accumulate mosquitoes and other biting insects. These simple preparatory initiatives can eliminate a lot of grief if conditions worsen.

Usable Materials

Remember that what a person carries is always the most easily accessible and the most dependable shelter material. If it is necessary to build a temporary emergency shelter, the first questions that must be answered are, "What is the primary element or factor that this shelter must protect me from, and what type of shelter is needed?" Is it cold, heat, rain, snow, insects, or something else? Function is more important than shape.

From an energy expenditure point of view, it makes sense to look for already developed sites or easily convertible resources, such as a hollow tree trunk or a fallen tree, so that with little effort a site can be turned into a serviceable shelter. A good example of this would be an exposed root ball from a tree that has blown down or eroded at the roots and fallen. In areas with no trees, you may be forced to build a shelter with nonconductive materials such as dirt, brush, sod or grass, and even leaves.

It is worth repeating that it is virtually impossible under typical emergency conditions to build a waterproof and windproof shelter from natural materials. To insure optimum protection, a person must have some type of man-made material readily available, such as a plastic bag, tent fly, tarpaulin, or coated tarp. If it is absolutely necessary to utilize boughs, leaves, or other natural materials, remember several important basic principles. When using natural materials, use them "as they grow in nature." This may be one bough stacked upon another with the butts pointing in the same direction—up. Using any natural materials in this fashion, like shingles on a house, is the only hope for effective precipitation protection. However, it will be marginal at best.

Basic principles of heat transfer (body heat loss or gain) and thermal conductivity (insulation) are the foundation for proper shelter building.

- Thermal conductivity and heat transfer is the measure of any substance's ability (or inability) to conduct heat. Comparisons of example substances are shown in **Table 6–2**.
- A lower value indicates a better insulator.
- In terms of survival, remember that the human body will lose or gain heat anytime it is in contact with a surface that is cooler or warmer than body temperature.

> **SAFETY**
>
> Shelters should always be kept small, dry, and well insulated. Less body heat will be needed to warm it and warmth will be retained longer.

Table 6–2	Thermal conductivity
Insulator	**Conductivity**
Air	1.0
Wood	3.5
Glass	7.0
Ice	7.0
Lead	145.0
Steel	1930.0
Aluminum	8600.0
Silver	17400.0

Trapped air is considered good insulation and is therefore a poor conductor.

Insulation Sources

Any man-made or natural materials that provide dead air space between you and the ground or environment can be considered an insulation source. While natural materials such as bark, deadwood, thick boughs, grass, or leaves do provide a measure of insulation, they are certainly not as efficient as most of the man-made products that could be available with any degree of preparation. In stalled transportation, any upholstery, carpet, foam rubber or other padding material would be considered good insulation. Many outdoorsmen prefer to carry a short section of insulated pad specifically for kneeling or sitting on when hiking in the outdoors. A small pad of this type can be a lifesaver in cold, wet, or snow conditions when used in conjunction with a plastic leaf or garbage bag.

Don't overlook your backpack or spare clothing items laid on the ground with some type of vegetation stuffed inside as insulation. Coiled rescue rope with a stuff sac filled with leaves or grass on top have been used successfully as an insulator from the ground.

Provided that you have adequate protection directly from the surface, snow is a great source of insulation in bitter cold winter environments. Snow can measurably enhance the efficiency of any natural material shelter by blocking the wind and adding dead air space to the walls of a shelter.

Fuel Sources

Gathering fuel for a fire and keeping it stoked costs energy and usually requires extended exposure to the elements. There may not be enough readily available fuels to warrant the effort to maintain a fire. A few hard and fast questions must be answered quickly. Are there adequate fuels? Should any shelter that I build be constructed to allow a fire inside or near the opening? Fire is a great morale builder, but is a fire really needed? A small, cramped, slightly uncomfortable shelter may be better with no fire.

Wind Direction

Check wind direction and exposure. Wind will generally blow down drainages at night and up during the day. If at all possible, a shelter entrance should be 90 degrees to the prevailing wind.

Water Sources

While having water nearby to an emergency bivouac may seem convenient or optimal, there are some drawbacks to being near water. Shelters right next to creeks, rivers, lakes, etc. will be damper and cooler in general and in most cases, much more prone to mosquitoes and no-see-ums. At certain times of the year, this can be particularly annoying or even dangerous. Drinking water sources, while convenient, should not really be a determining factor for shelter placement in any environment except extreme desert conditions.

General Considerations

The best shelter material and resources are the ones you carry with you. Keep it as simple as is needed. Natural materials can enhance and make any shelter more efficient, but don't count on utilizing natural materials exclusively. They may be in short supply when you most need them. Think and improvise more insulation materials to improve what you brought.

Improve on what is already there in nature. Enlarge a natural opening so it is possible to get in and out easily. Try to make enough room to stretch your legs, but this is not necessarily a prerequisite to an effective shelter.

Dirt and grass can be used for filling cracks or making the wall base. Snow can be used in the winter on a tarp or tent as an insulative cover, but this may require supportive pieces of wood or poles for the structure.

In hot weather, consider the following when building a shelter:

- Shade from the sun is the most important daytime shelter requirement. Materials or objects that produce shade will be a valuable resource.
- Moving air (convection) will be helpful. Beware of pockets or locations where there is little air movement.
- The principle of putting a shelter floor 12 to 18 inches above or below the ground level during the day reduces the temperature in the shelter substantially. However, the very real issues of energy

expenditure, availability of digging and construction tools, and the capability to dig if injured or while caring for a fellow rescuer or victim may make this impractical.

- Keep clothes on and the head covered to protect against sunburn.
- Do not stay in closed metal structures such as a vehicle without adequate ventilation. Temperatures can become intolerable and can cause hyperthermia.
- At night, when desert air cools considerably, better shelter and a fire might be needed. Work during cooler periods to improve shelter and general situations.
- Insects, snakes, scorpions, and the like are active at night. Protect your sleeping area, shelter, clothes, and shoes from easy access by these critters. Shake out clothing and shoes before putting them on again.

In cold weather, consider the following when building a shelter:

- Forested areas can provide overhead shelter, fuel for fires, and materials for insulation. A "downed tree shelter" can be the easiest natural shelter of all to exploit. It may already have a roof, floor, and one or both sides. If there is snow, a "tree pit shelter" may be a very real option and readily available.
- Scrape out a trench in the snow or ground on windblown prairies or exposed ridges. Pile rocks or other materials for a windbreak. Line the trench with limbs, grass, bark, stalled transportation materials, extra clothes, or any thing that will provide insulation. Put snow or dirt on top of a framework, crawl in, and close up.
- Snow at specific temperature gradients is a good insulator and gives good wind protection if used properly. However, it is hard to work with, requires a degree of practice and skill, and takes considerable energy. Digging a snow cave takes a long time and requires a tool. A large snow cave is not considered an immediate action survival shelter. Digging into a snow bank may use less energy. Work at a pace to minimize sweating, and try to keep clothes dry by utilizing plastic bags, tarps or some types of ground cloth material. Snow shelters must have adequate ventilation, especially with two or more people. A candle provides light, some heat, and is also an excellent indicator that oxygen is running out (you need to provide better ventilation). Avoid overheating the inside of a snow shelter, and as a precaution against getting wet, round and smooth inside surfaces so that any

moisture will run down the sides. If it melts, you may get wet. Protracted use of a snow shelter can cause the walls and ceiling to thaw and freeze into ice. If ice builds up, the shelter will become more of a conductor of heat rather than an insulator.

Firecraft

It is said by some that the ability to light a fire under a variety of conditions is among the most valuable of all survival skills. A number of years ago in the forested high country wilderness of Oregon, two teenage girls undergoing an Outward Bound experience got into trouble in a bad storm. Though they repeatedly tried to start a fire, they were not successful and the two young women died of hypothermia. In this case, the ability to start a fire literally made the difference between life and death.

Fire building is a skill that is only mastered by practicing in a wide spectrum of conditions with different materials. Proficiency requires a basic knowledge of how a fire burns and which tinders and fuels are best. If for no other reason, fire plays a vitally important psychological role in survival. Once having started a fire in difficult or emergency conditions, it provides a sense of achievement that to some extent replicates some of the most important elements of everyday life: the ability to cook or heat liquids to drink, to feel warm in the worst of conditions, and most of all, the ability to see in the dark. Fire can also provide dry clothing, a signal, a big boost to morale, and it can also be used to purify water.

Remember that if your clothing is inadequate, you will need a shelter. If your clothing and your shelter are inadequate, then you will definitely need a fire. Steep terrain, ground cover, availability of fuel, environmental conditions, and even time can all have an adverse impact on your capability to start a fire. Ask, "Is it worth the cost of energy expended to build and maintain a fire?" This is a realistic hard and fast decision that may have to be made. The smaller, drier, and better insulated your shelter is, the less heat is lost and the less need you have for fire.

Location of a Fire

Look for a location that is open and away from trees or other ground cover. Sandy or gravelly soil without grass or roots is best. The area should be protected from the wind, near potable water if possible, and near additional fuel supplies.

In forested or brushy areas, insure that the fire cannot spread out of control. In dry summer forest conditions, or even in dry grassy or low vegetation areas, it is

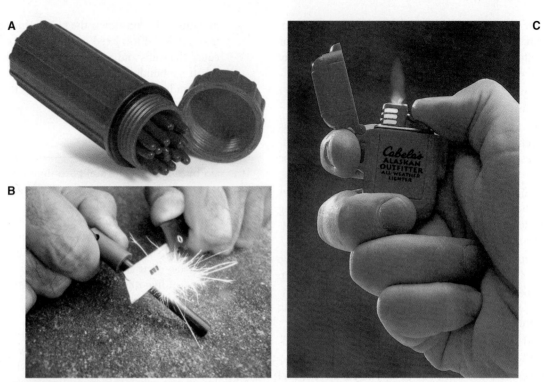

Figure 6–4 Any emergency survival kit should contain several methods of fire starting, such as (A) matches and striker in a waterproof container, (B) a magnesium bar and steel knife, and (C) a specialized survival lighter.

a good idea to clear a fire circle that is about five to six feet in diameter on sandy or gravelly soil and scraped down to mineral earth that is free of duff, grass, and roots.

A circle of dry rocks can contain the fire and is helpful for cooking and expanding the heat source. *Caution:* Do not use river rocks, as they contain moisture and often explode when heated.

Never build a fire:

- Near dry, flammable materials
- In very dry grassland
- Under overhanging branches
- In a very resinous (pitch-smelling), dry forest
- Under a snow-laden tree
- Directly on the snow
- On or near wet rocks

Fire Making Sources

There are two primary types of fire starting devices: friction (including wooden matches) and spark/heat producing (**Figure 6–4**).

Friction and Matches

There are many ways to start fires using friction, but the match is the most available and easiest to use. Wood matches carried in a waterproof container are one of the best and most reliable methods of starting a fire.

The "strike anywhere" type of matches are a myth and this type of match should not be chosen as a primary or backup system for starting a fire. Most matches are dependent upon both friction and a chemical reaction between the match head and the striker pad. While it is possible under certain circumstances to light some of these wooden matches with the fingernail or zipper from the trousers, it certainly is not reliable as a fire-starting source. If the specific striker pad for any container of matches gets wet, they become virtually impossible to light. Coating a match with shellac, varnish or other similar waterproofing material often makes it more difficult to light. Waterproofing a match with wax or paraffin tends to be much more reliable. Practical field trials and personal experience show that the best type of match to have in an emergency is the Recreational Equipment Inc. (REI®) Storm Proof Matches. They are reliable, readily available, waterproof, and they work incredibly well.

Primitive skill methods for starting fires such as bow and drill, hand drill, fire saw, plow board, fire thong, or South-Seas fire plunger are all methods developed in specific environments with specialized resources and all require a high degree of skill and practice to accomplish.

It is unrealistic to think that SAR volunteers or the average outdoors person could depend upon these methods as reliable and effective under adverse conditions. Acquiring primitive skills using friction takes a lot of time, practice, and energy. While some of these more primitive methods are great confidence builders, it is far better to carry matches in a waterproof container than to depend on these skills.

Spark/Heat Producing Devices

One of the best backup systems to have as a fire starter is a metal match (spark producing magnesium rod with a steel striker). Although not as easy to use as a wooden match, this device is second only to the wooden match as a reliable means of starting a fire, especially with the right tinder.

Using alternatives to matches and friction to start a fire generally requires good tinder (such as Vaseline™ and cotton balls) to capture the heat and/or spark produced, ignite the tinder, and subsequently ignite kindling. Unlike the use of matches and friction devices, using spark- and heat-producing devices is almost always reliable despite the presence of damp or wet conditions; they just take more practice to be effective. Examples of these devices include:

- Flint and steel (produce spark)
- Vehicle battery (shorting the terminals or live wires produces spark; vehicle cigarette lighter produces heat)
- Cigarette lighter (liquid fuel, wick, flint, and steel produce both spark and flame)
- Metal match (magnesium bar and steel striker produce spark)
- Magnesium fire starter (same as metal match)
- Chemicals (mixture of two or more chemicals to produce enough heat to ignite tinder)

Sporting goods and recreation stores often carry many types of spark/heat-producing fire starters. Any emergency survival kit should contain several methods of fire starting.

Fire Materials: Tinder, Kindling, and Sustaining Fuels

Fire materials should be gathered before attempting to start a fire. Try to use the driest possible materials that may be obtained from hollow logs, dead stumps, dead limbs on living trees, or dead twigs and limbs found away from the damp ground.

In very wet weather, dry wood can be found in the center of old stumps and the center of dead standing trees. Dry twigs can usually be found near the trunks of larger trees. Old burned out or broken off stumps (and any spires sticking up out of the stump) usually indicate high pitch concentrations ideal for building fires. Carefully plan, collect, and protect from the elements all of the necessary components: tinder, kindling and sustaining fuel.

Tinder

Tinder is anything that will ignite at a very low temperature, with a spark, small flame, or other heat source. It must be dry. Remember to start small and work up to larger combustible materials.

Consider the following for tinder:
- Vaseline impregnated cotton balls (this is absolutely the best)
- Dry grass, crushed
- Cotton or scraped cloth (not synthetic material)
- Fine, dry wood shavings
- Dry cattail fuzz
- Bird down
- Pitch wood, fine shavings or powdered wood
- Petroleum products
- Dry, reddish pine needles
- Seed down
- Shaved sticks
- Paper (shredded or rolled and tied into a knot)
- Inner bark of cedar or birch
- Dried moss or lichen
- Candle
- Oil- or gas-soaked cloth
- Flares or other pyrotechnics
- Birch bark

Kindling

The initial fuel stage is kindling. Find something that will ignite easily from the tinder. It needs to be relatively easy to burn material such as small diameter sticks and twigs, broken wood splinters, split or shaved pieces of wood to increase surface area and flammability. Or, it can simply be a material like congealed pitch that provides the increased heat to start larger sustaining fuel. Dry kindling can be split from larger pieces of dry wood using a knife and another piece of wood as a mallet.

Consider the following for kindling:
- Finely split wood
- Fuzz stick, carved with jackknife
- Small dry, dead branches and twigs
- Dry grasses twisted into bunches
- Congealed pitch that bleeds from conifers

Sustaining Fuel

Sustaining fuel is anything that will burn for an extended period of time. Generally it will not burn from the initial flame or spark and requires high temperatures for continued burning.

Consider the following for sustaining fuel:

- Dead wood (standing or recently fallen trees or shrubs)
- Dry peat
- Dried dung
- Rubber
- Green wood that is split
- Animal oil or fat
- Bundles of grass
- Pitch
- Petroleum or fuel, oil and soil mixture for improvised stove

Be cautious and do not use man-made products (e.g., plastics, upholstery, carpet, etc.) as many emit poisonous gases when burned and some may explode.

Starting the Fire

It is a good idea under virtually all conditions to start with a small platform of sticks or logs. This elevates the tinder up off the damp ground, vegetation, snow or other less than desirable base material. Place a larger log, bigger diameter branch or stick at one side of this small platform. This base serves as the foundation structure and will lend itself to the fire starting process (**Figure 6–5**).

Tinder should be arranged on the platform right next to the larger branch or log on the side. Kindling is then placed over the top of the tinder so that it rests against the larger log or branch much like the roof on a lean-to shelter. This ensures adequate oxygen flow to the tinder and can also allow maximum heat from the tinder or flame to rise through the greatest amount of kindling. When the kindling begins to burn well, add larger pieces of fuel. The platform provides several key functions. First, depending on which side of the platform the larger log or branch is placed, it provides a windbreak. It also provides elevation from the ground dampness, better oxygen flow to the tinder and kindling, and an excellent base for adding sustaining fuels. Be patient and do not smother the kindling flames with larger material until the flame has reached a good hot temperature. The second mistake often made in fire building is cutting off the flow of air (oxygen) to the flame by adding too much fuel too quickly.

All of the combustible components (tinder, kindling, and sustaining fuel) must be gathered before attempting to build a fire. Keep all materials as dry as possible. Remember that the heat from each successive stage in the process should rise through the maximum amount of material stacked neatly on top in the next stage. Properly built, a fire should gradually and steadily build in intensity throughout the entire process.

Fire Without Wood Fuel

A metal can, container or improvised container such as a headlight holder or battery box can serve as an emergency stove with a mixture of oil, gasoline and a cloth wick. Oil-soaked rags or shredded upholstery in a shallow pan of oil will also burn. Fill a container one third full of dry dirt or sand. Although it will improve the draft by making small holes on the sides, it really isn't necessary. Saturate the soil with a mixture of one part oil to 2 parts gasoline or diesel. Wait a few minutes and then ignite it with a match or spark. Stir occasionally when the flames die down. The wicking action up through the soil will pull the gas oil mixture up to the surface.

Firecraft Tips

- Conserve matches whenever possible by lighting a candle or fuzzy stick.
- Green wood will burn if finely split.
- Find dry wood for fire starting in the center of standing dead trees or large undergrowth. Small dry twigs are often available near the base of green trees.
- If you have no cutting tool sufficient for splitting wood, whittle a hard wood wedge, and drive it into weathering cracks in the end of the wood. A good knife and a wooden mallet (branch from a tree at least 2–3 inches in diameter) will serve as a good improvised splitting tool (see Figure 6–5).
- A reflector (metal, rock, wood) on one side of a fire makes it more efficient. For a fire site with a large rock surface on one side or at the base of a cliff, do not use the rock as a reflector. Build the fire far enough away from the rock so that you can sleep between the two. The rock will provide warmth on one side, while the fire warms the other.
- Fire supplements the body's heat-producing mechanism. In colder weather, several small fires built around you heat better than a single, larger fire.
- Cooking fires should be walled-in to concentrate the heat.
- If a fire must be built in deep snow, build it on a platform of green logs. Two layers of green logs 3 to 4 inches in diameter stacked in opposing

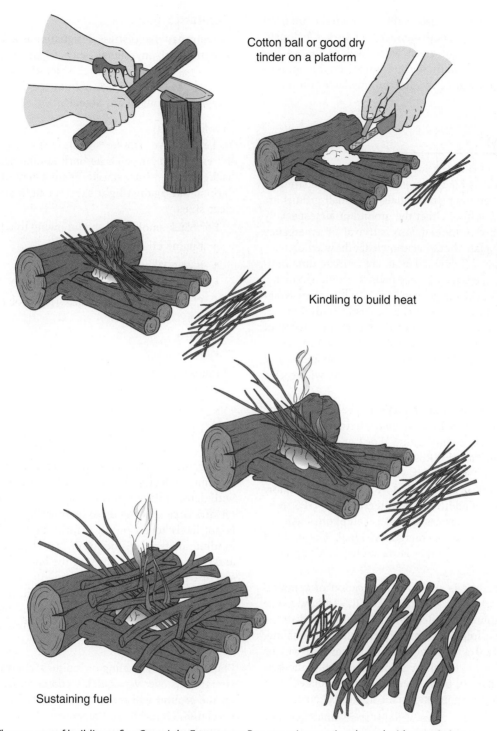

Cotton ball or good dry
tinder on a platform

Kindling to build heat

Sustaining fuel

Figure 6–5 The process of building a fire. Copyright Emergency Response International, used with permission.

directions will usually suffice to keep the fire from sinking for a good number of hours. Obviously, any platform of green wood will prolong a fire from sinking in these conditions. The thickness of the wood will be the determining factor on time.

Signaling

Emergency signaling is intended to make a person or persons more visible and most often implies distress of one form or another. Individuals and small groups are difficult to spot from either the ground or air, especially when visibility is limited. Any survival or emergency contingency plan should acknowledge how emergency situations may develop and at an appropriate time indicate how rescuers may be notified. The time factor before rescue depends largely on how effective distress signals are and how fast they can be made ready for use. Most successful rescues and/or recoveries are a result of individuals who are able to assist in their own rescue by getting the attention of someone who can help. The sooner you effectively signal, the sooner you will receive assistance.

In general, electronic signals or beacons are the most reliable and easily activated. There are three primary types: ELTs (Emergency Locator Transmitters) carried on aircraft, EPIRBs (Emergency Position Indicating Beacons) carried on watercraft, and PLBs (Personal Locator Beacons) carried by an individual in any environment. In addition, the integration of GPS technology into these devices as well as cell phones will enhance their value as an emergency signal. The use and operation of these devices is discussed in Chapter 2, SAR Systems.

Good signaling is really the application of common sense about what to use, when to use it, and how to use available resources to effectively communicate distress. Be ingenious, follow the basic principles of signaling, and your chances of being seen or discovered will be greatly enhanced. The more signals you make, the better your chances of being seen. The more isolated your environment, the more important signals become.

Although various types of flares and smoke generating devices (pyrotechnics) make excellent signals, they are heavy, require training in their safe use, and can be dangerous. The following signals are recommended for use by SAR personnel:

- Fire (smoke and light)
- Mirror (preferably glass not metal)
- Loud whistle, such as Fox 40® or Lifesaver #1®
- Colored signaling panels

Standard Signals

The international distress designation is a series of three repetitions of any signal, such as three loud sounds, three fires, three flares, etc. Voice distress is *Mayday, Mayday, Mayday* or *S.O.S.* Acknowledgment by rescuers is two repetitions of any signal.

Smoke Signals

To be effective, smoke signals need to contrast with the environment, such as dark smoke against a light background, white smoke against dark background, dark smoke against light skies, or light smoke against clear skies.

For black smoke add the following to a fire:
- Engine oil
- Rags soaked in oil
- Pieces of any rubber product
- Plastic or synthetic material (polyester, nylon, polypropylene, etc.)
- Pitch
- Pitch wood

For white smoke add the following to a fire:
- Green leaves or grass
- Moss, ferns, or other wet vegetation
- Green tree boughs
- A limited amount of water or wet cotton clothes

In some environments, an evergreen torch can be an extremely effective signal. Select a small evergreen tree with dense foliage, cut it down, and move it to the center of a large clearing or some other location where fire is not likely to get out of control. Place dry tinder and kindling material in the lower branches of the cut tree and secure it either by burying the butt of the tree in the soil or with a smaller stake driven into the ground. If an aircraft or other ground searchers are heard or seen, ignite the tree. In most low wind situations, this signal can punch smoke from 1200 to 1500 feet straight up.

Signal Mirror

Practice mirror-signaling techniques in advance because aircraft pass over very quickly and even distant rescuers on the ground will move out of sight if surrounded by vegetation (Figure 6–6). Prepare and be ready, as the opportunity may pass without someone seeing the signal.

Mirror flashes or reflections off of shiny objects have saved many lives. Use all of a mirror or small parts, a piece of shiny metal, or improvise a mirror from a food tin, belt buckle, or aluminum foil. Use your extended hand with two fingers held up similar to a rifle sight as an aiming device. Find the reflected sunlight on the ground from the mirror or shiny object and then position the mirror or object so that the reflected light passes

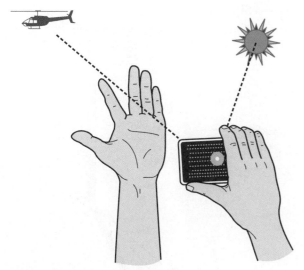

Figure 6–6 Aiming a signal mirror.

across your extended two fingers. Now, keeping the reflected light on your two fingers, move your arm so that your target (aircraft or rescue team) is centered between your fingers. Move the mirror or shiny object's reflected light back and forth across your fingers while keeping the target centered between them. It may be a good idea to continue sweeping the horizon even though no aircraft are visible. Mirror flashes can often be seen for many miles even on hazy days.

Shadows on Ground Signals

Shadows enhance, define, and make ground signal formations bigger and more easily seen. Use the sun to cast shadows from raised portions of the signal or into depressions in the ground. The signal should have the right directional orientation if optimum shadow effect is to be utilized. Near the equator, a north-south line gives a shadow at any time except noon. Further north or south, that same north-south line will also give the best results. Brush, foliage, rocks, or snow blocks piled in a line are effective methods of increasing the shadow size and emphasis. Remember, there are very few straight lines and right angles in nature, and the ultimate goal is to get someone's attention.

Color Signals

The right color attracts or grabs attention. White clothing on snow or green outer garments in forests are nearly impossible to see. Searchers can only see bright contrasting colors such as yellow-orange, light red, and white against green vegetation. Some have suggested that red disappears with distance on snow-covered terrain or backgrounds. If wearing dark clothes, change to a lighter color in a forested area. Use white underclothes as flags or change the color by turning it inside out.

Small signal panels or flags are more visible when moved slowly or waved. *Bright royal blue contrasts with virtually all environments and terrain.*

Other Signaling Methods

Repeated sounds coming from unusual places and at set times attract attention. Whistles, drums, gunshots, or anything audible such as using a big stick to bang on a tree or hollow log, can carry a vital message. If a whistle is not available, make one from a sapling or piece of metal. Yelling or shouting is only effective when a ground party is nearby. If searchers are looking, change your surrounding landscape. In brush, cut conspicuous patterns in the vegetation. In snow, tramp large side trenches or pile brush or rocks to spell out a message such as SOS or HELP. Place trenches or piles so the sun creates shadows to make obvious contrast to the normal scene.

Use available flares, two-way radios, or other signaling devices only when most noticeable. Small radios and emergency beepers have limited range and need to be on high ground for maximum effectiveness.

In the woods, spread colored tarps over treetops, or hoist a large white or colored flag on a pole lashed to the top of a tall tree.

At night use flashlights, strobe lights, recognition lights, or vehicle lights and flashers. Light can be seen several miles over water on a clear night. Electronic distress markers are also extremely effective.

A Cylume or chemical glow stick can be tied to the end of a string or rope and twirled around to make a large signal called a "buzz saw."

A whistle at night or in a fog can attract surface vessels, people on shore, or locate another separated raft.

Basic Principles of Signaling

- Have signals ready for immediate use.
- Use pyrotechnics in a manner that will not jeopardize safety.
- Use a ratio of 6:1 on letters or ground marks used. (Example: 3 feet wide and 18 feet long.)
- Fires are usually very visible at night or in reduced light.
- For maximum efficiency, place signal fires in open areas. Trees tend to disperse smoke.
- White or black smoke (depending on the surrounding/background terrain and vegetation) can be very visible.
- Moving or flashing lights attract attention in virtually any terrain.
- Shadows define, emphasize, and make larger any ground-to-air signal.

- Movement on a contrasting background attracts attention. Contrast is the key to effective signals.
- Colored flags, ground cloths, or bright clothing that contrast against the natural terrain, used with movement, are very visible. Bright royal blue is a very visible color in all environments.
- There are very few straight lines and right angles in nature. Therefore, they attract attention.
- Out of place formations, structures, vegetation, or color attracts attention. Do everything possible to disturb the "natural" look of the environment.
- Bigger is better.
- Choose a spot for signaling that is visible from 360 degrees, such as high ground, clearing, ridge, etc.
- Stay with your stalled or crashed transportation. If you must travel, leave a note and signs of your direction of travel.

Successful signaling can speed rescue and eliminate the possibility of a long, uncomfortable ordeal. Signals make you effectively larger.

Improvising Time and Direction

A situation may arise where SAR personnel may wish to roughly determine the time of day or general direction (relative to north). Although many methods exist for accomplishing this, only a few of the easiest and most reliable options will be described.

During the Day

Under normal circumstances, direction and time can be established and monitored with a compass, or a GPS and a wristwatch, for accuracy and dependable information. However, there may be circumstances where it is necessary to navigate without map and compass or tell time without the use of a watch. In these circumstances it is necessary to improvise and observe natural phenomena such as the stars or where the sun is, or even how a shadow falls. You can use the sun to find north (and any other direction, once north has been located) using a branch or stick placed in the ground to cast a shadow (Figure 6–7).

With a fairly straight stick about 18 to 24 inches long:
- Find a fairly level, brush- or vegetation-free spot. Push the stick into the ground, inclining it to get a longer, bigger shadow if necessary.
- Mark the tip of the shadow with the stick, stone, etc. Wait until the shadow tip moves a few inches (10 to 15 minutes with an 18 inch stick).

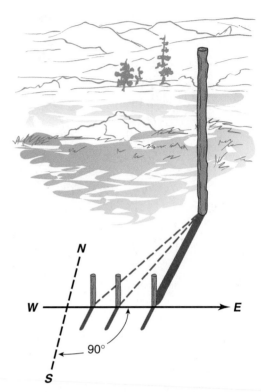

Figure 6–7 Stick and shadow method of determining direction.

- Mark the position of the new shadow tip.
- Draw a straight line from first marker (shadow tip) through, and about a foot past, the second marker.
- The line just drawn is an east-west line. The first mark made was toward the west end of the line. The last mark made is toward the east end of the line.
- A line perpendicular to the drawn east-west line is a north-south line.

This system works because the sun always travels precisely east to west, even though it might not rise and set at exactly 90 degrees and 270 degrees. The shadow tip moves in the opposite direction, so the first shadow tip mark is always west of the second, anywhere on Earth. Keep in mind that these improvised methods of determining direction are fraught with factors that do not allow accuracy. They are only general indicators and are far from providing the accuracy of a compass. However, they can provide enough data to establish a backup or check system.

An alternate method also uses a three-foot stick, this time pushed into the ground so it points directly at the sun, casting no shadow on the ground at the base of the stick. Wait 10 or 15 minutes and check the direction the

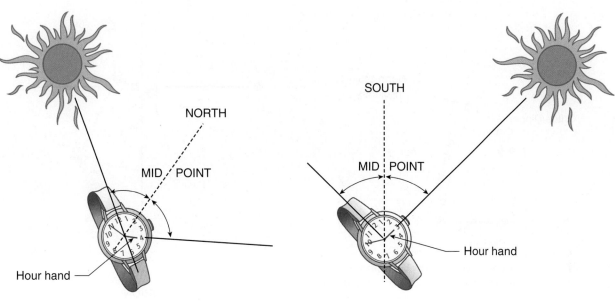

SOUTHERN HEMISPHERE

NORTHERN HEMISPHERE

If on daylight saving time subtract one hour from actual time

Figure 6–8 Finding directions using a wristwatch.

shadow falls. A line drawn through the tip of the shadow and the base of the stick is an east-west line. The narrower the stick is at the top, the easier it will be to determine general direction.

The shadow tip method used for finding direction can also determine approximate time of day:

- After drawing an east-west line, draw an intersecting, perpendicular north-south line. Push a stick into the ground at the intersection. The west part of the line indicates the position of the stick's shadow at sunrise (arbitrarily 0600 hours). The east part of the line indicates shadow position at sunset (1800 hours). The north-south line indicates shadow position at noon.
- The shadow of the stick becomes the hour hand of your clock and you can estimate time using the noon and 6 o'clock lines as guides.
- The shadow clock is not even close to being as accurate as a watch. However, it divides the day into 12 unequal hours, with sunrise always 0600 and sunset always 1800.

- Twelve o'clock shadow time is always true midday, but spacing of other hours varies somewhat with location and time of year.

An ordinary wrist- or pocket watch can help establish direction using either standard or daylight saving time (Figure 6–8). Point the hour hand at the sun and determine the halfway point between that hour hand and 12 o'clock or 1 o'clock (daylight time), and that will indicate a north-south line (south in the northern hemisphere and north in the southern hemisphere). On cloudy days, hold a small stick at the center of the watch so its shadow falls along the hour hand. A line drawn halfway between the shadow and 12 o'clock (on the side of the dial that contains the smaller numbers 1 to 6) indicates north in this hemisphere.

At Night

Determining direction at night will take a little knowledge of the constellations (Figure 6–9). On a clear evening you can find the North Star by locating the Big Dipper. The two stars forming the end of the bowl are

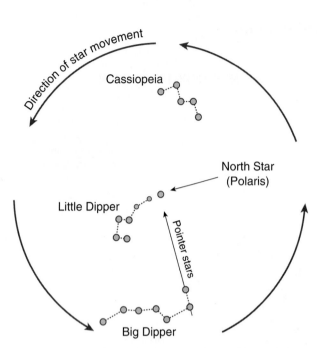

Figure 6–9 The relationship between the Big Dipper, Polaris, and Cassiopeia. In the Northern Hemisphere, a line drawn straight down from the North Star (Polaris) will be within 1° of true north. Find the North Star by locating the Big Dipper or Cassiopeia. The two stars on the outer edge of the Big Dipper are called pointers because they point almost directly to the North Star. If the pointers are obscured by clouds, Polaris can be identified by its relationship to the constellation Cassiopeia.

"pointers." Visualize a straight line drawn through the "pointer stars." Along this line, approximately five times the distance between the pointers is the North Star (Polaris), which is located above the Dipper lip. The Big Dipper rotates around the North Star, and is not always at the same position in the sky. When the Dipper is low in the sky and is obscured by trees or high ground, the constellation Cassiopeia (The Queen's Chair)—a group of five bright stars shaped like a lopsided "M" (or "W" when low in the sky)—can be used. The North Star is straight out from the middle star in Cassiopeia, at about the same distance as from the Dipper lip. Actually, a straight line from the middle star in Cassiopeia through the North Star will intersect the first star up the handle of the Big Dipper. Since Cassiopeia is almost directly opposite the Dipper, one constellation will generally be observable for finding the North Star.

Direction from Orion

The constellation of Orion consists of seven stars (**Figure 6–10**). The three central stars close together are called the Belt of Orion. The star through which the

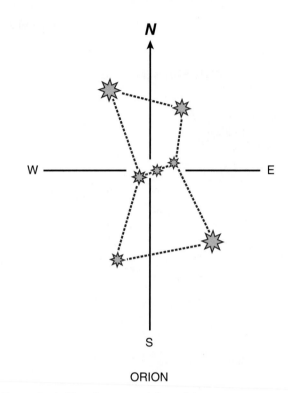

ORION

Figure 6–10 Direction to north from Orion.

north-south line passes is exactly on the Celestial Equator. No matter where on Earth you are, this star rises due east of you and sets due west.

Water Procurement and Treatment

The daily intake and output of liquids and certain chemicals by the body are essential for life processes and normal functions of vital organs. It is estimated that the body itself is approximately two-thirds water. The average daily body water requirement for proper biological balance and efficiency is two quarts per day. In any emergency, water can be critical. For instance, in harsh desert terrain, your life will depend upon your water supply and how well you manage and conserve your body water. The minimum daily requirement of two quarts per day can increase to a gallon or more in hot environments. Always carry enough water.

Improvised methods of water procurement such as transpiration bags, stills, catch basins, or seepage holes are really survival situation sources. They are usually marginal at best and should never be relied upon to supply enough water for field operations.

The Beach Well

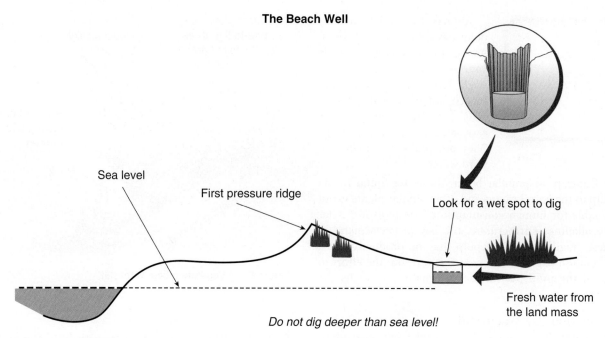

Figure 6–11 Water from a beach well. Copyright Emergency Response International, used with permission.

Along the Seashore

Along coasts, fresh water may be found in dunes above the beach, or in the beach itself well above the high tide line (Figure 6–11). Check hollows between dunes for visible water. Dig if the sand is moist. Otherwise, along the seashore on sandy beaches, dig a hole just over the first sand dune that is directly adjacent to the water. A damp area in a depression is a good place to dig. This is where rainwater and drainage from the local water tables collect. Dig until the hole begins to fill with muddy water; a deep hole is not necessary. (If you dig too deep, you may reach salt water, which is unfit to drink.) Shore up the sides of the hole with beach wood or brush. Let the impurities and suspended particles settle and the water clarify. Make the water safe by some purification method.

Desert or Arid Lands

Assess your water requirements. Will you be missed and can you expect someone to come looking within 12 to 24 hours? It may be wisest to sit and conserve body water while awaiting assistance.

Efforts to find water by search and digging will consume energy and water, and will increase your water requirements.

Do not rely on the sensation of thirst to indicate how much water you need. Drink plenty of water anytime it is available, particularly when you are eating. The main way to conserve your water is to control the amount you perspire.

How to control perspiration and conserve body water:

- Keep your clothes on. Clothing helps control sweating by not letting perspiration evaporate so fast. Clothing also prevents sunburn.
- Wear a hat, and cover your neck with a neck cloth.
- Light-colored clothing reflects light and heat.
- Keep in the shade and rest during the day.

> **SAFETY**
> Do not ever drink seawater or urine. The chemical makeup will actually cause dehydration and even toxicity.
>
> *SARTips*

Where to Look for Water

Water is more abundant and easier to find in loose sediment than in rocks. Look for springs along valley floors. Flat benches or terraces of land above river valleys may have springs or seepages along their bases, even when streams are dry. Signs of damp sand along the bottom of a canyon or base of a hill can be dug in as described in the previous seashore section. Dry streambeds may have water just below the surface. Try digging at the lowest point on the outside of a bend in the streambed channel.

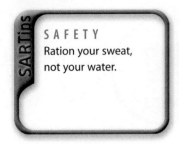
Animal trail forks usually point toward a source of water. As the animals move from their various habitats, they progressively converge as they approach water. Watch for animals and birds moving in the early morning or late evening. They are probably moving toward water.

Contrary to popular belief, the water found in the pulp of the barrel cactus and other similar plants is not suitable for human consumption. The moisture is far too alkaline. Furthermore, the law protects many of these fragile cacti. The pulp may be productive in a vegetation bag still (see next section), but the effort to get at the pulp from a cactus usually outweighs the benefit.

Vegetation Bag Water Still

Vegetation bag water stills are a relatively new innovation that appears to be superior to traditional desert solar stills (Figure 6–12). Water produced through vegetation bag stills tastes much like the plants used, but the idea is sound when poisonous plants are avoided.

How to build a vegetation bag still:

1. Cut foliage from trees or leafy plants.
2. Shake the branches thoroughly to eliminate dust, bird droppings and insects, because these will definitely taint the water source.
3. Seal them in a large, clear, plastic bag. Do not completely fill the bag.
4. Set the sealed bag in the sun to extract the fluids contained within.
5. Insert a piece of surgical tubing into the water reservoir if you have it so that the bag does not have to be dismantled to get at the water.

If a large, clear plastic bag is used and filled with approximately one cubic yard of foliage, the bag should yield a little less than a pint per day. Do not use poisonous or irritating plants.

Water produced by this method is normally bitter to taste, which is caused by biological breakdown of the leaves as they lie in the water produced and are heated in the moist "hot house" environment.

Water Transpiration Bag

One of the most efficient and easily constructed water sources in both desert and mountainous regions is the water transpiration bag (Figure 6–13). It is efficient because it capitalizes on a plant's capability to pull water

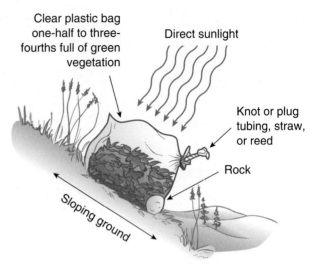

Figure 6–12 Vegetation bag water still.

from the ground. It also requires very little energy to construct and is easy to tap into.

How to construct a transpiration bag:

1. Place a plastic bag over a living limb of a medium size tree or large shrub. (Do this after shaking the branches thoroughly to eliminate dust, bird droppings and insects, because these will definitely taint the water source. A tube can be used to suck the water from the bag.)
2. Seal the bag opening at the branch and tie the limb down to allow collected water to flow to the corner of the bag.

The amount of water collected and the taste of the water procured by this method will depend on the species of trees and shrubs used. Without a doubt, the water transpiration bag method surpasses other methods (vegetation bag or solar still) in yield and ease of construction.

Conventional Desert Solar Water Still

Despite the fact that this method is portrayed in most survival books as a viable source in desert conditions, do not waste your time. This method is very costly in terms of energy, and hundreds if not thousands of outdoor "experts" have tried in vain to make this method work effectively. Again, the prevailing advice is: don't waste your time!

Mountains

A mountainous area is often the easiest geographic environment in which to locate water. The amount of difficulty will depend upon elevation, vegetation type in

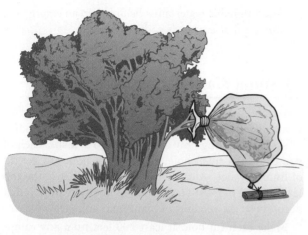

Figure 6-13 Water transpiration bag.

the area, geologic structure of the mountains, and annual precipitation.

Most canyons have streams, springs, or intermittent run-off flow during all or part of the year. Look in the very bottom of the canyon floor near catch pools and depressions of streambeds. Look for changes in vegetation, which are clues leading to a seep spring. If there is no water visible, often a small amount of digging will uncover water.

Where to Look for Water

- Look for large rock formations with green moss or lush vegetation and seek water at the base.
- Small clumps of isolated green vegetation in arid mountains is a good sign of a spring.
- Collect dew from leaves, plastic sheets, metal of the stalled transportation, or any wet surface. Sponge the water off with an absorbent cloth.
- Improvise rainwater collectors. Catch rain in plastic sheets or waterproof clothing.
- *Caution:* Water holes with few or no tracks nearby and no plants in or around them should be avoided.

Arctic and/or Extreme Winter Conditions

Water procurement and dehydration (lowering of the body's water content) are as great a problem in cold conditions as in the desert. In arctic conditions, all the available water is frozen and the extremely low humidity saps your body of water through respiration and perspiration.

Where to Look for Water

- Frozen streams and lakes may cover water.
- If the sun is shining, you can melt snow on black or dark colored plastic, a dark tarp, metal surfaces of any stalled transportation, or any surface that will absorb the sun's heat. Arrange the surface so that it tilts slightly or any fluid on the surface will run to a low spot and perhaps refreeze. The melted water can be directed to drain into a hollow or container at the edge of the surface.
- Whenever possible, melt ice rather than snow for water. You get more water for the volume with less heat and time.

If planning on flying over or traveling through arctic or winter environments, your emergency preparedness kit should contain a stove and pot to melt ice and snow. Do not eat ice or snow. A day or two of eating ice or snow results in swollen, raw mucous membranes in the mouth. Also, the expenditure of body heat and energy to melt the snow may be more detrimental to your health than the lack of water.

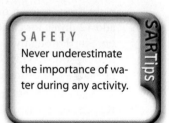

SAFETY
Never underestimate the importance of water during any activity.

SARTips

Preparation of Water Under Emergency Conditions

Symptoms of illness from contaminated water include nausea, vomiting, diarrhea, low-grade fever, vague feelings of discomfort, fatigue, and weight loss. Under emergency conditions, it might be necessary to filter and purify muddy, stagnant, or polluted water to drink. This type of water may not seem palatable, but if treated properly it can usually be made harmless and may save your life.

Clarification

Clarification is simply the act of removing or filtering sediment (dirt, debris, and such) from your water and should be done before attempting to purify it (killing bacteria, viruses, and parasites in the water). You can get water that is almost clear from muddy streams or lakes by digging a hole in sandy soil one to six feet from the bank. Allow water to seep in, and then wait for it to settle. Improvise a filter out of a can or cloth (sock, sleeve, etc.) using layers of sand at the bottom, then a layer of charcoal, then a layer of grass on top. Multiple layers of cloth make a good filter. If you have containers, let muddy or turbid water stand for a day. Be gentle when slowly pouring clear water off of the sediment.

Remember that even the clearest of water can be highly contaminated with germs and parasites that can cause illness and even death. Always clarify (if necessary) and purify all water procured in the field before consumption.

Purification

One of the best methods of purifying water is to bring it to a rolling boil and then let it cool. It will be safe to drink. Unless you are at very high altitude, all parasites, viruses, and bacteria in the water will be killed by bringing it to a boil.

Two percent tincture of iodine can also purify water by adding four drops to each quart of clear water or eight drops to each quart of cloudy water. For a gallon, add 12 drops for clear water or 24 drops for cloudy water. Stir thoroughly. Be careful, though, as iodine is a potent poison. Too much—and any amount of solid iodine crystals—can be toxic.

Water purification tablets are also available. The directions on the container's label should be followed precisely to be effective.

Table 6–3 shows the amount of commercial bleach solution (5.25% hypochlorite) to add to water for purification. Add the chlorine solution to the water, stir, and let it stand for 30 minutes. After this length of time the water should have a distinct taste or smell of chlorine. If not, then add several more drops of chlorine, and let the mixture stand for 15 minutes more. The slight taste or smell of chlorine in the water is a sign of safety. (Note: several drops of hydrogen peroxide will remove the smell of chlorine from the water, making it more palatable.)

If questionable water must be drunk in an emergency, seek medical attention as soon as possible.

Personal Waste Disposal

Campsite preparations should include arrangements for waste disposal. If your group is small (no more than five or six) and staying only a night or two at a site, each of you can dig a small hole, called a "cat-hole," to get rid of human waste. A cat-hole is efficient because the top layer of soil in most areas is full of microorganisms that decompose the remains of plants and animals.

Make each cat-hole at least 200 feet from any campsite, trail, or water source, and choose a location that isn't likely to be visited by others. With the heel of your boot or a small trowel, dig a hole about 6 inches deep, but no deeper than the rich, organic topsoil. After use, cover the hole completely with dirt, and in a few days the microorganisms will break down the waste. Bacteria essential for decay are found only in the top layer of earth.

A latrine is used for more permanent locations and should not be constructed away from base camp as a general rule. Use a cat-hole in the field.

When using a trench latrine, leave the shovel nearby for each person using the latrine to sprinkle a little soil into the trench to prevent flies from infesting the waste.

Bury nothing in a latrine or cat-hole except human waste. Animals will dig up buried garbage and scatter it around the forest, and materials such as plastic, glass, metal, and cardboard take years to decompose (**Table 6–4**). Take all trash home with you for appropriate disposal. If you packed it in, you must pack it out.

Personal Cleanliness

Good hygiene and cleanliness are essential in the outdoors. They safeguard good health by minimizing internal, and external, infection as well as infestation by parasites such as fleas and lice. The smallest abrasion of an unclean body can easily become infected and present a major survival obstacle. Make sure to keep hands as clean as possible, clean under fingernails, and wash face, underarms, crotch, and feet at least once a day.

It is very important to wash feet only after the day's travel is done. Do not rinse feet off at travel breaks. It significantly softens them and makes them more prone to blisters and injury.

While you probably won't wash as frequently as you do at home, frequent bathing is strongly encouraged in

Table 6–3	Use of a 5.25% sodium hypochlorite solution (commercial bleach) to purify water	
		Amount of Bleach
Amount of Water	Clear Water	Cloudy Water
1 Quart (1/4 gallon)	2 drops	4 drops
1 Gallon	8 drops	16 drops
5 Gallons	1/2 tsp	1 tsp

Table 6–4 — How long does litter last?

Item	Time to Decompose
Aluminum cans/tabs	80 to 100 years
Vibram soles	50 to 80 years
Leather	Up to 50 years
Nylon fabric	30 to 40 years
Plastic film	20 to 30 years
Plastic bags	20 to 30 years
Plastic coated paper	5 years
Wool socks	1 to 5 years
Orange peel	2 weeks to 5 months

Source: Data are estimates from a waste disposal expert.

the field. However, do not simply douse yourself in the nearest lake or pond. The best approach environmentally involves taking water away from natural water sources, washing, and then disposing of the wastewater in a cat-hole. All soap used should be biodegradable, but friction often works as well. Water is best taken from rapidly moving water as opposed to stagnant ponds or lakes, which helps avoid bacterial problems and limits involvement with leeches and the like. Water used for brushing teeth or gargling should be purified and safe for drinking.

When washing in water is impossible, "air" baths are better than none. To take an air bath, simply remove clothing, especially underwear, and allow air to circulate over the bare skin. This can help prevent chaffing and some skin problems.

Special Considerations

For most people, discussing personal physical problems with others can be disconcerting and often difficult. However, no one involved in SAR should hesitate to communicate unusual discomfort, pain, or malaise to coworkers because the result may affect both the outcome of the incident and the safety of others.

The responsibility for communicating relevant personal health information is shared by all SAR team members. In addition, SAR leadership involves kind and often discrete inquiry into any individual team member's difficulties. Responsible leadership includes the ability to deal with problems appropriately without exaggeration or overreaction. Situations unique to women are no exception to this rule.

SAR leaders should make it understood that any individual with problems that affect the team's effectiveness and/or safety will be treated sympathetically and knowledgeably, without undue embarrassment. If anxiety is involved, SAR leaders should be nonjudgmental and sympathetic. If rest is required, the group should adjust, just as it would for a team member with a blister.

Special Considerations for Women

The physical and mental stress related to search and rescue challenges, heavy physical exercise, or even the reduction of fat in the blood may all induce changes in a woman's menstrual cycle. Like many athletes in training, some women experience temporary amenorrhea, in which menstruation stops completely. If unexpected, it can be troubling; however, it can also be a welcome relief.

It is important to note that medical research indicates that women's strength and endurance are in no way diminished during menstruation. However, SAR leaders should know about and be willing to openly discuss these topics. For instance, women between menstrual periods, during ovulation, sometimes experience cramping. These "mittelschmerz," as they are sometimes called, cause a cramping pain on either side of the abdomen and/or lower back. However, most women who experience it can adequately identify and deal with it.

Vaginal infections can be particularly annoying in the field and are often caused by stress, the use of oral contraceptives, and as a result of excessive sugar intake. Therefore, SAR leaders and female SAR personnel should be aware that, in order to avoid vaginal infections during extended field operations, women should be encouraged to wash regularly, wear loose-fitting cotton underpants, drink excess water, and, when possible, keep their sugar and carbohydrate intake down.

High altitudes increase the risk of blood clotting for both men and women. Women who take oral contraceptives are already at a higher risk of clotting, so a woman who takes oral contraceptives and expects to spend much time above 12,000 feet (4,000 meters) should discuss the risks with her doctor. Also, due to the possibility of unrecognized or undiagnosed complications, a woman with a recently inserted intrauterine device should wait a few months before traveling deep into the backcountry or to high altitude.

Any SAR team member who is pregnant should advise her team leader. In addition, a pregnant woman would be prudent to advise her physician prior to participating in SAR operations so that both understand the extent and requirements of her involvement. Most physicians suggest that pregnant women consider not participating in the more vigorous field aspects of SAR during their third trimester. However, the same physicians are likely also to suggest that a woman's participation in SAR be limited by her comfort and health, keeping in mind the importance of nutrition, hydration, and rest during pregnancy.

Anyone with anemia problems should be sure to include several foods that are high in iron in their diets. Foods that meet this criterion and are easily carried in the field include dried prunes, dried peaches, raisins, dates, sesame seeds, pumpkin seeds, and wheat germ. It should also be noted that some of these foods when eaten in quantity could cause constipation, so their intake in the field should be carefully monitored.

In the field, used tampons and pads must either be burned in a very hot fire or carried out. Female SAR workers should be sure to add small plastic bags to their packs for this purpose. Crushing a few aspirin and placing them in the bag, or wrapping the tampons in fragrant leaves, can help eliminate the problem of odor. Extra care should be taken to keep a pack containing used pads or tampons out of the reach of animals. The odor of these items is particularly attractive to many animals and can lead to unwanted confrontations.

Although not just a consideration for women, SAR personnel should consider removing all jewelry before operating in the field. In cold weather metal jewelry can be dangerous because the metal can be cooled below freezing and cause a localized cold injury. In any type of weather, dangling jewelry from the ears, wrists, or neck can become entangled and cause traumatic injuries. In either case, SAR personnel should give serious consideration to removing all jewelry before becoming involved in field operations.

SAR Terms

Kindling The initial fuel stage.

Sustaining fuel Anything that will burn for an extended period of time.

Tinder Anything that will ignite at a very low temperature, with a spark, small flame, or other heat source.

Water clarification The act of removing or filtering sediment from water.

Water purification The act of killing bacteria, viruses, and parasites in water.

References

Auerbach, P.S., ed. (2001). *Wilderness Medicine*, 4th ed. St. Louis, MO: Mosby, Inc.

Cooper, D.C. (1998). *Aviation Survival Handbook*. Cuyahoga Falls, Ohio: National Rescue Consultants.

Farmer, K. (1976). *Woman in the Woods*. New York, New York: Stackpole Books.

Fear, E.H. (1979). *Surviving the Unexpected Wilderness Emergency*. Tacoma, Washington: Survival Education Association.

Fears, J.W. (1986). *The Complete Book of Outdoor Survival*. New York, New York: Outdoor Life Books.

Johnson, M. (2003). *The Ultimate Desert Handbook: A Manual for Desert Hikers, Campers, and Travelers*. New York, New York: Ragged Mountain Press/McGraw Hill.

Manning, H. (1986). *Backpacking: One Step at a Time*, 4th ed. New York, New York: Vintage Books.

Mears, R. (1993). *The Outdoor Survival Handbook*. New York, New York: St. Martin's Press.

Mears, R. (2003). *Bushcraft: An Inspired Guide to Surviving in the Wilderness*. New York, New York: Hodder & Stoughton.

Petzoldt, P. (1974). *The Wilderness Handbook*. New York, New York: W.W. Norton & Company, Inc.

United States Air Force. (1985). *Search and Rescue Survival Training*. AF Regulation 64-4. Washington, D.C.: Department of the Air Force.

United States Department of the Air Force. (1985). *Aircrew Survival*. U.S. Air Force Pamphlet 64-5. Washington, D.C.: U.S. Department of the Air Force.

United States Army, Marine Corps, Navy, Air Force. (1999). *Survival, Evasion, and Recovery: Multiservice Procedures for Survival, Evasion, and Recovery*. U.S. Army Regulation FM 21-76-1, U.S. Marine Corps Regulation MCRP 3-02H, U.S. Navy Regulation NWP 3-50.3, U.S. Air Force Regulation AFTTP(l)3-2.26. Washington, D.C.: Air Land Sea Application Center.

United States Department of the Army. (2002). *U.S. Army Survival Handbook*. Guilford, Connecticut: The Lyons Press.

Wiseman, J. (2004). *SAS Survival Handbook: How to Survive in the Wild, in Any Climate, on Land or at Sea*. New York, New York: HarperResource.

Chapter 7
SAR Clothing

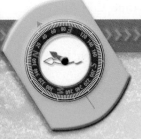

Objectives

Upon completion of this chapter and any course activities, the student will be able to meet the following objectives:

List at least three characteristics in the various natural and synthetic materials used in the construction of clothing as used in SAR. (p. 86-92)

List three of the factors concerning heat transfer due to clothing construction and/or design. (p. 92-93)

Describe the function of each of the following layers of clothing:
Underneath layer. (p. 94-95)
Wicking layer. (p. 95)
Clothing layer. (p. 95-96)
Insulation layer. (p. 96)
Shell layer. (p. 96-98)

Describe the proper SAR clothing to be used in various environmental conditions. (p. 87-103)

Describe some advantages and disadvantages of various types of outdoor footwear. (p. 100-101)

Dress for the Occasion

SAR operations pose unique clothing challenges for SAR personnel. History shows that lightly dressed SAR responders often become accustomed to working hard and traveling through varied environments with no thought of their clothing needs should they suddenly be forced to spend an undetermined amount of time in harsh conditions. Many do not carry or wear the clothes needed to survive. A simple rule before starting out is to ask, "Is what I plan to wear and carry adequate for the expected weather and environments in which I will be working? What about carrying just a bit more in case?"

Understanding clothing and clothing systems is essential for SAR personnel. To be comfortable, effective, and safe in a variety of environments, an understanding of clothing materials, designs, and systems is necessary.

Clothing Materials

Fibers that comprise clothing may be either found in nature (natural) or be "man-made" (synthetic). In addition, each of these natural and synthetic fibers has its own unique characteristics. These fibers may be hollow, oily, chambered, scaled, porous, long, short, thick, curly, straight, <u>hydrophobic</u> (repel water), and <u>hydrophilic</u> (absorb water), or any combination of these, depending on the material from which they are made. Enlightened textile and clothing manufacturers use the inherent characteristics of specific fibers to construct clothes that meet specialized needs. Durability, breathability, waterproofness, ability to wick moisture, insulation value when wet, resistance to burning or melting, etc., are all variables that are manipulated by the use of various fibers. Understanding the characteristics of a wide variety of fibers provides a foundation for understanding the principles of building a clothing system for SAR work.

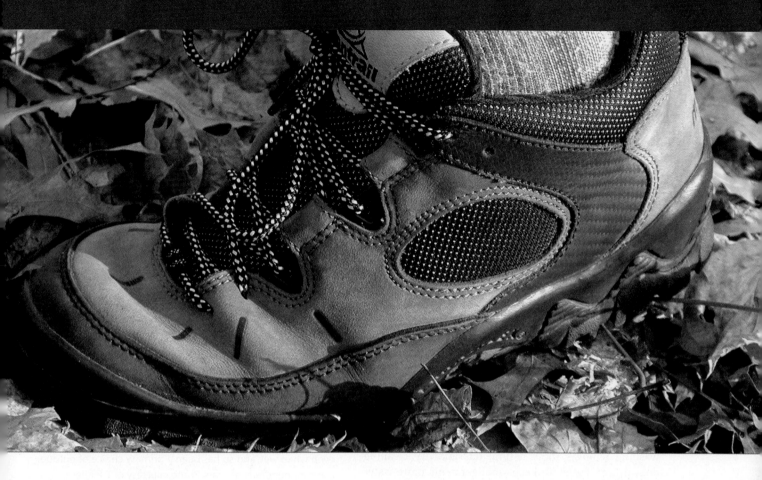

Natural Fiber Materials

"Natural" fibers are those derived from plants or animals. Cotton comes from the cotton plant, wool from the shorn fleece of sheep, silk from the web of the silkworm, and down from the feathers of waterfowl.

Cotton

In warm or moderate climates, cotton provides excellent properties for protection. For example, a light-colored, thin, cotton shirt protects from the damaging rays of the sun and quickly absorbs perspiration. This moisture then evaporates from the material, cooling the body. When kept dry cotton also affords excellent insulation against cold. However, when its gets wet from rain, snow, or perspiration, its insulation value drops to almost nothing. Since SAR operations usually involve physical labor, perspiration is always wetting one's clothing from the inside and the environment is often wetting it from the outside. Thus, the SAR mantra, "Cotton Kills," refers to when cotton is worn inappropriately in cold environments (Figure 7–1).

Cotton, especially the thicker variety, dries slowly because its fibers are hydrophilic and retain water. Because of this, it also pulls or "wicks" water rapidly from more wet areas to less wet areas.

Some types of cotton are better suited for use in SAR operations. Canvas, for example, is heavyweight cotton

used for items that require strength and durability. Other strong, durable cottons include denim, duck, and poplin. When tightly woven, these fabrics are abrasion resistant and can even protect against light wind and rain.

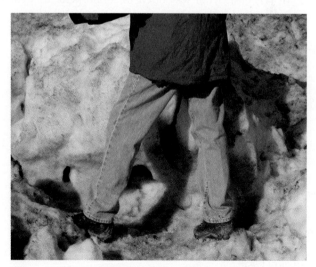

Figure 7–1 When kept dry, cotton affords excellent insulation against cold. However, when it gets wet from rain, snow, or perspiration, its insulation value drops to almost nothing. Thus, the SAR mantra, "Cotton Kills," refers to when cotton is worn inappropriately in cold environments. Cotton jeans are most often not well suited for field SAR operations.

Additional properties of cotton include:

- It burns easily but does not melt.
- Light-colored cotton is excellent for hot, dry climates because of its breathability and high ability to absorb water.
- It has very low durability unless blended with tougher synthetics, but rots under continued wet or hot and sunny conditions.
- Thick cotton dries slowly from the outside, which is a good characteristic in hot, dry weather.
- Tightly woven cotton makes a good windbreak and may be water resistant.
- It is a good insulator when dry, but poor when wet.
- It freezes solid when wet in extreme cold.
- When cut or torn into strips, it can be used as a bandage, cravat, sling, fire starter, and multiple other uses.

Wool

The principal advantage of wool over many other fabrics is its ability to insulate even when wet. The fibers are naturally curly and trap air in tiny pockets between them. Wool in its raw unprocessed state also contains oils such as lanolin, which repel water. Processing and washing removes these natural oils and dry cleaning does it even faster. To keep wool garments more water resistant and comfortable, they should not be laundered often. This should be balanced with the need to keep wool garments clean to maximize its air-trapping and insulation properties.

In the past, wool was often uncomfortable to wear against the skin because of its short, irritating fibers. Some individuals are even allergic to wool and wool blends. SAR personnel should be especially aware of this if wool is used in patient packaging materials (e.g., wool blankets, etc.). But, outside of the allergy to this fiber, wool remains one of the best insulating materials, even when wet, and so has been a primary choice of outdoor users for hundreds of years (Figure 7–2). Modern manufacturing processes have also overcome the scratchiness problem by marrying the wool to a layer of softer material, brushing the wool to make it less irritating, or otherwise using special wool and treatments to render the material extra soft and comfortable (e.g., Smartwool®).

Statistics show that people dressed in wool are more apt to survive in an outdoor environment than those dressed in cotton. However, the loose weave of some woolen fabrics does little

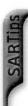

Figure 7–2 Wool remains one of the best insulating materials, even when wet, and so has been a primary choice of outdoor users for hundreds of years. Photo courtesy of T. P. Mier.

to stop the wind. A close-weave, windproof shell is essential over this type of wool in cold weather where wind is a factor.

Additional properties of wool include:

- Absorbs less moisture than any other natural fabric
- When wet, it is warm and retains nearly all of its insulation qualities.
- When wet, it will not freeze solid in extreme cold.
- It burns very slowly and is very resilient, breathable, and durable.
- In its pure form, it tears easily, so it is usually blended with other, stronger materials.
- It traps air well and is considered an excellent insulator.
- It gives off an unpleasant odor when wet.
- It can be purchased inexpensively at some surplus stores.

Silk

Silk is a natural fiber long recognized for its value in cold weather. It is the lightest, strongest, and softest of all natural fibers. It has hollow fibers that absorb and transport moisture away from the skin, making it a good insulator and useful as an underwear layer. Silk is noted for its comfort and higher relative cost, but the price has come down over the past few years. Silk blends are also now available that are more competitively priced and are as comfortable as pure silk.

Silk can be used alone or combined with synthetics or wool. It comes in several forms, the most common of which is spun filament silk consisting of several strands of monofilament fibers twisted around one another. Spun filament silk is heavier, softer, and even warmer than monofilament silk.

Additional properties of silk include:

- Silk is very comfortable against the skin, traps much air, and is very light.
- It is relatively expensive and tends to hold odors and stains.
- Silk is damaged by a hot iron, acids, sunlight, perspiration, strong soaps, and alkaline substances.

Down

Down is the soft, fluffy type of feather found underneath the larger, stiffer feathers of a duck or goose. It is an excellent form of insulation when dry because of its light weight and compressibility. Virtually no other insulation has the amount of dead air spaces pound for pound, and thus it is one of the best insulators available when it is clean and dry. This dead air space, which has the fluffy appearance in insulation, is called "loft." Down is used in sleeping bags, parkas, sweaters, gloves, vests, booties, pants, hats, and gloves.

According to U.S. federal regulations, "down" refers to a mix of down clusters, feather fibers, feathers, and residue. To be labeled "down," however, at least 80% of the mix must be down and down fibers, and no more than 20% longer feathers, feather fibers, and residue. Goose down is usually a better quality than duck down.

Nomenclature in the clothing industry refers to "fill power" with a number attached as a value of the quality of the down. Standard for the industry is "550 fill power" down, which means that one ounce of down will fill 550 cubic inches. There are some larger values available like 625 or even 700, but those are definitely not the norm and are probably used to sell products at a much higher price. The advantage of higher fill power is obvious: greater loft for less weight.

Anything labeled 80% down or even 80/20 down means that it contains 80% of the federal regulation, or at least 60% down and down fiber.

As a type of insulation added to clothing being worn in extremely dry, cold conditions, down is superior to almost everything else. However, when wet, down loses nearly all of its insulation properties and becomes almost completely useless.

Down must be sandwiched between layers of materials to stabilize it, that is, keep it from shifting to one corner of the garment. Therefore, some mention needs to made of the quality of the material from which a down garment is made: the stabilizing fabric. When this material is very thin (read, "cheap") and low-grade down is used, tiny feather quills can punch through the material and cause irritation of the wearer and loss of the down. This is undesirable but should be expected to some extent with most down garments.

Since SAR personnel frequently store gear for long periods of time, it should be noted that down-filled garments and gear (e.g., sleeping bags, overshoes, hats, etc.) should be stored uncompressed. That is, items with down in them should not be compressed during storage. They should be hung or laid out so that they are stored as close to full size as possible. Storing them with all the air squeezed out tends to reduce the "fluffiness" of the material and thus its insulation power over time.

Additional properties of down include:

- Light weight and very comfortable
- Maximum amount of dead air space in dry condition
- Absorbs moisture readily
- Clumps up with moisture and dampness
- Some people are allergic to down
- Loses nearly all of its insulation when wet
- Absorbs and retains odors, and will mildew when damp
- Requires a sandwich of extra baffles and seams to hold in place

Synthetic Fiber Materials

Synthetic materials are made from fibers that are produced by chemical synthesis. The wide variety of chemical compositions and fiber designs allow synthetic fibers to be an outstanding basis for materials used in outdoor clothing.

Nylon

Developed in the 1920s by the DuPont Company, nylon is stronger than cotton for an equivalent weight. It is also abrasion resistant, quick drying, long wearing, and nylon threads are almost completely impervious to penetration both by water and water-repelling compounds. This presents difficulty in two respects. First, perspiration stays on the surface and does not easily pass through the fabric. Thus, if nylon is worn as underwear, perspiration remains against the skin and is not wicked away. Second, waterproofing compounds do not unite with the nylon fibers as in cotton, and therefore must be "painted" onto the nylon material to fill in between threads.

One high-quality type of nylon, called "ripstop," is alternately stitched with thin and thick threads, giving it a checkerboard appearance (Figure 7–3). If torn, the tear allegedly will stop at the thicker cross thread—thus, the name "ripstop." Ripstop nylon is generally wind and abrasion resistant and is often used to make pants, shirts, and windproof shells.

Another variety of nylon, Cordura® (also developed by DuPont), is an abrasion-resistant, lightweight, and durable fiber available in various deniers (a measure of stitches per unit area). As examples, a lightweight version of the material (160-denier Cordura) is perfect for active and performance outerwear and a heavyweight version (1000-denier Cordura) is more suited for backpacks or boots. Many styles of alpine/outdoor technical outerwear also use high denier Cordura in high-impact areas such as knees, elbows, and around the ankles to help resist abrasion.

Nylon is manufactured into a variety of products, including parachutes and rope. It is also commonly used in conjunction with a waterproofing coating or membrane to make excellent shells. Nylon is also used in various blends (e.g., polyester/nylon) to make garments with characteristics of both materials.

The wide variety of colors in which nylon is available makes it easy for the wearer to be very visible (bright blue or orange), or very invisible (camouflage). The preference for SAR personnel is always to be more visible, and so camouflage and darker colors should be at best avoided, or at least used only when brighter colors are not available.

In general, nylon exhibits the following characteristics:

- High strength when wet
- Relatively resistant to alkali, mildew, and insect damage

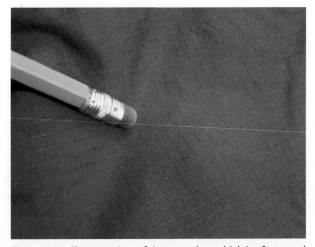

Figure 7–3 Close-up view of ripstop nylon, which is often used to make pants, shirts, and windproof outer shells.

- Excellent abrasion resistance
- Washes and dries easily
- Blends well with other fibers
- Low moisture absorption
- Can be damaged by sunlight
- Melting point of 263°C (505°F), but may become malformed (in a hot dryer or near a fire) well below that temperature
- Absorbs and holds perspiration and body oils
- Sparks and embers from a fire will easily cause holes and melting

Polypropylene

Polypropylene fiber was discovered in 1954 by two chemists at Phillips Petroleum Co., and became commercially available in 1960 under the name, Meraklon.® Synthetic undergarments fabricated from polypropylene dry rapidly and repel water, unlike natural fibers. In the language of physics, it is hydrophobic, that is, it will not absorb moisture. Polypropylene also has the lowest thermal conductivity of any fiber and, therefore, the highest insulation power. However, it should be noted that this property depends largely on the design of the material and garment made from the fiber. In the end, the thermal insulation quality of any garment is directly related to the quantity of its trapped, dead air space.

Besides drying rapidly, this synthetic fiber has great wicking properties, making it terrific for use in an underwear layer (see section below). In fact, polypropylene cannot hold more than 10% of its weight in water. This means that polypropylene will not only wick and insulate when wet, but will continue to wick moisture until the fiber is almost dry. It also has the lowest density of any other fiber and even floats. As a result, it is possible for polypropylene to be spun into clothing that has the bulk and air space needed for extra insulation without the weight. Additional attributes include:

- Quick drying; just wring it out and it is almost completely dry
- Easy care and very washable
- Non-allergenic
- High abrasion resistance

Polypropylene is available as sock liners, glove liners, long underwear, and in blends. Creative garment manufacturers also have developed double-layer underwear with polypropylene next to the skin and a layer of wool, cotton, or other material as an outer layer to help wick away moisture.

The least desirable characteristic of polypropylene may be that it melts (and shrinks) at relatively low temperatures (160°C or 320°F). Polypropylene from 20 years ago was often seen to shrink in a clothes dryer set to only moderate heat. Today's materials and blends, however, have been improved to the point where this is generally no longer a problem. Although many will not consider this a reason to avoid its use, aircraft pilots and passengers, fire fighters, and those who may be exposed to flash fires should choose another underwear material. For similar reasons, wearers of polypropylene should also avoid sparks and embers from a campfire or stove. Sparks can cause holes, and just the heat from a stove can melt the material of a sleeve to the skin and cause burns. Polypropylene also retains body odor, so those who perspire excessively may also wish to choose an alternative fabric.

Many new "blend" products on the market today claim they have retained polypropylene's good properties while minimizing its drawbacks. Some examples include: Capilene™, Chlorofibre™, Terelene™, Trantex™, and Thermax™. Many find these materials generally superior to polypropylene.

Polyester

Polyester is second only to nylon in use for outdoor clothing and equipment. It is strong, durable, and inexpensive, and now used to produce some of our most valuable outdoor garments.

Invented in Britian in the late 1930s by Calico Printers Association and developed simultaneously by the Imperial Chemical Company and DuPont in the 1940s, polyester is is used in the production of everything from floppy disk liners to hoses. Polyester fibers are softer and lighter than other synthetic fibers, giving it a softer, more comfortable feel. Polyester fibers are hollow, don't absorb moisture, and much like nylon are poor at wicking moisture. Polyester blended with cotton or nylon is often used in trousers and shirts. Ripstop polyester, similar to ripstop nylon, is also available. Variations of polyester are used to make underwear, clothing, insulation, and shell material.

Some examples of popular polyester insulation materials include Polartec®, PolarGuard™, Primaloft®, Dacron® Hollofil™ II, Quallofil™, Thinsulate™, and Sontique™.

Polartec®

Because of its warmth, comfort, and versatility, this type of polyester fleece or "bunting" has become increasingly popular as an insulation layer. This fluffy, soft, warm material is used to make everything from socks, gloves, and hats to underwear, jackets, and bodysuits.

Generally, Polartec® has the following characteristics:

- Resistant to stretching and shrinking
- Strong
- Quick drying
- Abrasion, mildew, and wrinkle resistant

- Melting point of 260°C (500°F)
- Resistant to most chemicals
- More costly than other synthetics
- Prolonged exposure to sunlight reduces strength

PolarGuard™

PolarGuard™ is composed of 100% polyester filaments, arranged into a thick, dense layer of continuous fibers forming a multitude of air-trapping pockets. A benefit of its continuous fibers is the virtual elimination of clumping and cold spots. It is moisture and rot resistant, non-allergenic, easily laundered, and proportionally less expensive than down.

There are numerous synthetic insulators on the market, but only PolarGuard™ has the continuous filament fiber and does not require a backing to stabilize the yarns. (The "backing" is a one-ply, non-woven polyfilament called scrim.) Quallofil™, Hollofil™, and the fiberfills (see below) are all short fiber insulators that require the scrim to stabilize their yarns. Short fiber insulators cannot be used in some construction techniques because there is no way to sew them down to ensure that the material will not shift, tear, or separate.

PolarGuard HV™ and PolarGuard 3D™ are two types of the PolarGuard™ family available on the market today.

PolarGuard HV™ is a "high void" (large, hollow inside) continuous filament fiber. Its design traps more dead air space than solid fibers and thus improves its insulation properties. Generally, the following are characteristics of PolarGuard HV™:

- Hollow, high-void fibers
- 25% lighter than standard PolarGuard™
- Continuous filament fiber
- Mildew, fungus, and moisture resistant
- Non-allergenic and odor-free
- Larger fibers give it a stiffer feel

PolarGuard 3D™ is similar to, and has all the qualities of, PolarGuard HV™ except its fibers are smaller by 40%. This creates a softer insulation that won't clump, but retains its loft and durability after years of use. In addition to the characteristics of PolarGuard HV™ (above), the following are characteristics of PolarGuard 3D™:

- Smaller and lighter fiber filament than PolarGuard HV™
- Retains loft for long periods

Primaloft®

Primaloft® was produced as a down imitator and possesses many of the qualities of down. But Primaloft® also insulates when wet. In addition, the fibers are treated with a water-repellent finish that does not allow water to penetrate, but allows moisture from the inside to pass through. Generally, the following are characteristics of Primaloft®:

- High loft insulation
- Soft "downy" feel
- Highly compressible, like down
- Easy to care for
- Durable

Dacron Hollofil II™

Hollofil II™ fibers are hollow and because of this are 8.5 percent larger than solid fibers. Softness in this insulation batting is the result of low friction between the fibers that have been treated with a special durable coating. Hollofil II™ is lightweight, non-allergenic, inexpensive, fast drying, easily compacted, and virtually nonabsorbent, but it does not seem to have the warmth or compressibility of PolarGuard™ or Quallofil™.

Quallofil™

Quallofil™ is made of "staple" fibers that are crimped in a zig-zag pattern, so they are oriented in many different directions to help them fill space and trap air. Each fiber is from 1 to 3 inches long when stretched out, hollow, and divided internally into four quadrants when viewed on the cross section.

The fibers have a silicone finish to reduce friction between adjacent fibers rubbing together. For this reason, Quallofil™ has a softer feel than many other fiberfills that are resin coated. Quallofil™ and several other fiberfills are made of polyester, with less than 0.1% moisture absorption. All the high-loft polyester fiberfills dry about 10 times faster than down.

Quallofil™ is a short staple fiber, so it requires scrim (a 1-ply nonwoven polyfilament backing) on both sides of the batting to stabilize it for sewing and durability. The scrim adds weight and stiffness to the raw fill. It is impossible to work with the loose fiber because it shifts around so much in sewing.

Quallofil™ has up to 25% more loft than Hollofil II™ or Polar-Guard™ when it is fresh from the factory, but after initial use it reduces to about 8% more loft than other fiberfills. The compressibility of Quallofil™ is about 20% to 30% better than Hollofil II™ according to its manufacturer (DuPont). Another way to look at compressibility is that Quallofil™ is about 80% as compressible as down, whereas PolarGuard™ is about 60% as compressible as down. Because Quallofil™ has no resin, it is softer and conforms better to the body, resulting in fewer draft spaces and more heat retention.

Thinsulate™ and Sontique™

Both Thinsulate™ and Sontique™ are a result of mixing synthetic fibers and reducing the size of the filaments themselves. Invented by the 3M Company, Thinsulate™ insulation is a blend of polyester and polyolefin fibers. What separates these insulations from all others is the fineness of the individual filaments, and the resulting entrapment of a "boundary layer" of still air along each fiber. What this means for the user is an extremely efficient insulation in terms of warmth per unit of thickness.

Sontique™ apparently has a larger proportion of the polyolefin fibers and thus retains a somewhat softer feel. Neither absorbs water, so both can be readily dried under field conditions. Manufacturers claim that these insulations have less than 1% moisture absorption and will dry ten times more quickly than down, which is not really saying much.

Because of their short fiber length, these insulations require a scrim layer to stabilize the fibers. Both also make ideal garment insulators for pants and other clothing articles because of their microfiber construction, where high loft products would interfere with function.

Heat Loss and Garment Features

Heat Transfer

The rate of heat transfer through clothing depends on three factors. First is quantity and thickness of dead air spaces trapped within the clothing and its layers. In addition, if the skin touches clothing, heat may be lost through conduction. For cold, still air conditions, thick layers of dead air spaces such as those found in dry down, or other fluff-filled clothing is needed for warmth.

Second is the amount of air that passes through a material: the more air that passes though the clothing, the greater the heat loss through convection and evaporation. Large knit, wool sweaters are fine in still air, but allow rapid heat loss in even moderate winds.

Third is water and moisture. Heat loss through wet clothing is generally very rapid since thermal conductivity of water is 24 times greater than still air. This means that wet clothing can extract body heat nearly 200 times faster than dry clothing, depending on the material from which the clothing is made.

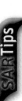

INFO

Waterproof: Material is impermeable to water, even water under pressure.

Water-repellent: Sheds water that is not under pressure; however, falling or wind-blown rain may penetrate the fabric.

Water-resistant: The material temporarily resists water under pressure.

Waterproof and breathable: Material is nearly impermeable to water droplets (waterproof) but allows water vapor to pass (breathable).

Garment Closures

Closures can be problems if they are not designed or applied properly. When choosing a closure, consider the environment in which it will be used. Most zippers offer little insulation or windproofness and necessitate some type of covering or at least some additional consideration. A second covering over the zipper usually does the job for warmth, but a second closure may be required for the garment to be <u>waterproof</u>. Waterproof zippers are also now available that do not require storm flaps or may have small flaps on the inside of the garment. Snaps and/or Velcro® are often used to close sleeves and storm flaps on jackets and parkas. Snaps are hard to work while wearing gloves and can get clogged in snow. Buttons also can be an annoyance and even painful if something applies pressure to it against the skin. Velcro® generally offers complete closure and versatility, and primarily protects against wind. However, mud and wet snow can "clog" the hooks and prevent it from closing properly.

Seams can be a problem, especially if waterproofness is important. Seams can be placed in a different area of a garment to help minimize its disadvantages, for example, away from the top of the shoulder in rain gear. Seams can also be sealed to prevent leaking. For shells, waterproof seams should be both taped and sealed. In higher quality shells, taped seams protect against abrasion or rubbing on the inside of the garment.

Vents may also be included in higher quality shell garments. These features are usually located in high heat and perspiration areas to allow moisture and heat to escape without having to remove the shell. Locations of vents are usually such that even when open the waterproof characteristics of the garment can be maintained (Figure 7–4).

In SAR, having quick and easy access to pocket items is a convenience that borders on necessity. Since many otherwise useful outer layers (shells, see below) are designed for recreation and not work, pockets are often missing altogether, minimally sized, or inappropriately placed. It is highly recommended that the placement and size of externally accessible pockets be a primary consideration when selecting and purchasing clothes for SAR work.

SAR personnel may also benefit from clothing specifically designed for active outdoor sports. As an example, trousers designed for snowboarding are often durable, loose-fitting, comfortable, warm, waterproof, and contain numerous pockets. Some have zip-off legs and their loose fit allows for additional layers underneath.

Many useful types, styles, and materials have been developed to help cross-country runners run in a wide variety of weather conditions. Lightweight, warm, long-sleeved shirts are common and wick moisture away

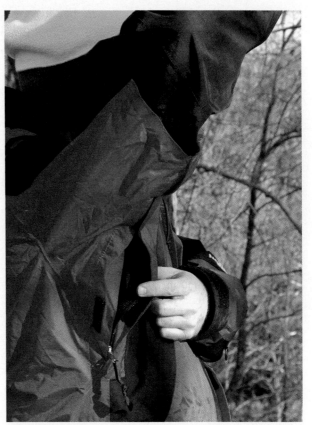

Figure 7–4 Vents are often integrated into higher quality shells to allow moisture and heat to escape without having to remove the garment. Photo courtesy of T. P. Mier.

from the skin while providing some wind and thermal protection. Of course, the same items are also available for the lower body. Some shirts have "glove" attachments to help protect the wrists and backs of the hands from sun, wind, and weather. Hats have been developed to block/reflect the sun while allowing perspiration to be wicked away and evaporate. Many of these features make garments expensive, but just knowing that these types of garments and features exist could be beneficial to SAR personnel.

The Layer System

Each of us is a heat-producing, homeothermic organism (able to maintain a constant body temperature) that depends on clothing to protect us from environmental extremes. However, each of us also has a different tolerance level or comfort zone for deviations from the body's normal temperature. So, a system of protecting one's body is needed that is versatile enough to work for different people in different conditions. One way to accomplish this has been termed the "layer system" and involves the use of clothing to regulate one's heat loss. This system uses multiple, adjustable layers of garments that can easily be added or removed to suit the environment, conditions, and desired level of heat loss. Multiple layers are used in lieu of one heavy layer to allow for fine-tuning of one's comfort. As physical exertion or the outside temperature increases, layers can be removed to facilitate heat loss and the movement of evaporating perspiration away from the body. As exertion decreases or the outside temperature drops, layers can be added to reduce heat loss. A primary principle of the method is that several thin layers of clothing will trap more air, and thus provide more insulation, than one massively thick layer. The ideal layering system seeks to establish a balance between breathability, wicking (movement of moisture away from the skin), quick-drying, insulation, durability, wind-resistance, and water-repellence while remaining light weight and offering freedom of movement with a minimum amount of bulk.

A five-layer system is suggested for SAR and consists of the following layers: underneath, wicking, clothing, insulation, and shell. The underneath layer is defined as the boxers-briefs/panties, bra/undershirt, and socks. The term "underwear" is not used here to allow for the distinction between the boxers, undies, and bra (underneath) layer from the wicking layer, that is, "underwear" such as long johns/long janes as named by most outdoor clothing manufacturers. The wicking layer is optional and worn against the skin but over the underneath layer for comfort and to pull moisture away from the skin in cold environments. The clothing layer is worn over the wicking layer to add insulation and allow for ventilation while protecting privacy. The insulation layer is worn to add warmth when needed. It can be heavier in colder environments and removed altogether in moderate climates. The shell layer is the outer covering of the system and protects the wearer from sun, wind, and water as necessary.

Generally, clothes for SAR operations should meet the "BUBU" criteria. The acronym means: they should be big (able to fit additional layer beneath), unconstricting (not tight, especially at the ankles and wrists), baggy (loose-fitting), and ugly (meaning not necessarily fashionable).

The Underneath Layer

For hygiene, discretion, and sometimes comfort, many prefer to wear undergarments such as briefs, boxers, a bra, panties, or an undershirt against the skin. These are often made of cotton for ease of cleaning, comfort, and low cost. But, they may also be of other materials at the discretion of the wearer. Some even prefer not to wear "underneath" garments at all. This is especially prevalent in hot environments where perspiration would quickly wet a cotton garment and lack of opportunity to dry would hold it damp against the skin. Over long periods, this could cause chaffing, irritation, and even injury. The option to wear this layer is, of course, up to the wearer. But, overall, undergarments are recommended if for no other reason than to extend the usable life of other clothing that would normally be worn over this layer.

Socks deserve more than just superficial consideration. Socks should not clump up against the feet or cause constriction or abrasion. They should provide comfort, promote circulation, and provide insulation in cold weather. Cotton socks, like cotton underwear in general, are not recommended for strenuous backcountry travel in any weather. They are poor insulators when wet, absorb and retain perspiration readily, stay wet, and hold the moisture against the skin. For constant, strenuous activities, including walking long distances, always wear two pair of socks: one thin layer against the skin (polypropylene, silk, nylon) to wick away moisture and one insulating layer (thickness dependent on environment). This helps keep the feet dry and minimizes the mechanical friction on the skin of the feet that leads to blisters (**Figure 7–5**).

Care for the feet daily. Wash and massage the feet at the end of every day and let them dry thoroughly. Do not rinse or wash the feet between long field exercises. This causes the skin on the feet to soften and become more prone to injury. Wait until the end of the travel day to wash the feet and change into clean socks at least daily. A preferable alternative to submerging the feet in

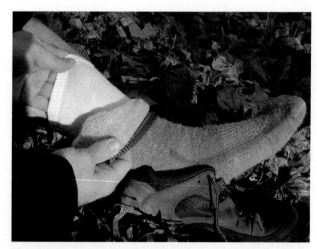

Figure 7–5 Wearing two pair of socks (one thin layer against the skin and one insulating layer, as needed) helps keep the feet dry and minimizes mechanical friction against the skin that leads to blisters. Photo courtesy of T. P. Mier.

water during SAR operations might be to use a damp towel or disposable towelette to wipe off the feet without getting them soaking wet. During long field operations when washing one's feet is not a simple option, changing into clean socks at least once per day should work in the short term.

The Wicking Layer

While this layer provides some insulation, its primary function is to control moisture and provide comfort against the skin. Functionally, the wicking layer should literally pull moisture away from the skin to the outer layers where it can evaporate. If moisture is not wicked away, it will remain on the skin and in the clothing. This will at least reduce comfort and potentially lead to either hypothermia (in cold weather) or hyperthermia (in hot weather).

Most modern cold weather garments that fall into the category of this layer (also known as "underwear" by many clothing manufacturers) comes in three weights: light weight, mid-weight, and heavy weight (also known as "expedition" weight). Since it is not easy to adjust this layer once donned, only the lightest or thinnest of these garments necessary to maintain comfort should be worn.

In cool weather, the warmth of dry, snug-fitting garments worn against the skin are often preferred. Although thin silk or wool may work fine, fabrics like polypropylene and variations of polyester (Capilene™, CoolMax®, and Polartec®) work very well at passing moisture from the skin to outer layers for evaporation. Rather than absorbing moisture like the natural fibers, the synthetics work by repelling water. Therefore, for maximum performance, synthetic underwear layers should be thin and in close contact with the skin so that perspiration moisture can be forced through it to outside layers. This is why a synthetic wicking layer is often recommended over its natural fiber counterpart when physical exertion is expected (e.g., skiing, SAR operations, etc.).

Clothing Layer

The clothing layer includes shirt, pants, sweater, gloves, and hat, and is the layer worn just outside of the wicking layer (if worn). The clothing layer should offer some insulation and absorb moisture passed from the layers beneath. It should also fit comfortably, not be too tight, and dry quickly. Multiple closures in this layer offer alternative methods of ventilation without actually removing the entire layer. For example, unbutton some buttons, unzip a zipper (partially or all the way), etc. In moderate conditions where a shell will not be worn and the clothing layer will the exposed to the environment, durability and snag/tear resistance should also be considered.

The use of cotton in this layer is more acceptable than in other layers because moisture won't be held close to the skin. But in cold temperatures where the clothes are likely to get wet, cotton may still not be a good choice. The wicking layer's material should wick moisture away from the skin while the loose-fitting clothing layer breathes, saturates, and aids in evaporation of moisture. Heavy-duty, reinforced cotton or blend trousers, such as army fatigues, are frequently used in this layer because of their loose, roomy fit and their multiple utility pockets. Brush pants with reinforcing material at the knees, seat, and leg fronts, are commonly used by bird hunters to handle thick, wet underbrush. These make excellent trousers for SAR operations in cool weather. Wool, flannel, and light/mid-weight synthetic shirts are durable additions to the clothing layer.

In wet and/or cold conditions, avoid cotton in the clothing layer. If the weather is cold enough, it may freeze, restricting movement and forming a vapor barrier, trapping moisture and creating a "refrigerator" effect. In the summer, on the other hand, cotton can be beneficial, offering breathability, evaporative cooling, and abrasion resistance. Wool and synthetics may be worn almost any time because they do not share the limitations of cotton especially when wet.

In hot weather, moisture-laden clothing close to the skin can prevent evaporation and reduce the body's ability to control its temperature—two bad things for the SAR worker. Thus, many prefer to wear loose absorbent clothing with minimal or no underwear so that air can flow freely next to the skin and promote evaporation, drying and cooling. Thin cotton, silk, and even fine grades of wool work well as a loose layer and may feel comfortable in the heat. Whatever the material, wearing very baggy clothing in hot environments will promote the "bellows effect" and keep the body cool. The same wind that can kill in a cold environment can save a life in very hot environments.

Fabric color is important. Dark colors absorb the heat of the sun and are generally a better choice in cold climates, but are hard to see at night and in wooded environments. Lighter colors, on the other hand, reflect more of the sun's radiant heat, are preferable in warmer climates, and are usually easier to see in environments that present dark backgrounds. Besides controlling temperature, colorful clothing has other benefits. SAR personnel wearing colors that contrast with the environment are easier to see. Bright colors like fluorescents or colors not commonly found in the outdoors should be worn unless stealth and camouflage are important (rare in land SAR). Studies have shown that royal blue is the least occurring color in nature. It also contrasts with many environments and is easily seen in most outdoor settings. Blaze or "hunter" orange is also a very visible choice that is hard to miss in most environments.

Short pants may work in some limited circumstances, but one should always keep a long pair available in case the weather changes or conditions call for leg protection. Cotton blue jeans, although popular and fashionable in the United States, are usually constrictive and possess all the limitations of cotton (cold when wet, absorb and hold water, etc). Therefore, cotton jeans are most often not well suited for field SAR operations.

Insulation Layer

The purpose and function of the insulation layer is to trap air between the wicking and shell layers. With very little exception, material thickness equates to insulation and warmth. But insulation is better achieved through multiple thin layers than one thick layer. Examples of garments that might work well as insulation include sweaters, fiber pile jackets and trousers, parkas, insulated vests, coveralls, mittens, face masks, or anything that might help prevent heat loss.

The style of the insulating garment is also important. Pullover, button-down, full-zip, and integrated systems (insulation that zips into a shell) are some of the options. Whatever style is chosen, the closure systems should be varied between layers for best results. For example, if zippers are present in both insulation and shell layers, a relatively uninsulated area exists in the center of the chest where the zippers overlap. Alternating the location of closures between layers can prevent this type of problem.

Many garment manufacturers suggest synthetic insulation layers because they retain much of their insulating ability when wet, wick better, and dry more quickly than natural fibers. Polyester fleece has become very popular for good reason. Besides being soft and lightweight, polyester fleece fibers trap dead air well and are hydrophobic. Also popular are synthetic, down-like materials such as are Primaloft® and the PolarGuard™ families, which are moisture resistant, non-allergenic, and quick drying.

Generally when dry, nylon fleece, polyester pile and batting, goose down, and wool all have similar insulation values for the same thickness. The exceptions to this rule include some high-density foams and synthetics like Thinsulate™, which provides nearly twice the insulation per unit of thickness. If insulation comparisons are made by weight only, however, dry, clean, high-quality goose down is unparalleled.

Insulation capability when wet is especially important when considering usefulness of a garment over a broad spectrum of environmental conditions. In this regard, synthetics are superior to most natural materials (e.g., down and cotton) because they retain more of their loft and insulation while absorbing less, and being less effected by, water.

Insulation of the torso is most important and may be accomplished with a fleece vest or jacket. Extremities, including legs, arms, hands, feet, face, and head are also important areas to protect from heat loss (covered below in special considerations). The insulation provided should be adequate for all climatic conditions the wearer may encounter. A heavy down jacket is probably not required in Florida and lightweight fleece, as the primary insulation, is not likely adequate protection against the cold of a Montana winter.

Technology also offers an interesting twist on warmth in outer wear. For example, Malden Mills, the makers of Polartec® fleece jackets, licensed a new technology to North Face®: battery-powered electric jackets. Unlike the electric blankets of the past that have the traditional wires running through them to produce heat, this garment uses lightweight lithium batteries to conduct heat through stainless steel microfibers thinner than a human hair. The fibers are flexible, washable, and as soft as the fabric through which they are woven. The high-tech version by North Face® does not look unusual, but it heats up to over 100°F on full power. It's expensive, but another great example of how technology can positively impact outdoor wear.

The Shell Layer

The shell layer is the layer that actually protects the wearer from wind, sun, sand, rain, and snow. As a minimum, it should cover and protect the head, neck, torso, and arms. In still air, an appropriate shell can keep the wearer 10° to 25°F warmer. In windy conditions, a good shell can provide an increase of up to 50°F in warmth.

There are many different kinds of shells available, ranging from pullover parkas to full-zip jackets. They may be lined, insulated, waterproof, water-resistant, water-repellent, or have a number of other characteristics. Their length may vary from short, waist-length (for ease of movement), to mid-thigh length (for improved wind and thermal protection). Some shells include hoods (highly recommended), and they too come in many styles ranging from detachable with zipper or Velcro® to permanent and/or stow-away styles. Of course, the material from which a shell is made also varies widely and is the key to its water resistance, wind resistance, and overall durability. In short, there are so many variables in shell garments that space prevents a comprehensive treatment of all the options. So, four of the most common types of shells and their characteristics will be discussed here.

Waterproof Shell

The first shell type is fully water- and windproof. It is usually made of coated nylon that is rugged, relatively inexpensive, and lightweight. But it may also be made of coated cotton ("cotton duck") or rubber. Coated nylon is nylon coated with a waterproofing agent. Seams in this type of garment may also be treated and/or taped to prevent the passage of water. Over time, the material used to coat the fabric and seams eventually wears off and may require reapplication. In addition, the same waterproof characteristics that keep water from getting into the shell also prevent moisture, like perspiration, from escaping. It is by definition a vapor barrier. So, any perspiration inside the shell produced during exertion must be vented to the outside through zippered or Velcro® vents or by opening the garment's fasteners. If strenuous exercise is anticipated and a waterproof shell is worn, ventilation must be assured to prevent a moisture buildup underneath.

A vapor barrier—a completely waterproof membrane inserted between or on top of layers—may be either beneficial or dangerous, depending on the environment in which it is used. In very cold weather, a vapor barrier strategically placed in one's layer system may increase heat retention significantly by all but eliminating the evaporation of moisture from the skin. However, in moderate and warm climates, the same principles can cause the layers under the barrier to get and stay very wet. This can pose a hyperthermia threat in the right conditions. In addition, since evaporation from the skin is reduced or eliminated, overheating (even in cold weather) can also be a real danger. This is why vapor barriers are generally not recommended in all but the coldest (arctic) weather.

Thin, inexpensive, waterproof, plastic, or vinyl emergency rain gear is also available but not recommended for SAR operations. They may offer limited protection from wet weather but they are generally too flimsy to withstand the rigors of nearly any SAR environment. Because they are so inexpensive, they may also include elastic at the wrists and sometimes hood and/or waist. This "feature" could cause a constriction problem and should generally be avoided in outdoor clothing. Because of their material, they may also become brittle and tear easily in cold weather. Next to footwear, purchasing high-quality rain gear (jacket and trousers) may be the best money spent by SAR personnel interested in warmth and comfort, especially during extended SAR missions (**Figure 7–6**).

No waterproof material or garment is suitable in all outdoor environments. When working hard outside in the pouring rain, you will get wet no matter what is worn, from both the inside and the outside. Even if it is

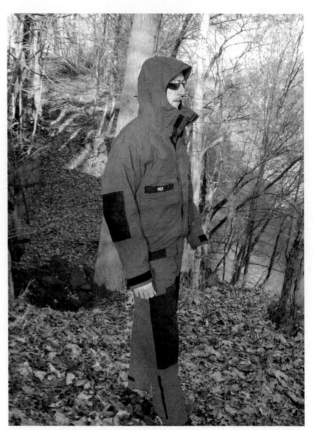

Figure 7–6 Next to footwear, purchasing high-quality rain gear (jacket and trousers) may be the most important investment spent by SAR personnel interested in warmth and comfort, especially during extended SAR missions.

impossible to keep dry in a given situation, it is possible to remain fairly comfortable by picking the right system to begin with, and properly adjusting the layers as necessary.

Water-Repellent Shell

The second shell type is an inexpensive, highly breathable, and <u>water-repellent</u> garment generally geared for the aerobic user. "Water-repellent" means that it sheds water that is not under pressure; however, falling or wind-blown rain may penetrate the fabric. The primary role of this garment is to allow moisture (perspiration) to easily pass through the fabric while maintaining an adequate windbreak. It is not intended to protect the user against extremely wet conditions. These garments are generally made water repellent by combining tightly woven synthetic fibers with a durable, water-repellent coating that penetrates the fabric and reduces the surface tension of the fabric. This combination causes water to bead up and run off the surface of the fabric rather than soak through.

Water-Resistant Shell

The third shell option is as breathable as its water-repellent cousin, but it resists the passage of water to a higher degree. "Water-resistant" means the material temporarily resists water under pressure. This shell usually combines a water-resistant membrane with some type of durable water-repellent finish. This combination works well when strenuous activity is necessary in more severe, wet weather. Gore Activent® is an example of a water-resistant fabric. Patagonia™ Pneumatic® and The North Face Hydreneline® are examples of this type of shell. These garments are moderately expensive and are not considered waterproof or designed to withstand severe wet weather conditions.

Waterproof and Breathable Shell

The last shell type is nearly impermeable to water droplets (waterproof) but allows water vapor to pass (breathable). This is achieved by marrying a durable, water-repellent outer material (often nylon or polyester) with a waterproof, laminated micropore membrane on the inside (Figure 7-7). The result is a shell, hat, footwear, gloves, or trousers that are completely waterproof and breathable.

The way it works is that the laminate material is constructed with very small pores (micropores); these pores are so tiny that water droplets cannot pass through but water vapor can. Functionally, this means that rainwater cannot pass into the shell, but perspiration and moisture in the form of water vapor can escape. Gore-Tex®, Mountain Hardware's Conduit™, and Patagonia's H2No® are examples of this type of fabric (see Figure 7-7).

Generally, these shells are expensive, with prices ranging from $250 to $450 (U.S.). The fabric also comes in two versions: two-layer (softer, more pliable) and three-layer (heavier and more durable). Since these types of garments may require a significant investment, all options should be examined prior to making a purchase.

If a shell is marketed as "waterproof," ask about a warranty. Many reputable outdoor clothing manufacturers offer lifetime warranties on their garments. The high cost of this type of garment is often prohibitive. But, with careful use and care, such a garment should last a long time.

When warmth is important, wear a windproof shell regardless of it being waterproof or not. The warmest wool clothing or insulation layers can be rendered all but useless in a high wind. An insulating garment that traps a great deal of air can lose that air in a high wind. A windproof shell is often all that is needed to provide comfort to the wearer in moderate temperatures and dry climates.

Since the shell layer is often the only layer visible, and SAR personnel should be as visible as possible (to each other as well as the lost subject), selecting a highly visible color is an important consideration in choosing a shell. Dark colors, and, of course camouflage are more difficult to see in many environments and should generally be avoided for use in SAR. SAR personnel need to be seen. So, pick a color that is highly visible in the environment in which you intend to wear it, and better yet, purchase a shell that integrates reflective material into it as well.

Additional Clothing Considerations

When dressing for the outdoors, certain parts of the body require special attention. There are also special considerations for women that are often overlooked, especially by manufacturers who design and construct most outdoor clothing for men.

Head

The unprotected head can be responsible for more than half of the body's heat loss in cold environments, and a similar amount of heat gain in hot environments, mostly by radiation. Since the head has relatively little insulation of its own, head covering of some type should be worn in both hot and cold weather: in cold weather to protect from heat loss (Figure 7-8), and in hot weather to keep from overheating (Figure 7-9). This may require more than just a hat. The neck, ears, forehead, eyes, and even the nose all require protection (covering) as well.

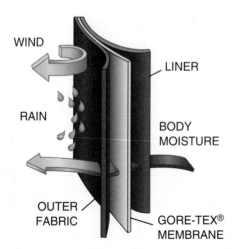

Figure 7-7 Gore-Tex® fabric and how it works. Courtesy of W. L. Gore & Associates, Inc.

In colder conditions, insulation fibers such as fleece or wool work well. Choose a fiber that is hydrophobic and wicks moisture away from the head and face. Protecting the entire face and head is important in cold weather. Balaclavas and face-mask type headwear are great for this task. Ear bands protect the ears but leave the top of the head—a major source of heat loss—exposed and uninsulated. In milder temperatures, lighter hats with a brim or vented ball caps allow air to circulate near the head while shading the head/face/eyes from the sun. Waterproof hats can even be used as improvised water containers.

In desert environments, the head still needs protection, but from external heat, not heat loss. To promote cooling, wear a light-colored, light material hat with a wide brim and plenty of ventilation. The idea is to reflect the sun's radiant heat away from the head, provide as much shade as possible, and promote the circulation of air beneath the hat so that perspiration evaporates quickly. Hats with extended bills, mesh sides (for ventilation), drawstrings (to hold them on), and drapes to cover the neck have been specifically designed for desert use (see Figure 7-9).

Many do not realize that constriction can also be a problem with hats. This can lead to impeded blood flow to the ears and scalp and predispose one to cold injuries. Make sure that whatever type of head protection worn is not too tight, and make sure to remove it and massage the scalp when possible and safe to promote circulation.

Many recognize that sunblock and sunglasses (high UV protection) should be used in very sunny and high altitude environments. However, the need for eye protection from flying debris, small tree limbs, brush, and other hazards is often overlooked. Walking through a wooded area, especially at night, is a serious hazard to the eyes. High winds, especially in sandy environments can also be a significant problem. Glasses may be needed to protect not only from the sun's rays, but also from hazards in the environment, and reading glasses may not be enough. Not only should sunglasses be worn in sunny and high altitude environments, but clear safety glasses may be needed in wooded environments, especially at night, and goggles may be needed in high wind situations.

Hands

The fingers are very often affected by extreme cold and, therefore, deserve special attention in such climates. Since SAR work often necessitates dexterity, the hands are

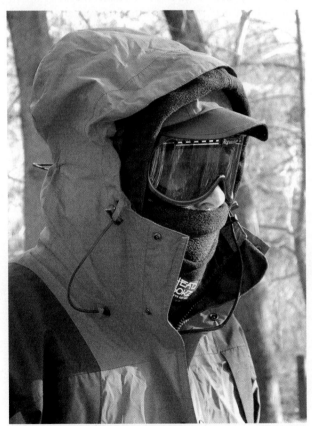

Figure 7–8 In colder conditions, fleece or wool hats work well to wick moisture away from the head and face. Balaclavas and face-mask type headwear are great for protecting the entire face and head. In addition, do not overlook the importance of protecting the eyes in cold weather Photo courtesy of T. P. Miei.

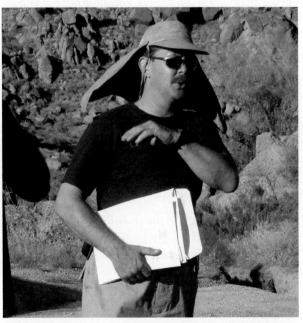

Figure 7–9 In hot weather, wear a light-colored, light material hat with a wide brim and plenty of ventilation. As a minimum, it should shade the head, face, and neck from the sun. Photo courtesy of F. Wysocki.

important tools. Mittens generally keep the hands warmer than do gloves, but they may impair dexterity. Overmits (a second, larger pair of mittens worn over other gloves or mittens) may be necessary in very cold environments or where snow or slush might be encountered. Leather gloves may be required in SAR work, but they should not be exclusively depended upon for warmth in very cold environments as leather tends to absorb water and offers minimal insulation by itself. Leather does a great job of protecting the hands from abrasions and wind while improving traction and grip. In cold weather where leather gloves are needed, consider wearing larger ones with wool or fleeces gloves underneath. Also, do not forget to protect the wrists. A great deal of heat can be lost in cold weather through wrists exposed to the wind, rain, snow, and cold. Generally, make sure to overlap all adjacent garments in cold weather (e.g., gloves and jacket, jacket and trousers, jacket and head wear, etc.) to prevent the exposure of bare skin.

Wearing a thin pair of gloves under mittens can keep the hands warmer in extreme cold. Thin gloves (polypropylene, silk, nylon) allow heat to pass easily, allowing the heat from the fingers to heat each other. In addition, perspiration can pass through the gloves and into the insulating mittens to keep the hands dryer and, in turn, warmer. Antiperspirant applied to the hands and feet can also reduce perspiration in those areas and, thus, keep hands and feet warmer in cold environments.

Where bodily fluids may be encountered, latex or vinyl gloves (some people are allergic to latex) should be worn for protection. If additional gloves are also necessary for protection from abrasion or cold, latex or vinyl gloves can be worn underneath to keep them from being torn during use.

Feet and Footwear

The feet are in constant contact with the environment, and foot problems can incapacitate SAR personnel. Therefore, both the feet and footwear require special attention.

Preventative maintenance is half of the battle to having comfortable feet. In terms of foot care, here are some suggestions:

- Examine the feet at the end of every day and clean them thoroughly.
- Tend to any hot spots immediately. (A hot spot is a reddened, slightly tender area on the skin of the foot that is evidence of rubbing or pressure from footwear and is an early sign of an impending blister.)
- Massage the feet regularly.
- Always wear clean, dry socks.
- Always wear two pair of socks for field work.

- Avoid folds or seams in socks while they are in use.
- Air dry the feet often, but do not soak or rinse them until the end of the day.
- Keep toenails trimmed, but not too short.
- Tighten footgear on inclines and loosen them a bit on flat ground.
- Have footgear properly sized by a professional.
- Keep the feet dry!

Important factors when selecting footwear for SAR work is fit/comfort, stability/support, durability, traction, and protection from the elements.

Proper fit is the most important aspect of any footwear. Something as seemingly insignificant as a blister from ill-fitting footwear can eventually incapacitate an individual to the point of not being able to travel, a potentially dangerous situation in many environments. In addition, SAR personnel can hardly be effective when their feet hurt.

Fit is directly related to comfort, and properly fitted footwear by definition is comfortable. Because of the many subtleties of properly fitting footwear and the high cost of making a mistake, having footwear properly sized and fitted by a professional is highly recommended. Before seeking a professional, however, it is also recommended to be familiar with the terminology of the shoe trade. Terms like upper, lower, mid-sole, tanning, gusseted tongue, bellows tongue, shank, and welt (different types) will likely be used. One should also be familiar with the various types of footwear before venturing into the marketplace. These include: running, hiking, light hikers, mountaineering, climbing, walking, tennis, cowboy, arctic, snow, cross trainers, and many more. The best choice will depend on the types of specific environments and SAR operations one is likely to encounter. A boot designed for use in the mountainous terrain of Colorado may not be suitable for the desert terrain of south Texas. Similarly, an insulated, waterproof boot may be desirable in Maine in autumn, but the same boot may not be suitable for use in Georgia in July. Even though a pair of cowboy boots may be quite appropriate for a mounted search team in California, and deck (boat) shoes may be perfect for use by a water rescue team in Florida, neither type of footwear may be safe in mountainous terrain.

Footwear for SAR work must also provide stability and support. That is, it must neither allow one's ankle to turn easily in rough terrain nor allow the wearer to feel the rough terrain through the sole. It must also be durable enough to withstand many uses (without damage) and offer a superior return on investment. Traction is also a consideration. The sole of the footwear must provide adequate traction in the terrain in which it is intended to be used without causing undue damage to the environment or the wearer.

Footwear must also protect the wearer from the elements. Automatically putting on additional socks in cold weather is not a good idea because it will constrict the feet (more than when they were sized), impede blood flow, and cause the feet to get cold. Wear two pair at all times (see the underneath layer section for more about socks). An adequate amount of insulation should be integrated into the footwear to protect the wearer from temperature extremes. In cold weather, insulation can also be added to the outside of the footwear (e.g., mukluks, overboots, etc.) as long as the feet do not get constricted. Footwear should be improved if it no longer provides enough warmth.

For most SAR operations, high-top, mid-height hiking shoes or light mountaineering boots should be adequate (**Figure 7–10**). However, in technical terrain (e.g., high altitude, vertical rock, snow/ice, etc.) specialized footwear should be worn after seeking professional advice.

Properly cared for, expensive boots like those often necessary for SAR should last for many years. To help assure longevity, clean and dry them after every use, and then store them in a cool, dry place away from sunlight, insects, and vermin. Never dry boots over or near a fire or in the dryer. Overheating can damage the material and weaken stitching. Boots should be dried at room temperature but may be placed near a radiator or forced air heating vent. Applying conditioners and/or sealers to boots may also help protect them. Products like mink-oil (leather protector), Sno-Seal® (leather treatment), Seam Seal (a waterproofing liquid by Aquaseal®), silicone spray, and beeswax all provide some level of protection for leather and rubber products. Be aware that using these and many similar products may eliminate breathability and thus could void the warranty on the footwear. For best results, instructions provided by the manufacturer for boot care should be followed.

Once the purchase is made, "break in" any footwear before wearing it into the field. While wearing the same socks that will be used outdoors, wear them around the house, walk stairs, and test their fit. If there is a problem, some manufacturers will exchange boots that were only worn inside for replacements. However, the best reason to break them in is to work out any problems—including pressure points, arch support, and the like—before going into the field.

Footwear should be worn snug, but not tight, during travel on tracks, trails, and level ground. When walking uphill or downhill, tighten the laces a bit to remove any possibility of movement of the footwear. Loosen them again once back on flat ground. Overly-snug footwear is a primary cause of cold feet among outdoor travelers. Keep footwear only as tight at necessary to maintain comfort, minimize blisters, and promote safety.

Generally, when hands and feet are cold, one should check for constriction problems and then put on a hat. Much of the body's heat is lost through the head and neck. So, when the feet and hands are cold, it could be because the blood flowing to them is not being warmed enough due to heat loss elsewhere. Use the BUBU approach to dressing for the outdoors: Big, Unconstricting, Baggy, and Ugly.

Gaiters

Gaiters applied to the lower legs prevent and protect against dirt, debris, snow, ticks, and chiggers from getting in the boots and on the legs. They can also keep snow and water from wetting the trousers and subsequently promoting heat loss in cold environments. Snow can melt quickly in the trousers and wet the garment. Walking through dew-covered grass or weeds can wet the lower trousers very quickly.

Gaiters usually attach with a small hook to a lower lace towards the toe of the shoe or boot. Some boots actually provide a small hook for this purpose. Some gaiters connect to the boot by a tight, wide rubber band that is especially designed to adhere to the welt of the boot (perimeter of the sole). All also have some method of attaching around the lower leg.

Gaiters are usually constructed with Cordura® or heavy ripstop polyester or nylon. Most are coated with

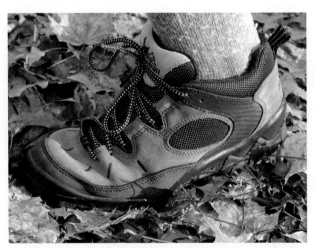

Figure 7–10 For most SAR operations, mid-height, light hikers (shown) or light mountaineering boots should be adequate. Photo courtesy of T. P. Mier.

some waterproofing agent. They may use Velcro®, zippers, snaps, or a combination of closures. There are two sizes of gaiters; the smaller size, six inches or so, primarily protects and prevents entry of foreign matter into the boot. It simply wraps around the ankle/collar of the boot. The larger gaiter runs the length of the shin and provides a broader range of protection. It attaches underneath the boot with strap and buckle or cordage, and is usually used in conjunction with elastic or a small strap to keep secure on the shin. Not only does the larger gaiter protect against foreign object entry, it may also help as a windbreak and protects the lower leg against abrasion, insects, plants, and even snakes. Use them with caution, though. Constriction may be a problem, especially if worn improperly, and waterproof gaiters can cause the same problems as a vapor barrier; that is, condensation under the layer can wet the garments underneath.

Constriction

Elastic at the wrists, ankles, waist, head, or feet can cause a problem with blood flow. These constriction problems impede the flow of the blood that warms the extremities. As the blood flow decreases to the extremities, the risk of cold injuries increases.

From these considerations, some general guidelines can be derived: elastic should generally be avoided in outdoor clothing; use a strap to hold on a hat, suspenders instead of a belt, and—bottom line—avoid all tight and constricting clothing of any kind (Figure 7–11).

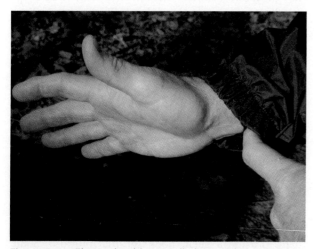

Figure 7–11 Elastic should generally be avoided in outdoor clothing; use a strap to hold on a hat, suspenders instead of a belt, and—bottom line—avoid all tight and constricting clothing of any kind. Photo courtesy of T. P. Mier.

Clothing for Women

Women have needs that are not always addressed by clothing manufacturers, who often simply repackage clothing designed for men. Although offerings specifically designed for women may be difficult to find, the search is usually worth the effort.

To start, clothing and footwear are available that are sized and designed specifically for women. Seek them out. Women should not settle for clothing designed for men. For example, pants and underwear layers are available that have full front to back crotch zippers. This can be incredibly important in colder climates when a great deal of heat is lost when exposing the entire lower half of the body is necessary to answer the call of nature.

Here are some examples of sources of clothing and wetsuits for active, outdoor women. Many more undoubtedly exist or will come into existence after this book is published, but these offer examples of what is available for women.

- Isis for Women
- Altrec.com Outdoors
- Title 9 Sports
- Mountain Equipment Coop
- Sahalie
- Northwest River Supplies

Survival Tips on Clothing

In summary, there are some fundamental guidelines/issues concerning dressing for the outdoors that must not be overlooked:

- When your feet are cold, put on a hat.
- Do not overheat so that clothing becomes wet by perspiration.
- Use the layer system.
- When sleeping in harsh, cold conditions, arrange dry, spare clothing around the neck and shoulders with padding and insulation added to each kidney region, as these areas are more susceptible to cold. Also, wear a knit stocking cap because if your head is warm, chances are your feet will be, too.
- Dry wet clothing by allowing it to freeze and then beating ice crystals from fabric.
- Wearing darker clothing in winter to absorb the sun's heat energy may be a good idea, but beware of not being visible enough. SAR personnel must be very visible.

- Clean clothing allows proper ventilation through clothing layers. Dirty clothing inhibits ventilation and causes moisture buildup on clothing layers. Wear clean clothes.
- Light-colored clothing reflects the sun and heat in warm weather.
- In hot weather, wear clothing that promotes circulation of air beneath layers.

Suggestions for Outdoor Clothing Purchases

One of the first questions asked in basic SAR skills classes is, "Where/how do I purchase appropriate outdoor clothing without spending a lot of money?" Indeed, it is possible to find inexpensive, quality clothing that will provide them with the protection and comfort needed for SAR. Here are some suggestions:

1. Plan ahead and buy winter/outdoor clothes/items during spring and winter clearance sales.
2. Using this same "reverse season" purchasing thought process, check various stores/catalogs/Internet sources other than the stereotyped label of "outdoor stores" to purchase clothes and all sorts of equipment that can be used for SAR. Consider the following (catalogs and stores):
   - Ski shops for winter gear, waterproof pants, gloves, eyewear, undergarments, etc.
   - Cross-country running specialty stores for lightweight breathable clothes, layers that wick, water bottles, socks, hats, etc.
   - Snowboarding specialty stores for waterproof pants, socks, eye wear, gloves, undergarments, neck gaiters, face fleece, etc.
   - Parachute supply houses for socks, gloves, eyewear, pouches that can be attached to packs, wrist altimeters, etc.
   - Recreational vehicle stores for environmentally biodegradable toilet paper, glow sticks, 12-volt portable water heater, folding tables, 12-volt lights, etc.
   - Rafting supply stores for waterproof bags and containers, light weight tarps, folding tables, folding cots, etc.
   - Forestry supply for colored flagging tape, orange vests with pockets, compass kits, reflective tape, etc.
3. Try the clearance sales offered by name brand outdoor shops and Web sites (L.L. Bean®, REI®, etc.)
4. Stores such as Sierra Trading Post® specialize in selling seconds from all sorts of companies.
5. Use the "reverse season" thought process when checking at the local Salvation Army store or secondhand stores.
6. Even though the military surplus stores really don't have an "off season," it's good to rummage around in the store just to see what is available at least twice a year.

SAR Terms

Hydrophilic Refers to fabric that absorbs water.

Hydrophobic Refers to fabric that repels water.

Hyperthermia Condition or illness caused by the body's core temperature being significantly higher than normal (which is 98.5°F/37°C).

Hypothermia Condition or illness caused by the body's core temperature being significantly lower than normal (which is 98.5°F/37°C).

Waterproof Material that is impermeable to water, even water under pressure.

Waterproof and breathable Material that is nearly impermeable to water droplets (waterproof) and yet allows water vapor to pass (breathable).

Water-repellent Sheds water that is not under pressure; however, falling or wind-blown rain may penetrate the fabric.

Water-resistant The material temporarily resists water under pressure.

References

Cox, M., & Fulsass, K. (eds.) (2003). *Mountaineering: Freedom of the Hills,* 7th ed. New York, NY: Mountaineers Books.

Farmer, K. (1976). *Woman in the Woods.* New York, NY: Stackpole Books.

Johnson, M. (2003). *The Ultimate Desert Handbook: A Manual for Desert Hikers, Campers, and Travelers.* New York, NY: Ragged Mountain Press/McGraw Hill.

Manning, H. (1986). *Backpacking: One Step at a Time,* 4th ed. New York, NY: Vintage Books.

McManners, H. (1998). *The Complete Wilderness Training Book.* New York, NY: DK Publishing.

Petzoldt, P. (1974). *The Wilderness Handbook,* 1st ed. New York, NY: W.W. Norton & Company, Inc.

Rawlins, C., & Fletcher, C. (2002). *The Complete Walker IV,* revised ed. New York, NY: Alfred A. Knopf, Inc.

Chapter 8

Safety in SAR Environments

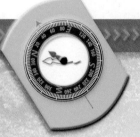

Objectives

Safety Basics

Search and rescue teams throughout the nation are called upon frequently to solve complex problems in a wide spectrum of environments. Search and rescue personnel, whether at the end of a long search or responding directly to a person in distress, should realize that most such incidents are solved by well-trained specialized resources, not just by dedicated responders.

Because of the critical need for these specialized skills and the absence of any up-to-date, widely accepted technical manuals, each agency, rescue squad, or volunteer organization, has developed its own training standards, capabilities, and techniques. While some are credible and technically correct, many have undoubtedly contributed to the death of would-be rescuers. The entire process of rescue (locating, accessing, stabilizing, and transporting) must have continuity, consistency of nomenclature, and most of all, a firm foundation in training and planning.

Some of the specialized environments and associated problems that SAR team members may have to deal with are included in **Table 8–1**.

While each of these present different problems to SAR personnel in the field, the rescue scene manager's job may change very little. Identification and proper use of specialized skills and resources are the key factors in each case.

Regardless of the type of rescue environment the following general rules should be followed:

1. Technical personnel should be used for technical rescue.
2. If the subject is deceased, evacuate only if and when there is no risk to fellow team members, or at least when the hazards have been assessed and justified.
3. Stabilize the subject before evacuating, if possible; continue stabilization procedures during transport.
4. Decide on the easiest route before traveling.

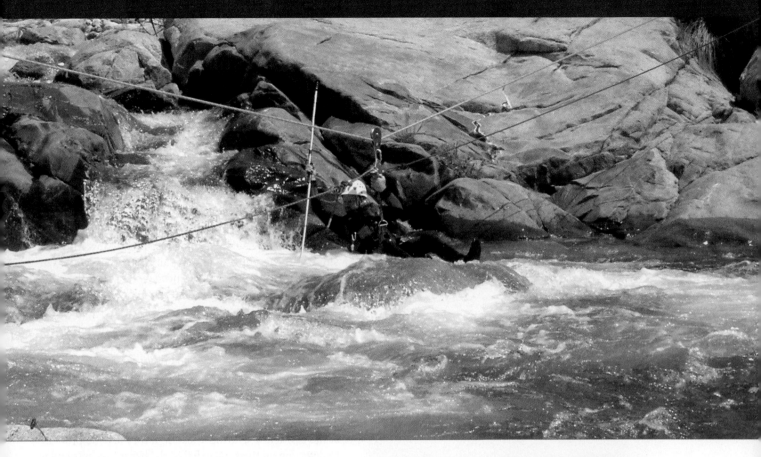

5. Appoint someone to serve as route-finder, who with a radio and markers can report potential hazards, problems, etc.

6. Litter teams of at least 6 to 8 personnel (3 teams minimum) should be used in no more than 20 minute shifts. Others may also be required to carry equipment.

7. Use accepted procedures to care for and protect the subject.

8. A radio operator should follow the litter team.

9. If using a helicopter for evacuation, make sure that:

   • The subject is informed and briefed.

   • The subject is protected.

   • Someone goes with the subject who knows what has been done medically for the patient.

Special SAR Environments

Specialized SAR environments bring on a diverse set of problems and potential complications for rendering aid to injured and/or stranded subjects. Each environment holds its own set of obstacles to increase the complexity and difficulty of a particular mission.

Table 8–1	Specialized SAR Environments and Challenges
Mountain	Air shafts
Vertical rock	White water streams
Vertical ice	Coastal white water surf
Flat ice	Flash floods
Avalanche	Slow rising floods
Crevasse	High winds
Cave	Sea and lake
Mines	Snow and blizzard
Wells	Booby-trapped stills
Hazardous material dumps	Confined spaces
Urban/city	Trenches

Technical Rock Rescue

Mountaineering, rock climbing, and casual scrambling have created the need for specialized SAR expertise (Figure 8–1). Individuals and groups involved in rock rescue have refined and developed techniques for most

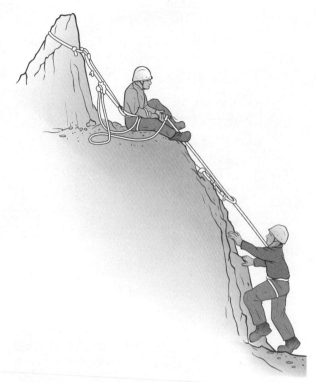

Figure 8–1 Specialized SAR expertise is necessary for technical rock rescue in mountainous terrain.

situations. The hallmark of a technical rock rescuer is the ability to improvise and modify tools or techniques to meet any crisis. He or she must be comfortable using climbing gear and being exposed to heights.

Once an individual has been located in this environment and the situation surveyed, it will become necessary to gain access. Local groups familiar with a particular area already will have solved this problem. The solution may involve either climbing or descending to the subject. Safety for all persons involved is paramount because an accident during a rescue is almost always catastrophic. Climbing up to the subject requires a knowledge of rock climbing techniques, possession of the proper equipment, and familiarity with their use. Local clubs or mountaineering stores can be contacted for more detailed assistance. Specialized technical rock rescue teams, such as those sanctioned by the Mountain Rescue Association, routinely practice climbing techniques and the solving of vertical rescue problems.

The decision to go up, down, or sideways to reach a subject will depend on ease of access to both the top and the bottom. Fast moving water at the bottom, for example, may preclude an approach from below. Conversely, a brush-filled approach to the top may preclude a top-side approach. Helicopter availability, adequate landing sites, suitable anchor sites, and ease of climbing are also

considerations when deciding whether to approach from the top or bottom.

Descending necessitates good technique and proper anchors. Rappelling, or descending via rope, allows more control by the descending rescuer, but "ties up" his or her hands. Because of this, the incident commander may elect to lower the rescuer in a sling rather than allow him or her to rappel. Lowering necessitates greater communication between the top and the rescuer, but allows the rescuer's hands to be free. Lowering also usually takes more rescuers to perform.

If the subject is able to assist him- or herself, lowering a rope to the subject, and subsequently lowering the subject to the bottom, may be all that is necessary. On the other hand, if the subject needs to be placed in a litter, the assistance of additional rescuers and equipment undoubtedly will be required.

Steep inclines, cliffs, bluffs, and similar terrain features that involve elevation differential may require specialized skills and equipment to ascend and/or descend. SAR personnel should not attempt traveling over this type of terrain without expert guidance and the proper equipment and training. When these are not available, SAR personnel should travel around the area, note it, and present it at the debriefing. During a search, it may also be prudent to determine if the subject fell in the hazardous terrain by carefully searching likely "landing" spots.

Cave and Mine Rescue

Standard obstacles in this underground environment include poor communications, difficulty in lighting, and cramped, wet spaces. In addition, reduced visibility often mandates lighting the rescue scene beyond the normal limits of a flashlight or headlamp.

A water cave or live cave involves a moisture range inside the cave from mud to rivers. In the United States, western caves are generally drier than eastern caves. However, humidity, wetness, and cold temperature create a potential for hypothermia greatly underestimated by the average caver. Flooding is often a great problem, and many cavers have died because of inattention to the weather on the outside. Caves become natural drains for streams during heavy rains and thus can provide problems for both caver and rescuer. Wind and temperature are other underestimated problems associated with cave and mine emergencies. Extreme movements of air often develop along passages, which intensifies convective air chilling.

Confined passages, low crawls, and squeezes pose unique problems for the rescue of injured cavers. The use of standard items such as litters, backboards, and splints may not be possible in such places. Confined passages with varying, often toxic, constituent gases can also lead to difficulties for victims and rescuers alike. Occasionally, self-contained breathing apparatus (SCBA), surface supplied air (SSA), and/or self-contained underwater breathing apparatus (SCUBA) may be required. Nevertheless, the potential alone justifies extensive atmospheric monitoring while operating in the underground environment.

An essential part of any cave and mine rescue operation involves a thorough orientation to the specific hazards known to be associated with a particular underground area. This involves pinpointing the locations of pits, waterfalls, siphons, canyons, and other difficult formations that may pose extrication, search, or safety problems. Many caves have been mapped by the National Speleological Society and the National Park Service.

Once a subject has been located, the real difficulties may begin. The goal is to move that person rapidly and comfortably to the surface, but without practice underground, that task will be virtually impossible. Neoprene exposure bags similar to body bags have been used for this purpose and serve well to keep the individual dry and protected during what may be a very long and slow evacuation.

From a medical aid standpoint, procedures must be performed smoothly in dark, cold, and muddy conditions. Experienced cave rescuers agree that repackaging supplies and equipment for underground use is essential. Streamlining kits, packs, and containers is a must for unobstructed passage through crawlways and tight spaces in the cold, damp conditions.

Team members often carry a minimum of 24 hours of light in a helmet-mounted lamp, two additional sources of light with spare bulbs and batteries, and waterproof matches and candles. Other equipment needed in this environment might include:

- High-quality helmet with chin strap and headlamp attachment.
- Sturdy, warm clothes, including gloves, for damp, dirty conditions for up to 24 hours (i.e., wool material, fit that allows good mobility).
- Lug-soled boots that are light, warm, inexpensive, and drain water.
- Non-stretch, specialized caving rope that is highly resistant to abrasion.
- Neil Robertson style wraparound litter (or even an old conveyor belt) that can aid in dragging an injured person through small passages. A common Stokes Litter may work fine.
- Wetsuits for longer missions in extremely wet caves.
- Durable harnesses and slings that are resistant to both chemicals and water.

- Plastic sheeting to divert water and waterfall around a subject during evacuation.
- Small portable pumps, siphon hose, and plastic to divert, dam, or pump water around areas during operations.
- Warm food and drink carried in thermally insulated containers.

Essential caving skills include all of the capabilities and proficiencies that exist in rock climbing, including vertical rope technique, ascending, rappelling, belaying, and being comfortable while working at the end of a rope. All of these must be practiced until they can be done well in cold, wet, and dark, confined spaces. Team practices should be conducted both on the surface and underground with participants being forced to work in mud, suffocating tight squeezes, soaking waterfalls, and occasional blinding darkness. Under these conditions, all team members should be aware of the possibility of hypothermia during training.

If a cave is found in one's assigned search segment, the following guidelines should be followed:

1. Examine the area near the opening for evidence of the entry of others (e.g., tracks, sign, etc.).

2. Do not enter the cave beyond the "natural light zone" near the opening of the cave. Safely going past this area requires specialized equipment and skills.

3. Note the cave on a map and make sure to mention it, along with the likelihood someone would/could have entered it, at the debriefing.

River and White Water Rescue

There are dozens of potentially dangerous problems in the river SAR situation. Log and debris piles at various bends in the river can become not only strainers to the recreational victim, but death traps for the would-be rescuer. The banks of the stream may be deeply undercut with treacherous overhanging debris and snags that can catch on clothing, equipment, and skin. These factors combined with muddy and rapidly rising water render river rescue difficult and unpredictable.

In fast moving water situations, the single greatest problem associated with the environment is that responders underestimate the power and threat of moving water (**Figure 8–2**). Foolhardy heroics and overzealous enthusiasm frequently lead to further tragedy. Cold water immersion coupled with wind and cold temperatures

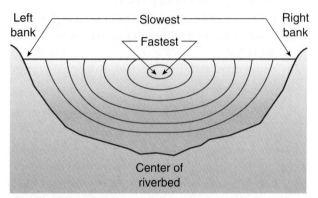

Cross Section of River

Left bank — Slowest — Right bank

Fastest

Center of riverbed

Figure 8–2 Example of how the cross section of river affects the velocity of moving water.

may predispose anyone to hypothermia. Then, wet clothing, darkness, and injury may add to the danger. Noise associated with moving water may obviate clear communications. Poor contact between the victim and rescuers, or between rescuers and other rescuers, is confusing and dangerous.

All potential responders in this environment must know how to read the water for capsize points and other dangerous phenomena. The hydraulics formed by low head dams, collapsed bridges, or other submerged structures can be drowning machines for unsuspecting individuals. Rescue team members must know how to protect themselves in fast moving water at all times. Mandatory skills in this environment include good judgment, strong swimming capability, knowledge of all types of technical systems and equipment used in climbing, and a thorough understanding of river dynamics and hydraulic influences.

River rescue is a very specialized training area that requires specialized equipment and skills. Entering the river environment, including walking near moving water, should only be attempted by specially trained personnel. If properly trained and equipped personnel are not available, the river/moving water environment should be carefully avoided. SAR personnel without specialized training who come across moving water during a search should note or confirm the location on the map, be careful not to approach too closely, and make sure to mention the water during the debriefing. Do not attempt to cross moving water deeper than mid-thigh or moving very fast. Chapter 12, Foot Travel for SAR Personnel, contains more information on how to cross moving water.

General Water Precautions

A fundamental understanding of certain techniques and hazards applies to all water situations. Survival swimming is a technique that may be useful in warm water

and immersion hypothermia will definitely come into play in cold water.

Survival Swimming

Most swimmers don't realize that if they are injured but conscious they can survive in all but the coldest and roughest seas. A simple technique called "survival floating" or drown proofing, was developed during World War II. The technique is based on two premises: (1) Almost everyone will float while their lungs are full of air, and (2) it is much easier to float vertically than horizontally. To perform the survival float, after taking a deep breath, float vertically with hands limply held at the sides, allowing the body to relax in the water with the chin tucked to the breast. As the need to breathe arises, exhale through the nose slowly while raising arms and crossing them in front of the face. Now, as if parting a curtain, extend arms and push downward with thumbs toward the sides and at the same time tilt the head back. As the mouth comes out of the water, take a breath, lower the head and relax again. If relaxed with this technique, alternately switch between a slow, horizontal movement toward shore and survival float. Even with a cramp it is possible to stay afloat and relax the muscle by slowly massaging it between breaths of air. The only place where survival floating is not recommended, and indeed may be dangerous, is in cold water where hypothermia is a consideration.

Immersion Hypothermia

All boaters, swimmers, and people who work on or near water should understand the factors that determine the body's cooling rate while immersed. Properly used, this vital water safety knowledge can extend survival time from minutes to hours. In terms of rescue, this could be the difference between life and death.

As discussed in the section on survival physiology, hypothermia is cooling of the body's inner core. In immersion hypothermia, this rate of cooling is greatly accelerated because, submerged in water, the skin and peripheral areas cool very rapidly due to the increased surface area in direct contact with cold water.

Sea water freezes at 28° to 29° Fahrenheit (F), depending on impurities in the water. Fresh water is usually about 32°F when it freezes, but, like sea water, a high level of impurities will lower the freezing point. Depending on clothing worn, a person falling into water at or near freezing will quickly exhale, shiver violently, and then go into a spastic fetal position with hands and knees under the chin, usually with no control of skeletal muscles.

A body immersed in water near its freezing point will cool very rapidly. Upon submersion, reflex contractions of smaller blood vessels will give a fleeting increase in

Table 8-2 How Hypothermia Affects Most Adults

	Survival Time after Immersion	
Water Temperature Degrees F (°C)	Exhaustion or Unconsciousness	Expected Time of Survival
32.5° (0.3°)	Under 15 minutes	15–45 minutes
36.5–40° (0.3–4.5°)	15–30 minutes	30–90 minutes
40–50° (4.5–10°)	30–60 minutes	1–3 hours
50–60° (10–15.5°)	1–2 hours	1–6 hours
60–70° (15.5–21°)	2–7 hours	2–40 hours
70–80° (21–26.5°)	2–12 hours	3 hours to indefinite
Over 80° (Over 26.5°)	Indefinite	Indefinite

Survival times for average adult holding still in water while wearing a PFD. *Source:* U.S. Coast Guard.

blood pressure and heart rate, but subsequently both will reduce to near death levels. In such a situation, the subject is usually unconscious in 5 to 7 minutes, and often dies in only 10 to 20 minutes.

Survival Time

Varying circumstances in every situation will affect individual cooling rates. Body energy levels, type of clothing, metabolic rate, and circulatory problems all affect survival time. In addition, body fat, physical size, age, and gender influence survival time in cold water. **Table 8-2** shows general survival times for an average adult holding still in water of varying temperatures while wearing a standard personal flotation device (PFD) and light clothing.

Activity and Warmth

Exercise increases body temperature and expends calories. Exercise is an accepted way to maintain body temperature in open air, but this is definitely not the case in water. Increased activity in water substantially increases the rate of inner core cooling due to increased circulation to the arms, legs, and skin. Cooling is caused by continuous movement of water over the surface of the body (convection); this cooling effect is similar to convection losses in wind but is much more severe. The average person swimming or holding still in moving water while in a PFD cools 35% faster than if merely suspended in still water. A subject or rescuer turned swimmer should consider how far it is safe to swim in cold water. The average

person can swim about 0.85 miles in 50°F water before being incapacitated by hypothermia. As a rule, subjects finding themselves in water 50°F or colder should not try to swim to safety unless well within one mile of shore or rescue.

Personal Flotation Devices

A personal flotation device (PFD) is designed to serve one primary purpose: to help keep the wearer's head above water. Because no PFD is capable of keeping one's head above the water all the time, some compromises usually have to be made in terms of mobility, comfort, and flotation. It is critical that all rescuers wear PFDs when working near or on the water to guard against the hazards of hypothermia and drowning.

PFDs should always be approved by the United States Coast Guard (USCG) or similar authority in other countries. There are five types of USCG-approved PFDs in the United States and each type is designated with a Roman numeral (**Table 8-3**). Generally in SAR, such approved PFDs should be made out of foam, have a torso and/or crotch strap, be brightly colored, be of the correct size for the wearer, have a nylon (rather than a metal) zipper, and have a whistle (for signaling) attached. A small knife, in a sheath, may also be attached to the PFD for use when cutting line becomes necessary, and river rescue personnel often attach a length of webbing or prusik loop with one or two carabiners.

Type I PFDs are required on commercial vessels and provide the maximum buoyancy. They are brightly

Table 8–3 — Types of USCG approved Personal Flotation Devices

Number	Description
Type I	Maximum buoyancy, bulky, will turn an unconscious wearer face-up
Type II	Horse-collar type, easily donned, will turn an unconscious wearer face-up
Type III	Minimum safe buoyancy, comfortable, will NOT turn unconscious wearer face-up, but will keep conscious wearer upright
Type IV	Throwable devices, designed for grasping and holding, not for wearing
Type V	Specific activity or hybrid (inflatable), will turn unconscious wearer face-up

colored and designed for use in rough water where they should turn an unconscious person into the face-up position. Because they tend to be large, bulky, cumbersome, and come in only two sizes (adult and child), they are usually not recommended for most SAR work. However, where rough waters are anticipated and maximum flotation is required, a Type I PFD may be the best tool for the job.

Type II PFDs are the relatively inexpensive "horse collar" style devices that are made to be donned easily in an emergency. Although not as effective as the Type I, the Type II is also designed to turn an unconscious person into the face-up position. Their relative low cost and other features cause it to be best suited for general boating and quick rescue activities.

Type III PFDs contain the minimum amount of buoyancy required for safety, will usually maintain a conscious person in an upright position, but will not necessarily turn an unconscious person face-up. These characteristics allow flexibility in design to match the needs of specialized and general boating activities such as fishing, skiing, canoeing, and kayaking. In general, these devices are comfortable, pliable, easy to swim in, provide some thermal protection, are brightly colored, come in various sizes, combine both zippers and torso straps, and provide an excellent choice for most water rescue activities.

Type IV PFDs are throwable devices such as ring buoys and flotation seat cushions that have a minimum of 16 pounds buoyancy. These devices are not designed to be worn, but grasped and held until rescue.

Type V PFDs are divided into two classes: specific activity and hybrid. The specific activity devices are designed and restricted to the specific applications indicated on the label. Examples include water skiing, board sailing, work vests, and commercial white water rafting. The hybrid class of Type V PFD, on the other hand, is inflatable and contains a minimum of 7.5 pounds buoyancy when uninflated and 22 pounds buoyancy when inflated. These devices have an oral inflation tube, often have an automatic CO_2 inflation cartridge, and are designed to turn an unconscious person the same as a Type I or II. For USCG acceptability, however, these hybrid PFDs *must* be worn (except when the vessel is not underway or when the user is in an enclosed space).

In summary, USCG-approved Type I PFDs are best suited where rough waters are expected and maximum flotation is required (i.e., rescue on the open sea). Type II PFDs are useful where ease of donning is important and a quick rescue is anticipated (i.e., flat water rescue or sudden boating accident). Type III PFDs are best suited where comfort and mobility is important, but where maximum flotation is not (i.e., river rescue). Type IV PFDs are useful for throwing to a victim during a rescue, but should not be worn as flotation to affect a rescue. Type V specific activity PFDs are appropriate when the particular device has been specifically designed for its intended use. Type V hybrid PFDs, on the other hand, should be used as flotation only in an emergency.

PFDs offer more than just flotation; they also act as a cushion to protect the user from a fall, debris in the water (i.e., rocks, logs, etc.), or other trauma. In addition, they provide a layer of thermal protection. For instance, Type I and II PFDs offer limited thermal protection, but well-designed Type III and V PFDs may offer 50% to 75% increases in the predicted survival time. In the end, one point needs to be emphasized: No protection is offered by a PFD to the individual who is not wearing the device.

Dry suits (neoprene suits that trap air against the skin providing both warmth and buoyancy) are expensive and bulky; however, they are useful in cold water or ice situations where hypothermia is a primary concern. The "Gumby" suit is an example of a type of dry suit that is designed for use where a clothed rescuer could quickly don the suit and affect a surface rescue in cold water. The Gumby suit is an oversized, one-piece garment, not designed for underwater use, which offers substantial flotation. However, this device and others like it should always be worn beneath an approved PFD when used in a water rescue.

Three options are open to a person in cold water without a life jacket: swim to safety, survival float, or tread water.

With the first option, swimming, distance to safety is the primary consideration and water temperature is the secondary consideration. If there is no refuge within a safe swimming distance, or the water temperature is too cold to swim for it, only survival floating or treading water remain as choices. If the survival floating or drown proofing method of conserving energy and staying afloat is used, the primary heat radiating area of the body—the head—is repeatedly immersed. Thus, survival floating causes body cooling 82% faster than a person holding still in a life jacket. The third option, slowly treading water, loses heat 34% faster than holding still in a PFD (substantially less than survival floating). Treading water slowly, therefore, is definitely the best option to extend survival time when without a PFD.

Increasing Survival Time

The body's primary heat loss areas are the head, neck, sides of the thorax (chest), groin area, sternum, and wrists (Figure 8–3). Therefore, it makes sense to concentrate primarily on insulating these areas if immersed in cold water. The Heat Escape Lessening Position (HELP) was designed to provide just such protection and is performed by hugging the arms close to the sides of the chest to insulate the rib cage, crossing the legs, and assuming a semi-fetal position with the head out of water (Figure 8–4). This HELP position can increase survival time up to 50% in cold water. If more than one person is involved, they should all huddle together to conserve energy by wrapping their arms around each other's shoulders and pulling each other close while keeping their legs crossed. This is called the "huddle" position (Figure 8–5).

Cold, Snow, and Ice SAR

Perhaps no other type of SAR environment requires greater diversity and broad-based foundation of personal and team skills than that of winter snow and ice. These include downhill and/or cross-country skiing, snowshoeing, technical climbing, winter survival, and a good understanding of snow and ice physics. Unlike climbing on rock, snow and ice conditions change on a monthly and minute-to-minute basis. The effects of gravity, wind, temperature, slope, heat exchange, load factors, and avalanche continually impose problems for missions under these conditions. Technical and non-technical SAR problems in snow and ice environments are longer, more taxing, technical, and complex. Combined with shorter days, extremes in weather and the ever present threat of hypothermia and frostbite, techni-

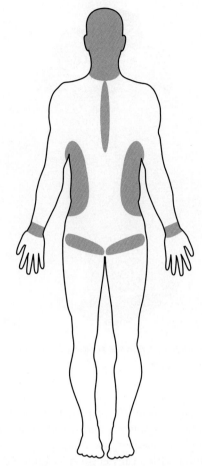

Figure 8–3 Body zones of heat loss. Gray regions depict areas of greatest heat loss in the body.

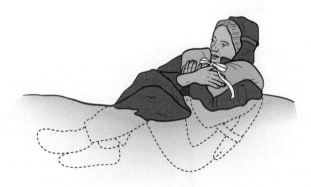

Figure 8–4 Heat Escape Lessening Position (HELP) for keeping yourself warm in cold water.

cal missions of this type are unacceptable for all but the most experienced team members.

Versatility and improvisation are essential components of the overall strategy that must be used in snow

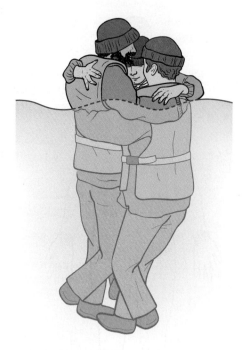

Figure 8–5 Huddle position for keeping more than one person warm in cold water.

and ice. Transportation of the patient is often one of the most difficult problems, and it can be all but resolved through detailed preplanning. Innovations like covering a litter with a canvas cover or improvising an attachment to cross-country skis provide some clever solutions to common winter problems. Commercial products like the Sked® Litter have streamlined the laborious task of transporting injured people in snow and ice conditions.

Immersion Through Ice

Large sections of the United States lie in latitudes far enough north for low temperatures to freeze most still bodies of water. Every year unsuspecting travelers and outdoor enthusiasts fall through ice and drown or die from hypothermia. While it is impossible to detail all conditions or indicators for safety on ice, there are some basic considerations and actions that could save a life when someone falls through ice.

There are many specific types of ice, each with distinctive characteristics. The first type of ice to form is called frazil ice. Frazil ice is formed by the collection of disk-shaped crystals suspended in water, forming a thin, opaque film that floats to the surface. As the temperature drops, these crystals combine to form a solid sheet. Frazil slush is soft collections of frazil crystals that form in moving water where a current prevents a solid freeze. Clear ice is new ice formed by a long, hard freeze. It often reflects the color of water beneath and so can be many colors. It is considered the strongest ice. Snow ice is opaque or milky-colored ice that is formed from the freezing of water-soaked snow. This low-density ice is porous and is considered to be very weak. Layered ice has a striped appearance and is formed from many layers of frozen and refrozen snow. Candle ice forms into finger-like structures in an ice surface as it rots or disintegrates. Candle ice resembles many candles bundled together and is commonly found in late winter or early spring. Rotten ice is old ice that is honeycombed with pockets of air bubbles that in advanced stages of disintegration looks black as it becomes saturated with water. Old, rotten ice may appear to be quite thick, but may crumble under the slightest pressure.

Ice thickness is only one factor that determines its strength. Weather, water depth, size of the body of water, and obstructions all affect the strength of ice. For instance, pure water freezes faster and deeper than water containing chemical or pollutants, and large, deep lakes take longer to freeze but are slower to decay. New ice is usually stronger than old ice, and a light wind tends to speed up ice formation while a heavy wind slows it down. Water rising through the cracks, warm temperatures, and rain can all cause slush to form on ice. Slush should be avoided because it is a sign that ice is no longer freezing from below, and water or slush on ice erodes it. River ice is considered weaker than lake ice due to the current, and smooth, straight stretches of river ice are stronger than river bends because the current is slower. Obstructions such as rocks, logs, decomposing vegetation, and piers produce heat, which also slows ice formation.

Waterfowl and fish can also hinder ice formation. Waterfowl often gather to try to keep an area of open water for feeding. If they leave, the area will have far less ice over it than surrounding areas.

Ice Safety

The only absolute regarding ice safety is to *stay off of it*. To be properly equipped to judge ice dangers and potential rescue techniques, one must possess knowledge of how ice is formed, the types of ice, and factors affecting its strength. However, as a general guide to indicate what kinds of activities good, clear, solid ice can support, use the following:

2 inches = walking
4 inches = fishing
5 inches = snowmobiles
8–12 inches = vehicles

Self Ice Rescue

The first reaction after going through any ice is panicky groping or chopping at the edge of the ice to get out. There are often no handholds and victims exhaust themselves without making headway toward escape. A normal person will not have the energy to break ice to shore unless the distance is very small. To escape, extend arms and hands as far as possible up onto the ice, then kick your feet up and extend them to the rear as if swimming. Continue until you slowly work yourself up onto the ice. Anything sharp such as a knife, keys, belt buckle, or pen, may help get a hold on the ice. The key is to distribute your weight over the widest possible area and move slowly and deliberately—avoiding quick, panicky moves. Once solid ice is reached, roll away from the weak areas as far as possible before trying to get up. If ice cracks or starts to give way, lie down quickly, spread out, and roll away from the area.

Ice Rescue for Others

As with all water- and ice-related rescues, the phrase "Teach, Reach, Throw, Row, Go" should be used to indicate the order in which various types of rescues should be attempted. "Teach" means that the rescuer attempts to talk the victim into self rescue. When dealing with ice, the first four options (teach, reach, throw, and row) are often ineffective, especially if the victim has become hypothermic. However, they should still be attempted. Before attempting a "go" rescue on ice, a rescuer must be completely familiar with self rescue, hypothermia, and the various techniques, along with their associated hazards, for ice rescue. Traveling onto the ice to affect a rescue can be extremely dangerous and should not be attempted without proper training and equipment.

After removing the subject from the ice/water, beware of hypothermia. If snow conditions are dry, a wet subject can be rolled in the powder to absorb as much moisture as possible. If there is no snow or other way to absorb moisture, wet clothing should be removed and replaced with dry as soon as possible. Hypothermia associated with sudden immersion can incapacitate a subject very rapidly. So, rescuers should improvise a shelter, build a fire, or share clothing with others in order to protect the subject from further heat loss. In such a situation, immediate decisions and utilization of resources could mean the difference between life and death.

Avalanches

Although they represent one of the most catastrophic forces of nature, avalanches are not well understood. Basic avalanche ingredients—snow and slope—exist in mountains all over the world. Every year hundreds of thousands, possibly millions, of avalanches occur. While most have no direct effect on human activity, the remainder constitute a significant threat to life and property.

SAR in potential avalanche areas can be hazardous because it requires that SAR personnel be able to recognize and identify avalanche hazards. This is a specialized skill that requires additional training above and beyond conventional SAR training. Although this is not intended to serve as a comprehensive description of avalanched hazards and rescue, selected information is provided to illustrate some of the important issues involved.

Causes and Types

Snow undergoes very little change at constant cold temperatures and therefore usually remains unstable under these conditions. It settles and stabilizes rapidly when temperatures are near, or just above freezing. Stabilization is a metamorphic change dependent on a number of variables, with temperature being the leading factor. However, storms starting with low temperatures and dry snow, followed by rising temperatures, are more likely to cause avalanches than continued constant cold. Rapid weather changes cause snow pack adjustments that may affect stability of snow and cause an avalanche.

The two principal types of avalanche are loose snow and slab. Loose snow avalanches usually start at a point and spread "fan shape" down a slope. They grow bigger and the quantity of snow increases as they descend. Loose snow moves as a formless mass with little internal cohesion. Slab avalanches, on the other hand, start when a large area of snow begins to slide at once. There is a well-defined fracture line where moving snow has broken away from stable snow. There may be angular blocks or chunks of snow. If snow cracks and these cracks run, slab avalanche danger is high.

With ice avalanches, the principles and practical aspects are significantly different from snow avalanches. However, both kinds of avalanche occur in glacier-clad mountains and threaten human activities. On some steep mountain flanks, both snow and ice avalanches fall from the same slopes.

Ice avalanches occur when material is released abruptly from perennial ice deposits, usually mountain glaciers, above steep slopes. Massive blocks of ice break free and fall down the mountainside, sometimes touching off secondary rock and earth slides.

Sustained winds of 15 miles per hour or more cause the danger to increase rapidly. Snow plumes (cornices) from ridges and peaks indicate that snow is being moved

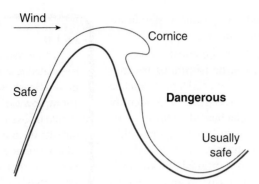

Figure 8-6 Avoid disturbing cornices from below or above. Gain ridge tops by detouring around cornice areas.

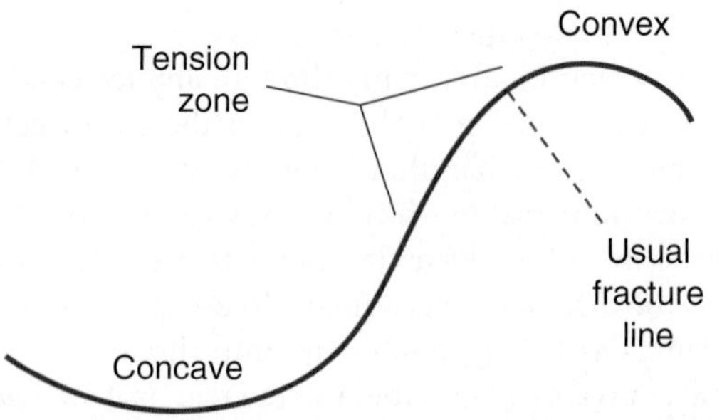

Figure 8-7 Slope profile. Dangerous slab avalanches are more likely to occur on convex slopes, but may also occur on concave slopes. Short slopes may be as dangerous as long slopes.

onto leeward slopes, which can create dangerous conditions (Figure 8-6).

When Can They Happen?

As previously stated, sustained winds of 15 miles per hour or more can increase danger rapidly. About 80% of avalanches occur during and shortly after storms. Loose, dry snow slides easily. Airborne powder avalanches travel very fast and are slowed little by minor obstacles in their path. The rushing, highly destructive snow cloud is preceded by a strong blast of air that may or may not contain snow particles.

Snowfall rates of one inch per hour or more increase avalanche danger. Small crystals comprised of needles and pellets are more dangerous than the more common, star-shaped snow crystals. Moist, dense snow settles rapidly, but during windy periods can be dangerous.

Slope location, steepness, and shape are significant factors in avalanche formation. During spring, slopes facing noon sun receive the most energy and begin to melt first, thereby increasing snow avalanche activity. Shaded slopes are more subject to dry snow avalanche activity.

Dangerous slab avalanches are more likely to occur on convex slopes, but may also occur on concave slopes. Short slopes may be as dangerous as long slopes (Figure 8-7).

Humans and animals are very effective avalanche triggers. Severe ground vibrations, such as earth tremors or explosions, are powerful avalanche starting agents. Loud noises from explosions and supersonic booms can also start snow slides.

Where Can They Happen?

Avalanches are most common on slopes of 30 to 45 degrees (60%–100%), but large avalanches occur on short or long slopes ranging from 25 to 60 degrees (Fig-ure 8-8). An avalanche need not be spectacular to kill. People have been killed by local, very small slides, including roof-top-slides.

Avalanches are very prone to recur in the same locations. Pushed-over small trees and those with limbs broken off indicate old slide paths. The nature of the slide path affects direction, speed, breadth, and density of an avalanche. Large rocks, trees, and heavy brush help anchor snow. Smooth, grassy slopes are more avalanche prone. Leeward slopes (direction toward which the wind blows) can create hollow-sounding slabs where avalanche danger is present. Windward (opposite leeward) slopes are usually strong enough to resist movement.

Old snow surface is important. Rough surfaces aid stability; smooth surfaces are unstable. A loose underlying snow layer is more dangerous than a compacted one.

What Specific Dangers Do They Represent?

While snow avalanches can occur wherever there are deep accumulations of snow on steep slopes, hazards develop only when people and property come into proximity with slide areas. The single most disastrous avalanche accident in the United States occurred in 1910 when three cars from a snowbound train were swept into a canyon in the Cascade Mountains, causing about 100 deaths.

For centuries mountain dwellers have stubbornly built and rebuilt in avalanche paths, and even added to their peril by cutting protective forests.

Catastrophic ice avalanches may descend unexpectedly from a glacier tongues long considered stable. In January 1962, in Peru, the greatest avalanche on record occurred when three million tons of ice broke from a hanging glacier near the summit of North Huascaran. Falling over 3,000 foot cliffs, ice tore out great chunks of rock and touched off a secondary avalanche as it

Avalanche Slope Angle

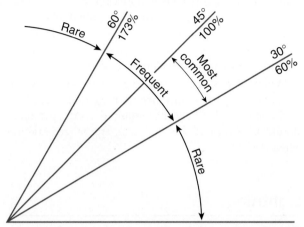

Figure 8–8 Avalanche slope angles and their effects. Avalanches are most common on slopes of 30 to 45 degrees (60%–100%), but large avalanches do occur on slopes ranging from 25 to 60 degrees. The diagram shows the slopes where avalanches are most common.

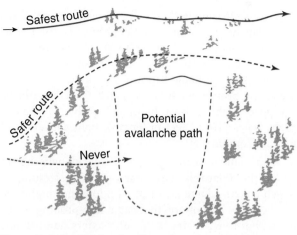

Figure 8–9 Potential avalanche path.

bombarded a lower glacier. The avalanche destroyed seven villages, killed 4,000 people and 10,000 head of livestock during its 15 minute, 10 mile journey.

Safety Procedures and Actions to Take

"Test skiing" has been adopted as a formal safety measure in major ski areas. Selected steep slopes are traversed by groups of two or more trained and experienced patrollers to release small avalanches to limit the potential for development of large avalanches, remove unstable snow for a time, and stabilize snow cover.

When test skiing fails to release snow slides, explosives are often used to check stability of slopes and release avalanches at selected times. These explosives are hand-placed or projected from a number of different types of guns.

Backcountry skiing should only be practiced in groups and when avalanche conditions are considered stable. Safest routes are in valleys far from the bottom of slopes. If dangerous slopes must be crossed, stay high and near the top, and avoid avalanche fracture lines (Figure 8–9). If it is necessary to ascend or descend a dangerous slope, proceed straight up or down and not back and forth across the slope. Snowmobiles should not cross the lower part of slopes.

People caught in an avalanche zone can immediately try to get out of the slide path or to catch hold of trees, shrubs, or other anchorages. If escape is impossible, one should try to discard skis or other impediments and "swim" in hope of staying near the surface and/or working toward edges. It may be possible to get clear of the slide path by escaping to the sides, but the chances of directly outrunning an avalanche are poor to none. Avalanche victims are usually either carried away by the slide from its starting zone or hit by the front of a developed descending avalanche. After one-half hour, a buried victim has only a 50% chance of survival, and suffocation is the principal cause of death.

Avalanche Search

Avalanche cords, around 50 feet long, are common pieces of equipment that skiers attach to their belts and let trail behind them in hopes that, should they become buried in an avalanche, the cord, or some portion of it, will come to rest on the surface. Then, rescuers can follow the cord to find the victim. The problem with the cord concept is that, although they have worked, they may not work all the time and may end up completely buried. Whether they work or not, SAR personnel must be aware that avalanche cords may be visible, and therefore useful, at an avalanche search.

The "hasty search" party of three to seven trained personnel may be a victim's best hope for survival in a regulated ski area, but a trained avalanche dog and handler also can be invaluable. In the backcountry, a victim's only hope may lie in help from companions or

> **SAFETY**
> If it is necessary to ascend or descend a dangerous slope, proceed straight up or down and not back and forth across the slope.

SARTips

onlookers. When used, the hasty search party posts an avalanche guard, forms a "scuff line" (a single row of people marching shoulder to shoulder), and then moves back and forth across the slope or up and down the fall line, probing beneath the snow with their avalanche probes. Such hasty search teams should be equipped with at least light, collapsible, avalanche probe poles (10–12 feet in length), light shovels, and first aid equipment.

An avalanche search party must decide whether to adopt the relatively fast coarse-probing technique, which covers a large area fast with low thoroughness, or the slow but more thorough fine-probing technique. For fine-probing, a line of rescuers stand shoulder to shoulder at the foot of the slide facing uphill with toes up to the guide cord. On a given command, the group drives probes vertically alongside their left toes. On further command, probes are driven alongside the right toes. The guide cord is moved forward one foot and searchers bring toes up to the new line and repeat probing. Because fine-probing is very slow, the risk of missing the victims in coarse-probing must be weighed against decreased survival chances in time needed for fine-probing. Historically, the probability of finding a subject alive after the first few hours is quite low.

The use of avalanche beacons, or transceivers, is also common around the world. When used properly, the avalanche beacon is a fast and effective method of locating buried avalanche victims. They come in older low-frequency models (2275 Hz or 2.275 kHz), newer high-frequency models (457 kHz), or a combination of the two (both high and low frequencies in one unit). However, high- and low-frequency transceivers do not transmit and receive with each other.

Avalanche beacons work in pairs: one transmitting a signal that carries about 100 feet, and another set to receive the signal of the other. In use, all members of the party keep their beacons set on transmit. Should an avalanche search be required, untrapped members of the party switch their beacons to receive and perform sweeps until they pick up the signal from the buried beacon (still set on transmit). In actual practice, the use of avalanche beacons to locate a buried victim is difficult and takes practice. Experienced and skilled practitioners can usually find a victim in a matter of minutes if they are properly equipped.

Priorities

Search techniques at present are getting better all the time and are beginning to incorporate newer, faster sensing devices, since speed is essential for survival. Knowledge can help people avoid being caught in an avalanche and it can assist in survival for those who become buried. If a person witnesses a slide, he or she should mark the last point where an individual was seen and give that information to rescuers. The Ski Patrol, local sheriff, or Forest Service should be immediately called for assistance in avalanche situations.

When SAR is necessary in cold weather, snow, and ice environments, additional training and specialized equipment will likely be required. SAR personnel should be aware of this and seek specialized training when necessary.

Lightning

This section summarizes recommendations of Lightning Safety Group of the American Meteorological Association included in their paper "Updated Recommendations for Lightning Safety-1998" as published in the *Bulletin of the American Meteorological Society*: Vol. 80, No. 10, pp. 2035–2041 (October 1999 issue). Used with permission.

Lightning is a release of light and energy produced by discharge of atmospheric electricity. This discharge may occur within a cloud, between clouds, or between cloud and ground. This last form of lightning poses the greatest threat to life and limb. On a very minor scale it is easy to produce our own lightning by walking across a rug or carpet and reaching out to touch something. The flash of light, spark, and pain that results is similar to what happens when lightning occurs.

Lightning powerful enough produces a distinct crackling, explosive sound called thunder. Thunder is sound caused by expansion of air heated by the intensity of the lightning stroke. Thunder can tell us approximately how far the lightning flash was from us. We can estimate distance in miles to the lightning by counting the number of seconds between lightning and thunder and dividing by five. For example, if we see a stroke of lightning and count to ten before hearing the thunder, the lightning flash was about two miles away.

How To Protect Yourself

Lightning causes more casualties annually in the United States than any other storm-related phenomena except floods (Figure 8-10). The seemingly random nature of thunderstorms cannot guarantee the individual or group absolute protection from lightning strikes, however, being aware of, and following proven lightning safety guidelines, can greatly reduce the risk of injury or death.

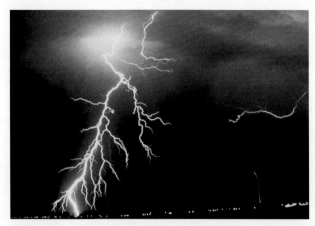

Figure 8–10 Lightning causes more casualties annually in the United States than any other storm-related phenomena except floods. Photo Courtesy NOAA National Severe Storms Laboratory (NSSL).

Safer Locations During Thunderstorms and Locations to Avoid

No place is absolutely safe from the lightning threat; however, some places are safer than others.

- Large enclosed structures (substantially constructed buildings) tend to be much safer than smaller or open structures. The risk for lightning injury depends on whether the structure incorporates lightning protection, construction materials used, and the size of the structure.

- In general, fully enclosed metal vehicles such as cars, trucks, buses, vans, fully enclosed farm vehicles, etc., with the windows rolled up provide good shelter from lightning. Avoid contact with metal or conducting surfaces outside or inside the vehicle.

- *Avoid* being in or near high places and open fields, isolated trees, unprotected gazebos, rain or picnic shelters, baseball dugouts, communications towers, flagpoles, light poles, bleachers (metal or wood), metal fences, convertibles, golf carts, and water (ocean, lakes, swimming pools, rivers, etc.).

- When inside a building, avoid using the telephone, taking a shower, washing your hands, doing dishes, or any contact with conductive surfaces with exposure to the outside such as metal door or window frames, electrical wiring, telephone wiring, cable TV wiring, plumbing, etc.

Safety Guidelines for Individuals and Groups

Generally speaking, if an individual can see lightning and/or hear thunder, he/she is already at risk. Louder or more frequent thunder indicates that lightning activity is approaching, increasing the risk for lightning injury or death. If the time delay between seeing the flash (lightning) and hearing the bang (thunder) is less than 30 seconds, the individual should be in, or seek a safer location (see above). Be aware that this method of ranging has severe limitations in part due to the difficulty of associating the proper thunder to the corresponding flash.

High winds, rainfall, and cloud cover often act as precursors to actual cloud-to-ground strikes notifying individuals to take action. Many lightning casualties occur in the beginning, as the storm approaches, because people ignore these precursors. Also, many lightning casualties occur after the perceived threat has passed. Generally, the lightning threat diminishes with time after the last sound of thunder, but may persist for more than 30 minutes. When thunderstorms are in the area but not overhead, the lightning threat exists, even when it is sunny, not raining, or when clear sky is visible.

When available, pay attention to weather warning devices such as NOAA weather radio and/or credible lightning detection systems; however, do not let this information override good common sense.

Remember, lightning is always generated and connected to a thundercloud but may strike many miles from the edge of the thunderstorm cell. Acceptable downtime (time of alert state) has to be balanced with the risk posed by lightning. Accepting responsibility for larger groups of people requires more sophistication and diligence to assure that all possibilities are considered.

An action plan or protocol must be in place and known in advance by all persons involved in a SAR mission. This plan should be conveyed to SAR field personnel in their assignment briefing.

Some Environmental SAR Challenges

It has already been established that mental and physical functions of the body are virtually inseparable. Both can impact our ability to effectively deal with the emergency environment. Although injury will be the greatest and most immediate physical concern, environmental stresses can produce equally dangerous but more subtle, insidious results.

This section is not a complete instructional manual on wilderness medicine at any level, nor is the information meant to replace field training by competent medical instructors, or to replace actual experience in treating and managing injuries and illness. It is recommended that all SAR personnel attend competent, prehospital medical training relevant to the environments in which operations are expected.

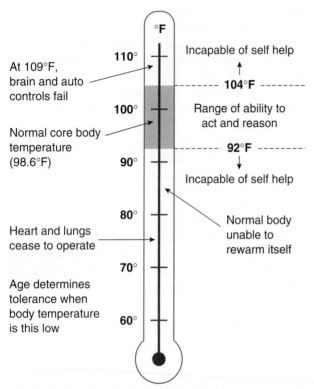

At 109°F, brain and auto controls fail

Normal core body temperature (98.6°F)

Heart and lungs cease to operate

Age determines tolerance when body temperature is this low

°F

110°

100°

90°

80°

70°

60°

Incapable of self help

‑‑‑‑‑‑ 104°F ‑‑‑‑‑‑‑‑

Range of ability to act and reason

‑‑‑‑‑‑ 92°F ‑‑‑‑‑‑‑‑

Incapable of self help

Normal body unable to rewarm itself

Figure 8–11 The normal temperature range for the human body is between 92° and 104°F.

Training in specialized prehospital medical issues should be undertaken by all SAR personnel. Several organizations specializing in this type of training offer outstanding programs in wilderness medicine and first aid.

Hypothermia

Hypothermia is defined as a medical condition or illness that is caused by the body's inner temperature being lowered so far below normal as to cause a person to become ill (**Figure 8–11**).

Hypothermia is sometimes called "exposure," although exposure is actually the method by which an individual becomes hypothermic. Hypothermia is also often called "the killer of the outdoors" because it has been established as a major cause of death among outdoor travelers. Causes of hypothermia include: falling into cold water (immersion hypothermia), traveling in cold weather while wet, alcoholic beverage consumption, drugs, improper dress, and even lack of funds for payment of utility bills (urban hypothermia). For SAR personnel and the subjects of their toil, hypothermia should be considered the most potentially important outdoor danger that is likely to be encountered.

A person can be considered hypothermic when their core temperature is found to be below 95°F (35°C). External (environmental) causes are related to the four primary ways in which heat can be transferred: radiation, conduction, evaporation, and convection (see Chapter 7 for definitions and details). Internal causes are usually related to the body's ability to produce heat required to maintain a constant body temperature. Heat is produced by movement of muscles (voluntary or involuntary), metabolism, and food. A failure or impairment in any of these systems can lead to hypothermia.

Hydration also plays a significant role in temperature regulation, as a small amount of dehydration (decrease in body water) can cause a decrease in thermal control. Dehydration occurs at a faster rate in cold and dry environments, and at elevation. Other topics that play an important part in thermoregulation include physiological control of body temperature and nutrition. These topics are not specifically addressed here, but deserve study on the part of every SAR worker.

A special "hypothermia" thermometer is required to diagnose hypothermia. Regular rectal thermometers do not register low enough. Since these are not always available, other methods of field diagnosis may be necessary.

Mild hypothermia should be handled immediately so that it does not progress into severe hypothermia, which has a much worse prognosis. A mildly hypothermic person (core temperature of 97° to 91°F) may show the following six signs:

1. Complaining of feeling cold with extremities showing "goose bumps."

2. Frequently wet from rain, snow, or other sources.

3. Usually shivering to some extent, which may become intense; this may be unapparent while walking.

4. As hypothermia progresses, the patient may develop problems with muscular coordination, most often beginning with clumsiness in detailed hand movements.

5. An inability to keep up with others in the party, later followed by stumbling and clumsiness.

6. Approaching 90°F core temperature, they may have difficulty in speaking, sluggish thinking, amnesia, or signs of depression.

Dr. William W. Forgey, in his book *Hypothermia: Death by Exposure*, suggests that a person who is unable to walk a 30-foot line properly should be presumed to be hypothermic until proven otherwise.

As hypothermia becomes severe (core temperature of 90°F and below), the following signs may become evident:

1. At lower than approximately 90°F, shivering may stop altogether.

2. Exposed skin may appear blue or swollen.

3. Unable to walk, with poor muscular coordination.

4. Confusion, incoherence, or irrational behavior. However, the patient may be able to maintain posture and appearance of psychological contact.

5. The subject may become careless about protecting him- or herself from the environment.

6. At less than 87°F core temperature, the muscles become severely rigid.

7. Semiconscious, stupor, loss of psychological contact, slow pulse and respirations as well as pupil dilation.

8. At less than 83°F core temperature, unconsciousness, heart beat and respirations are erratic, the pulse may seem absent.

9. At less than 79°F core temperature (and possibly before this level), cardiac and respiratory arrests occur.

If a subject is unable to protect him- or herself from the cold or understand the gravity of the situation, and certainly if the individual is unconscious, the core temperature is probably below 90°F and the situation should be considered an emergency. Because of hypothermia's ability to so precisely mimic death, no one should be considered dead until they are warm and dead.

Before treatment can be rendered to the hypothermic patient, mild hypothermia must be distinguished from severe hypothermia. Severe hypothermia is a medical emergency that necessitates advanced medical intervention as soon as possible. Do not try to rewarm a victim of severe hypothermia in the field. Evacuate them as soon as possible, jostling them as little as possible, and gently transport. Remove wet clothes during this procedure, but do it gently.

Mild hypothermia is treated primarily by preventing further heat loss. To do this, one must understand how heat is transferred and how to minimize these effects in the field. Remove wet clothes and replace with dry. Place the victim in a warm environment, if available (i.e., tent, near campfire, in a vehicle, in a sleeping bag with another person, etc.). Add dry insulation to the victim's clothing system. Make the person more comfortable.

Prevention of hypothermia is directed toward reducing heat loss and increasing heat production, both or either as needed. Reducing heat loss can be achieved almost entirely by appropriate dress (see sections on Clothing in Chapter 7). Proper nutrition and hydration are also important to staying warm. Beware of caffeine, alcohol, and "downer" types of drugs that may promote hypothermia. Hypothermia is much easier to prevent than treat, so know how to prevent it.

Freezing Injuries

Localized cold injuries include: frostbite, which is the general term used for frozen tissue; frostnip, a very superficial frostbite; trench foot (immersion foot), caused by exposure of tissue to wet, cold conditions; and chilblain (pernio, kibe, chimetlon), caused by the exposure of dry skin to cool or cold temperature.

Frostbite and Frostnip

Toes are most often affected by frostbite, but fingers and hands are also common sites. Frostnip occurs on the ears, the tip of the nose, and cheeks. Pain in the associated tissues is the earliest symptom of frostbite. As the tissue freezes, the pain disappears and the only symptom that may be apparent is the lack of feeling in the area. Affected tissue may turn pale or white, but usually it is not recognized because the areas are normally covered. Frostbitten tissues may also be cold and hard.

In the field, frostnip can be readily rewarmed, but a person with frostbite should be evacuated before rewarming is attempted. Rewarming frostbitten tissue and allowing it to refreeze can cause much more damage than simply leaving it frozen. The general treatment considerations for frostbite include:

1. Remove all constricting clothing to promote circulation to the injured area.

2. Do not allow a frostbite patient to walk on a frostbitten foot or to use a frostbitten hand.

3. Elevate the injured area during transport.

4. Smoking and alcohol use are strictly forbidden by frostbite patients.

Other Cold-Related Injuries

Immersion foot is a non-freezing injury that usually strikes the feet after being immersed in cold water for an extended period. It usually presents as redness of the skin that eventually leads to swelling and blisters. Numbness and pain may also be present; aspirin may help alleviate the pain. Treatment includes removing the involved area from the environment that caused the injury, rewarming it in warm water (100°–108°F), drying the area, and keeping it dry.

Chilblain is uncomfortable, but usually causes little impairment. Affected skin may be red, tender, warm, swollen, and itchy. Treatment is the same as for trench foot: remove from the cold environment and warm the area.

All cold injuries can be prevented by proper nutrition, hydration, and clothing. Never touch metal outside when the temperature is below freezing. Avoid getting organic liquids (gasoline, solvents, alcohol, etc.) on your skin in cold environments as they can immediately cause frostbite.

Heat-Related Problems

Important heat injuries for SAR workers include heat cramps, heat exhaustion, and heat stroke. It is unusual for a person to suffer only one of these maladies.

Generally, but not always, heat cramps occur before heat exhaustion and if not treated can lead to heat stroke. One is usually not stricken with just heat stroke. Heat exhaustion has probably been present, and may still be to a certain extent. It is important that these problems be recognized and treated immediately or, better yet, prevented.

Heat Cramps

Heat cramps are muscle pains which may occur when an individual exercises in environments of high humidity and temperature to the point of profuse sweating (fluid loss) and salt depletion. An otherwise healthy person may complain of sudden cramping in their lower extremities, abdomen, or both. They probably will be sweating and most likely have been working in a very warm environment. Treatment is aimed at eliminating the exposure and replenishing the lost water and salts. Immediately remove the affected person from the exposure. Salt tablets are not usually recommended, but sports-type drinks, such as Gatorade, are good. Rest, water, and electrolyte replacement usually allow for a quick recovery.

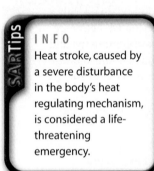

INFO

Heat stroke, caused by a severe disturbance in the body's heat regulating mechanism, is considered a life-threatening emergency.

SARTips

Heat Exhaustion

Heat exhaustion (sometimes called heat prostration) represents a somewhat more severe response to the same environment described in heat cramps, and is also related to water and salt loss. Heat cramps are a local (single area) affliction, whereas heat exhaustion is a generalized (whole body) problem. Heat exhaustion is more likely to have associated dehydration and may be first apparent by sudden unconsciousness. A person with heat exhaustion most often complains of headaches, fatigue, dizziness, nausea, and sometimes related cramping (see section on Heat Cramps). This person is usually sweating profusely and the skin is cool to the touch. This coolness of the skin is evidence of the body's evaporative heat transfer mechanism at work. The body temperature is usually normal, or slightly elevated, and the pulse may be rapid and weak. If heat exhaustion is minor and has just occurred, the treatment is the same as for heat cramps. If heat exhaustion is more severe, intravenous fluids may be required, which means advanced medical care. In the field, keep the person comfortable and cool while evacuating to advanced medical treatment (or bringing the care to the patient).

Heat Stroke

Heat stroke is caused by a severe disturbance in the body's heat regulating mechanism and is considered a life-threatening emergency. Generally, the sweating mechanism, one of the primary methods with which the body cools itself, fails in heat stroke and the body temperature increases. The temperature of the body can reach 106°F and higher within minutes. If the situation is not corrected quickly, then serious damage can occur to the vulnerable cells of the brain and central nervous system. This frequently strikes older persons, especially those with drinking problems, but it may occur at any age. When heat stroke occurs, someone has probably ignored the warning signs. The skin is hot, reddened, and dry in heat stroke, as opposed to cool and moist as in heat exhaustion. In addition, this person will probably have a strong, full pulse. A person with heat stroke may experience headache, dizziness, dry mouth, and go into a coma and have seizures. This person may be aware of the heat, but then quickly becomes confused, uncoordinated, delirious, or unconscious. The body temperature would be high, probably very high and should be treated immediately. Almost all untreated cases of heat stroke lead to brain damage and eventually death.

Treatment is aimed at lowering the body temperature as soon as possible by immersing the body in cool water, making sure not to cause shivering, or applying cold packs to pulse points until the core temperature drops to normal. Remove clothing immediately and place the patient in a cool area with low humidity, if possible. Massaging the extremities during the cooling process may help. Sprinkling or spraying cool water onto the patient while fanning is an easy way to cool a person quickly. Avoid causing shivering while cooling. A person suspected of experiencing heat stroke, even if his or her temperature is brought back into normal ranges, should be seen immediately at a medical facility.

Prevention of nearly all heat injuries can be assured by knowledge of the body and how it works in hot environments. Clothing systems appropriate for the environment must be used. The body should always be covered when in direct sunlight, and this includes the head. Generally in a hot environment the clothing should be very loose, thin, and light colored.

Solar Injuries

Sunburn
Sunburn and "snow blindness" can be problems for SAR personnel. Sunburn is a first degree burn (least severe thermal burn) that causes reddening and pain of the skin after being exposed to sunlight. Swelling might accompany the reddening, and more prolonged exposure to sunlight might cause severe pain and blistering. Chills, fever, and headache may also develop and, if the lips are sunburned, cold sores (herpes simplex) can occur. Everyone has a different sensitivity to sunlight; in general, blue-eyed redheads and blondes are more susceptible to sunburn than brunettes, and children are more susceptible than adults.

Some drugs, soaps, creams, cosmetics, and even ingestion of certain vegetables can vary one's ability to fight off the damaging rays of the sun. Ultraviolet light from the sun is the cause of sunburn and can cause burns even on cloudy days. The sun's effects can be intensified by elevation, wind, and lack of clouds; however, none of these are necessary to receive a burn. Cold, wet dressings may relieve the pain of sunburn, and soothing lotions may help discomfort. Preventing further exposure and relief of pain is the basic treatment plan. Severe sunburn that affects a large portion of the body or includes blisters should be treated as any other major burn and should not be taken lightly.

Sunburn is best prevented by wearing clothing when exposed to the sun. This should include covering for the entire body; the head, too. Some chemical preparations are available that can block the harmful rays of the sun. These must be reapplied frequently. Preference should be given to preparations that block out all of the sun's rays (those labeled SPF 30 or higher).

Snow Blindness
Snow blindness (photopthalmia) is simply sunburn of the eyes. Symptoms may not occur for many hours after the injury and at first may feel like the eyes are simply irritated and dry. Snow blindness may persist for several days. Later, the classic sensation of sand in the eyes may develop with associated pain when the eyes are moved or opened. Light alone may produce discomfort. Eyes will look red, the eyelids may swell, and excessive tearing is probable. Cool, moist coverings for the eyes might relieve some discomfort, but the condition should clear up within a few days if the eyes are allowed to rest while kept closed.

This condition can be prevented by simply having and wearing sunglasses or goggles that block no less than 91% of the damaging band of ultraviolet (UV) sunlight. Some method of preventing reflected light to enter the eyes from around the glasses must be provided (i.e., side shields, dirt on face, etc). Protection is just as important on cloudy days, and snow blindness has occurred during snowstorms. Improvised protection can be made from pieces of cardboard with small slits in them.

Altitude Related Problems
Occasionally SAR personnel are called upon to work at altitudes to which they are not accustomed. Some individuals may become ill if they travel to over 8000 feet and do not ascend slowly or take time to acclimate. The exact reasons for such illnesses are probably related to lower oxygen pressures at elevation, but no one knows for sure. At 18,000 feet elevation, there is approximately half the oxygen available than at sea level. Acute mountain sickness (AMS), high altitude pulmonary edema (HAPE), and high altitude cerebral edema (HACE) are three specific problems that can occur at elevation. SAR personnel must at least know of their existence and how to recognize them.

> **INFO**
> AMS – acute mountain sickness
> HAPE – high altitude pulmonary edema
> HACE – high altitude cerebral edema
>
> *SAR Tips*

Mountain Sickness
Mountain sickness (also called "acute mountain sickness" or AMS if sudden in onset) is not a disease, but a collection of symptoms that commonly occur to people that travel to over 8000 feet in altitude without acclimating (taking time to reach that altitude). Generally, the symptoms begin with fatigue, loss of appetite, sleepiness, weakness, apathy, headache, and sometimes nausea and vomiting. Headache is by far the most common and most irritating symptom. Headache may be blamed for the loss of sleep, but sleeplessness is another symptom of the illness. After a few days at altitude, the headache may be complicated by memory lapses, ringing in the ears, and difficulty in walking. Severe indicators include: difficulty in walking, loss of consciousness, hallucinations, HAPE, HACE (see below), and impaired judgment. If recognized immediately, treatment includes rest, fluid ingestion, and pain medication for the headaches. Sleeping aids may make the problem worse. If recovery is not quick, the patient

needs to seek medical help at a lower elevation. Evacuation to a lower elevation is the best course of treatment. Never travel to higher elevations if a member of your team has AMS symptoms.

Prevention is accomplished by attaining higher elevations slowly. First, spend time resting at lower elevations then progress higher at a slow rate. Descend at the first signs of illness. Some medications (acetazolamide and dexamethasone) may be helpful in preventing AMS when they are administered by a physician familiar with altitude problems.

High Altitude Pulmonary Edema

High altitude pulmonary edema (HAPE) is fluid in the lungs brought on by ascending to an elevation exceeding 8000 feet too rapidly. This can compromise a person's ability to breathe and, therefore, is considered dangerous and possibly lethal if not treated. Signs and symptoms include those of AMS plus coughing that produces white or red (bloody) mucus, weakness, shortness of breath, confusion, cyanosis, loud breathing sounds, and rapid heart and breathing rates. The victim of such an illness will die if not evacuated to lower elevation (less than 5000 feet) quickly.

Treatment includes evacuation to lower elevation quickly after the first signs occur. Do not allow the patient to walk down, especially alone. Prevention is assured by never traveling above 8000 feet.

High Altitude Cerebral Edema

High altitude cerebral edema (HACE) is fluid on the brain that occurs from exposure to altitude without acclimating. HACE causes progressive neurological deterioration such as change in consciousness, inability to walk a straight line, impaired judgment, hallucinations, and coma. Treatment and prevention are the same as for HAPE.

Water Deprivation

Dehydration is a condition that results from the excessive loss of body water. It is most often recognized by thirst, but thirst may be a late symptom. At elevation, thirst may be absent and water consumption must be continuous, because thirst is not always an accurate indicator of dehydration. At elevation, fatigue, weakness, and lightheadedness may be the first indicators. A person with severe dehydration will have a dry mouth and eyes, "loose" skin that stays pinched when pinched with the fingers (tenting), and may progress into unconsciousness and eventually death.

Treatment for dehydration is aimed at rest and consumption of liquids. If a person is unconscious, liquids cannot be consumed and immediate evacuation will be required. Preventing dehydration is one of the keys to health in the outdoors. Drink plenty of fluids, especially when working hard and sweating. Water needs increase at elevation and in both cold and hot climates. Push fluids at elevation and consume at least 4 liters of water per day in extremely cold or hot environments. Chapter 5, Physiology and Fitness, contains more information about hydration and health.

Blisters

Blisters are highly underrated and are the bane of SAR personnel. Blisters are fluid-filled pockets under the surface of the skin that are caused by friction against a particular part of the body (usually the feet), and are usually caused by ill-fitting footwear. They should be treated as soon as they are recognized, hopefully before the blister has completely "matured." The reddening of an area on the skin prior to becoming a full-blown blister is termed a "hot spot" and is simply red and irritated. In addition, the skin on a hot spot may feel like it moves easily over the underlying tissue.

Treatment of a hot spot is to apply some moleskin or tape over the area to decrease the friction being caused to the area. The shoes or other responsible garment should be adjusted so that friction is minimized. If a fluid-filled blister has occurred, cut a hole in the moleskin or tape the size of the blister and apply enough layers so as to keep all pressure off of the blister itself. Do not rupture the fluid-filled pocket unless travel is impossible otherwise. If a rupture is necessary, then pierce the corner of the fluid-filled sack with a sterile (or as clean as possible) needle. The puncture may become infected, so apply a topical antibiotic or wash the area with soap and water to make certain it is clean, and cover it with a bandage or gauze.

Prevention of blisters is usually accomplished by acquiring and using properly fitted footgear. Some degree of success has been attained by always wearing two pair of socks, a thin layer against the skin, and a second insulation layer with the thickness depending on the temperature. Massaging the feet at least daily promotes circulation and may decrease blisters. In addition, massaging may aid in the search for hot spots and is, at the very least, pleasurable. Chapter 7 has more information about appropriate clothing.

Snakes

Snakes have long been the stuff of nightmares but rarely a real problem for SAR personnel. Simply put, snake bite is quite rare. There are approximately 45,000 snake bites

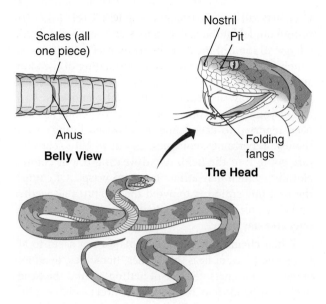

Figure 8–12 Positive identification of pit vipers (*Viperidae*).

Scales (all
one piece)

Nostril
Pit

Anus

Belly View

Folding
fangs

The Head

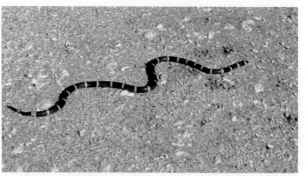

Figure 8–13 Identification of coral snake (*Elapidae*). Note that coral snakes can vary greatly in color. In the United States, however, consider any red, black, and yellow banded snake a coral snake, especially if the red band touches the yellow (or white) band.

in the United States yearly but only about 9000 bites are made by venomous snakes (**Figures 8-12** and **8-13**). Twenty to thirty percent of the bites will not have envenomation even when fang marks are present. In the end, there are only 12 to 15 deaths per year in the United States due to snake bite. To put it more plainly, one is far more likely to be injured or killed by a "domestic" animal such as a cat or dog than they are likely to be envenomated by a poisonous snake.

Following certain guidelines substantially reduces the chances of having problems with snakes and their associated bites. Never stick your arm, hand, or finger in a hole; use a stick or branch. If a snake is sighted, stay clear of it and do not back it into a corner. Avoid contact with snakes or wild animals of any kind, especially if the exact type is unknown. Any snake bite where the snake type is unknown should be considered poisonous until proven otherwise.

If bitten by a snake, retreat and identify it before it gets away. If unable to identify it, kill it with a long stick and carry it in a bag to the hospital with the patient. Seek medical attention after any snake bite. Certain treatments of bites in the field are not recommended, including incising the wound(s) and applying ice to the area.

A person who does get bitten by a snake almost always has plenty of time to get appropriate treatment. Death following significant envenomation generally takes 5 to 10 hours.

If envenomation from a poisonous snake is suspected, the affected area should be immobilized (splint extremi-

ties) and the patient should not be allowed to move about any more than necessary. Many physicians feel that oral suction should not be applied to any snake bite; ingestion of some venom can be poisonous or cause problems to the "sucker." For instance, infections around the mouth from some venom can cause severe scarring. Although there is no evidence that this will help, many experts will suggest constricting bands be placed above and below the bite. If this is done, care should be taken not to occlude arterial blood flow beyond the site (assure there is pulse distal to the site after application of band).

In summary, if a snake bite patient is simply transported directly to the nearest medical facility, no further prehospital treatment may be necessary.

Some safe practices and helpful tips when doing SAR work in snake country include:

- Do not place any part of your body in a position where it would be within striking range of a poisonous snake.
- Always watch where you put your feet. A walking stick may be used to probe areas where snakes may be hidden, such as under leaves or in rock crevices.
- Do not step over obstacles such as logs or large rocks. In snake country, the proper way to clear an obstacle is to step on top of it and checking below before moving forward.

> **INFO**
> Identification of coral snakes in the U.S.:
> *"red touch yellow, kill a fellow*
> *red touch black, venom lack."*
> Also, if every other band is yellow (or white), it's a coral snake.

SARTips

- Use caution when walking, searching close to high banks, rock ledges, rock walls, and other high places where a snake may be resting.
- Try to select a clear space in which to land when jumping across streams, ditches, etc.
- Do not sit on stumps, logs, rocks, etc. without carefully looking over and around the spot.
- Wear gloves.
- Keep your eyes and ears open.
- If you see a snake, freeze, and estimate the situation. Try not to block a snake's exit.

Insects

Stinging and biting insects can be a nuisance or even dangerous, so SAR personnel would do well to study the different insects in their area and follow some general guidelines regarding their management.

Insects most commonly confronted in field SAR situations include: honeybees, wasps, ants, caterpillars, spiders, ticks, scorpions, and beetles. There are many different types of each of these insects, many of which have specific treatments unique to the particular insect. So, if insects are a serious problem, further study will be required. For many insects stinging and biting is most often a defensive action. When their home or life is threatened, they can be provoked to attack. Therefore, avoid such provocations and you will likely avoid their potential result.

Generally, when a bite or sting is suspected (probably will be obvious) remove the patient from further exposure and apply cold to the area. If any debris is left on the skin, such as a stinger, scrape, do not pull the object from the surface. Make sure all debris is removed completely. Wash the affected area with soap and water.

If a lethal bite or sting is suspected, or if severe symptoms occur, seek medical assistance immediately. If the patient is allergic to the sting or bite, or if symptoms consistent with an allergic reaction arise, medical assistance is needed immediately. This is a medical emergency. Serious symptoms include: difficulty breathing, severe hives and/or rash, swelling in mouth or around eyes, unconsciousness, etc. When these signs and symptoms occur, no time should be wasted. Seek medical assistance immediately. Apply the specific treatment to a particular sting or bite if it is known.

Prevention of bites and stings is directed at proper dress and the use of repellents. Keep the head and neck covered in areas of high insect populations. The use of slippery materials is usually better (silk, nylon, etc.) than loose weave materials (cotton, wool, etc.). Tie clothing at wrists and ankles to prevent entry of bugs.

Use chemical repellents containing DEET (N,N-diethyl-m-toluamide) as the active ingredient. Some people are allergic to some of the ingredients in insect repellents, so watch for allergic reactions (e.g., reddening of the skin, skin irritation, etc.). Apply repellents in liquid form to the skin, spray the repellent on clothes, and keep both out of your eyes. Avon's product, Skin-so-Soft, has also been reported to keep some insects from biting. Avoid the use of perfumes, colognes, and deodorant soaps before going into the field. Avoid wearing bright colored clothing, which may attract bees and wasps. Of course, the best prevention is to avoid the creatures altogether by being able to recognize their nests and other hangouts and stay away.

When chemical insect repellents do not seem to affect some types of fleas, black flies, horseflies, deerflies, chiggers, and gnats, the use of netting around the head, neck, and hands may be the only option available. Minimizing exposure in, or simply getting out of, highly infested areas is also prudent, when possible.

Ticks

A special word on ticks: they run a close second to mosquitoes as vectors of human disease. Tick-borne illnesses pose a potential threat to anyone who works or recreates in wilderness, outdoor areas. Tick-borne disease in the United States includes: Lyme disease; Rocky Mountain spotted fever; Colorado tick fever; relapsing fever; and tularemia. The Wilderness Medical Society suggests the following for ticks:

Prevention:
- Wear protective clothing in tick-infested areas, especially long pants cinched at the ankles or tucked into boots or socks.
- Spray clothes with an insect repellent. While the standard repellent, DEET, may repel ticks, it won't kill them. A relatively new repellent, Permanone®, kills ticks upon contact and lasts for weeks on clothing and tents. It also works on mosquitoes, gnats, chiggers, and biting flies.
- Inspect all parts of the body at least twice daily for tick infestation.

Removal:
- Grasp the tick as close to the skin surface as possible with forceps, tweezers, or protected fingers. Pull with steady pressure; do not crush or squeeze the tick's head or body.
- Ineffective removal methods, such as applying kerosene, fingernail polish, isopropyl alcohol, a hot match head, or a heated piece of metal, do not affect tick detachment and may induce the tick to push deeper into the skin, salivate or regurgitate into the wound, increasing chances of infection.

- After removal, wash and disinfect the site of the bite.
- In general, prophylactic (preventive) antibiotics are not recommended.

Poisonous Plants

Poison ivy, poison sumac, and poison oak are well-known examples of plants that do not truly poison, but can be extremely irritating to the skin.

Poison ivy is a climbing vine with three serrated-edged, pointed leaves that grows in the eastern, mid-western and southern United States. In the northern and western states, poison ivy grows as a non-climbing shrub (Figure 8–14). Poison oak also has three leaves. It grows in the sandy soil of the southeast as a small shrub. In the western United States, poison oak is a very large plant that grows as a standing shrub or climbing vine. Poison sumac is a shrub or bush with two rows of 7 to 13 leaflets, and is found most commonly in the peat bogs of the northern United States and in swampy southern regions of the country.

The sap of these plants contains urushiol, a clear, sticky, oily resin that causes rashes and itching of the skin. Urushiol resin remains stable, even in dead or dried plants, and therefore is equally hazardous in the winter and summer. The resin can be carried by smoke that can be inhaled and affect the lungs if the plant is burned. Ingesting any part of the plant can cause a reaction in the oral cavity and gastrointestinal tract. Urushiol even stays stable in the necrotic blister, if it was not washed off completely, and can continue to irritate the skin and initiate new lesions.

Different people react to the resin differently, but much success can be achieved by simply washing the suspected contact areas with soap and water as quickly as possible after exposure. The rash is not contagious after the resin has been washed from the skin, but if the resin has not been completely removed from the skin or clothing, submerging the affected area in a bath can spread it to other areas of the body.

Estimates show that up to 85% of the U.S. population is allergic to urushiol and would acquire the rash on casual contact. The reaction ranges from mild to severe, and sensitivity can develop later in life. If you are allergic to poison ivy, you are also allergic to poison oak and poison sumac, and may be allergic to cashew nut shell oil, mango fruit peels, and Japanese lacquer. A person is not allergic to poison ivy the first time they touch it, but can become allergic as the skin sensitizes to the resin.

Treatment for these irritating plants includes drying (with lotions such as calamine) and itching control (by

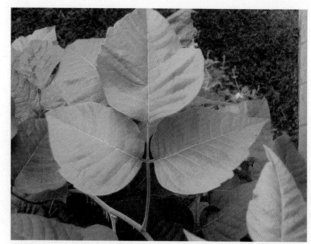

Figure 8–14 Poison ivy.

calamine and antihistamines). Alcohol, bleach, and topical steroids may do more harm than good and should not be used.

Other plants commonly found that can cause skin irritations include buttercup, daisy, mustard, radish, crown-of-thorns, milkbush, daffodil, hyacinth, dogwood, barley, prickly pear, primrose, geranium, tulip, and some nettles (stinging). Some of these actually involve hair-like projections that get caught in the skin, so mere washing does not always help. Washing with a rough towel or specific treatments may work, though. Irritations that occur from the plants listed generally should be treated as an irritation from poison ivy.

In the field, contact with these plants is usually not suspected or even considered until symptoms arise. This is the time to wash the affected area thoroughly. Learn to recognize these plants and avoid contact if at all possible.

General Considerations for Handling a SAR Casualty

In SAR work, medical help may be miles away and total medical ignorance can be dangerous or even fatal. When common sense is paired with basic knowledge of what to do, and what not to do, an acceptable outcome is possible.

Common sense is the most important component of necessary medical knowledge for SAR. Most problems arise by people not heeding warning signs or just ignoring the obvious. Heed the advice of those who know. Be prepared for the unexpected emergency. Be prepared physically, emotionally, knowledge-, and equipment-wise. Prepare for situations of risk by developing skills in less dangerous conditions. Do not tolerate horseplay in less than ideal conditions.

It is of utmost importance that the aid giver remains calm. If the rescuer panics, he/she can lose control of the situation. Acting calmly and purposefully establishes authority and reassures everyone. Do not further endanger yourself, the injured party, or others. Send for help (or more help) immediately, if necessary. You (the rescuer) are more important than your partners, your partners are more important than the victim, and the victim (injured party) is number three on the list of absolute priorities in SAR. Without you and your partners, there is no rescue, first aid, or search at all. The victim is not the last priority, just the third on a long list. The rescuer and his/her partners must have the skill, knowledge, and confidence that allow them to concentrate on the third priority: the patient. When this skill, knowledge, and confidence is lacking, the patient is not getting the care required.

Always hope for the best, but presume the worst. For instance, a victim of trauma has a broken neck until proven otherwise. Consider the worst that a problem could possibly be and treat it correspondingly. Never administer medicines or perform procedures if you are unsure of what you are doing. Never exceed your level of training. Know your limitations and do not overestimate your abilities. Follow the rule, "first, do no more harm." Seek appropriate medical advice as soon as possible.

Never move a seriously injured person(s) unless he/she is in danger from the environment or needs to be moved for medical reasons. This is usually a moot point in SAR, because SAR work is rarely required where a person is not endangered by the environment or doesn't have medical problems. Do not allow a person to "walk it off" until lack of injury has been proven.

Never approach an injured subject from above. Approach from the side or below and travel to the subject from a safe position. Debris falling (this includes rescuers) on the patient can be detrimental to his or her health.

Re-evaluate the condition of the injured party at regular intervals. A change, for better or worse, can mean a change in approach to the incident and its urgency. This information is also valuable to the definitive health care personnel that will deal with the subject. Keep a written record, if possible, of everything that occurs with regard to treatment rendered and medications given. This may serve to protect the interests of the rescuer as well as the patient. This can also be valuable to the definitive health care personnel that will deal with the patient later.

If you must remove constricting clothing or jewelry to make the patient more comfortable, have a witness and place the objects in a safe place.

SAR Terms

Acute Mountain Sickness (AMS) A collection of symptoms that commonly occur to people who travel to over 8000 feet in altitude without acclimating (taking time to reach that altitude).

Candle ice Resembles many candles bundled together and is commonly found in late winter or early spring.

Clear ice New ice formed by a long, hard freeze; considered to be the strongest ice.

Dry suits Neoprene suits that trap air against the skin to provide both warmth and buoyancy while in the water.

Frazil ice The first type of ice to form; a thin, opaque film that floats to the surface.

Frazil slush Soft collections of frazil crystals that form in moving water where a current prevents a solid freeze.

Hypothermia The condition or illness that is caused by the body's inner temperature being lowered so far below normal as to cause a person to become ill.

Layered ice Formed from many layers of frozen and refrozen snow.

PFD Personal flotation device designed to maintain the wearer's head above water.

Rotten ice Old ice that is honeycombed with pockets of air bubbles; may crumble under the slightest pressure.

Snow ice Opaque or milky-colored ice that is formed from the freezing of water-soaked snow; considered to be very weak.

References

American Meteorological Association, Lightning Safety Group. (1999). "Updated Recommendations for Lightning Safety-1998." *Bulletin of the American Meteorological Society 80,* 10, 2035–2041, October 1999.

Auerbach, P.S. (2003). *Medicine for the Outdoors,* 4th ed. Guilford, CT: The Lyons Press.

Auerbach, P.S., ed. (2001). *Wilderness Medicine,* 4th ed. St. Louis, MO: Mosby, Inc.

Auerbach, P.S., Donner, H.J., & Weiss, E.A. (1999). *Field Guide to Wilderness Medicine.* St. Louis, MO: Mosby, Inc.

Cox, M., & Fulsass, K., eds. (2003). *Mountaineering: Freedom of the Hills,* 7th ed. New York, NY: Mountaineers Books.

Forgey, W.W. (1989). *Hypothermia: Death by Exposure.* Pittsboro, IN: ICS Books.

Isaac, J. (1998). *The Outward Bound Wilderness First-Aid Handbook: Revised Edition.* Guilford, CT: The Lyons Press.

Johnson, M. (2003). *The Ultimate Desert Handbook: A Manual for Desert Hikers, Campers, and Travelers.* New York, NY: Ragged Mountain Press/McGraw Hill.

Manning, H. (1986). *Backpacking: One Step at a Time,* 4th ed. New York, NY: Vintage Books.

McManners, H. (1998). *The Complete Wilderness Training Book.* New York, NY: DK Publishing.

Petzoldt, P. (1974). *The Wilderness Handbook.* New York, NY: W.W. Norton & Company, Inc.

Rawlins, C., & Fletcher, C. (2002). *The Complete Walker IV,* revised ed. New York, NY: Alfred A. Knopf, Inc.

Schimelpfenig, T., & Lindsey, L. (2000). *NOLS Wilderness First Aid,* 3rd ed. Lander, WY: Stackpole Books.

Warrell, D., & Anderson, S., eds. (1998). *The Royal Geographical Society Expedition Medicine.* London, UK: Profile Books, Ltd.

Wilkerson, J.A., M.D., ed. (2001). *Medicine for Mountaineering,* 5th ed. Seattle, WA: Mountaineers Books.

Chapter 9

The SAR "Ready Pack" and Personal Equipment

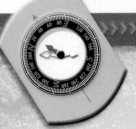

Objectives

Upon completion of this chapter and any course activities, the student will be able to meet the following objectives:

Describe the importance of having an adequate pack for SAR. (p. 128-131)

List the general contents of a 24-hour ready pack. (p. 128-130)

Describe the importance of body protection equipment. (p. 131-132)

Describe factors to consider when selecting the following equipment for use in SAR:
Ground protection. (p. 132)
Sleeping bags. (p. 132-134)
Shelters. (p. 134-135)
Water containers and systems. (p. 136-137)
Boots. (p. 137-138)
Walking/tracking sticks. (p. 138)
Flashlights/headlights. (p. 138)
Knives. (p. 139)

Packing Right

The decision regarding what equipment should be included in a SAR ready pack is mostly a personal one. However, some basic equipment is necessary if the pack is expected to meet the needs of SAR personnel. Details on some of the gear contained in the pack can be found in Chapter 11.

Carrying the appropriate equipment is an essential part of field preparedness for the SAR. SAR personnel must be responsible for their own ability to provide for personal safety and comfort in the field. SAR personnel are also expected to provide their own personal gear, clothing, and improvisational tools for use on SAR missions.

A 24-hour pack is the minimum that SAR personnel should carry during a mission (Figure 9–1). Its contents allow SAR personnel to be self reliant and comfortable for a period of time should a bivouac become necessary. If a subject is encountered, the contents can also be used by SAR personnel to assist until further help can be procured.

The 24-hour pack can be supplemented for longer missions. Appropriately, the supplemented packs are called "48-" and "72-hour" packs. In many regions where field SAR work can take personnel far from the safety and comfort of camps, 48- or 72-hour packs are minimum requirements. "Ready pack" is the generic term for any 24-, 48-, or 72-hour pack.

The contents of a ready pack can vary greatly from one area to another. Generally, however, certain components should be considered standard. Every ready pack should supply at least the following, which are explained in detail later in this chapter:

1. Equipment adequate to meet medical and survival needs for the individual SAR operator

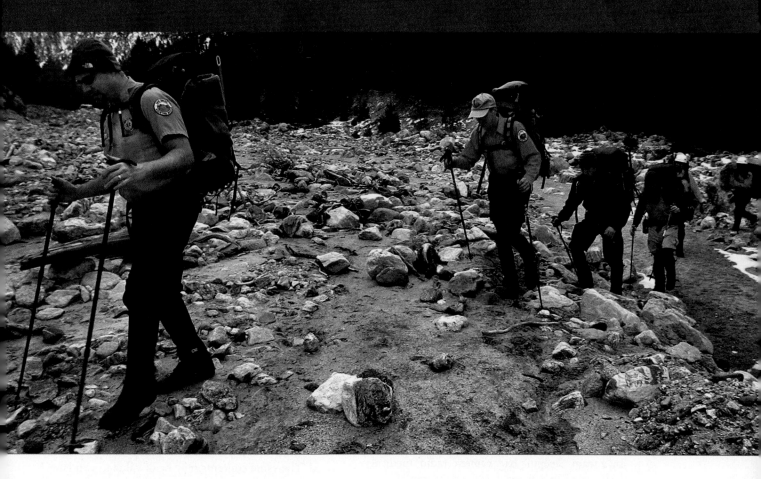

A small combination personal first aid survival kit should be part of any ready pack. Included should be small bandages, dressing, and material for cleansing small wounds as well as material that can be used to treat specific common wounds and illnesses such as blisters, headaches, indigestion, and splinters. Treating injuries and illnesses before they become bigger problems should be a goal.

2. Additional clothing appropriate for anticipated environment to supplement what is worn

   When deciding what is appropriate, consider that it WILL rain, it WILL snow, and it WILL be cold. Preparing for these potential problems can prevent an error in omission. In desert environments, do not think that it can't get cold as well as hot. At the very least, extra socks, gloves, and a hat should always be carried.

3. Bivouac or shelter material

   Something that can be used to protect SAR personnel or the subject from the environment (i.e., tarp, plastic, etc.) is useful as shelter. Tents can be adequate, but other material may be lighter, cheaper, and better suited for improvisation.

4. Water and food appropriate for mission duration plus "bivy" supply

Always carry more water than you expect to need. For extended field encounters, variance may be required from standard practice. For instance, water purification gear may be necessary rather than carrying large quantities of water (water is very heavy to carry).

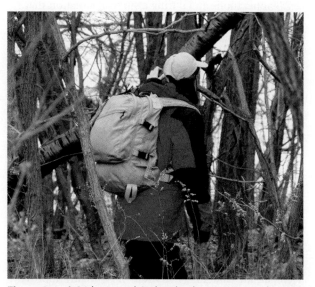

Figure 9–1 A 24-hour pack is the absolute minimum that SAR personnel should carry during a mission.

Generally, food should not be "meal" type; it should be of a type that can be eaten continuously to maintain strength and energy, rather than that which requires special preparation and a "meal" period. Food should be nonperishable and nutritionally sound. Candy may be nice for snacking, but it does not supply needed nutrients. Foods that are high in salt or caffeine should be avoided, and alcohol, tobacco, and recreational drugs should be prohibited.

5. Personal safety and comfort gear
   Flashlight, whistle, goggles, tissue, towelette, sunglasses, sunscreen, bug repellent, bandana, etc.

6. General SAR equipment (as required for situation)
   Flagging tape, compass, paper/pencil, personal ID, tracking stick, etc., should be included.

7. Improvisational tools
   Wire, twine, rope, tarp, leaf bag(s), knife, razor blade, safety pin(s), etc., should be included.

8. Team equipment (optional)
   This is defined as equipment that may not be required by an individual, but may be needed by a team. Sleeping bag, camera, radio, medical gear, string line, map(s), etc., are examples.

9. The pack itself
   A fanny or day pack works best, but a larger backpack may be required, particularly in harsh environments.

10. Inducement to drink hot/cold liquids
    Consumption of fluids is so important in SAR operations and during a survival situation that the additional weight and bother of carrying something that would make drinking water enjoyable is justified. Lack of fluids (dehydration) has been implicated in so many deaths and injuries that anything that might promote fluid consumption is encouraged. Examples include powdered drink mixes, tea bags, instant coffee, and bouillon cubes. The user of these products, however, should realize the effects that the contents might have. For example, coffee and tea contain caffeine, Gatorade® mix contains valuable electrolytes, but sweet drink mixes usually do not, etc.

The specific recommended contents of a ready pack (see Appendix 6) should be carefully chosen to supply the general needs of both the user and the mission. Here, all kit contents have been chosen with improvisation in mind. All pieces can be improvised in at least two ways, and most in many more.

Since the ready pack is meant to be carried at all times by SAR personnel, weight was also a consideration. Many pieces of equipment that were borderline (that is, questionable as to their value in such a pack) were deleted from the list in favor of lightness. Improvisation is more thought-reliant than it is equipment-reliant, so, even without some gear, SAR personnel should have the ability to meet any challenge.

Expert Advice

The following advice from experienced outdoor and SAR instructors relates directly to carrying equipment in the field.

Keep the Pack With You No matter what gear is collected and transported to the SAR mission site, it is all worthless if it is not where it's needed. Since there is not always warning before survival or improvisational skills are required, the ready pack needs to be with you all the time. Never set it down to go do something. Always have the pack with you. Do not respond to an incident without a ready pack (whether working in the field or not). Make it a habit to carry your ready pack with you everywhere.

Do Not Share When you are in the field or at a mission site, your ready pack is your home. Do not offer ready pack contents to others unless they are in dire need. The same contents may be of value to you later.

Care for Your Ready Pack Take care of your pack and its contents and give it the respect you would give any object that has the power to save, or maintain, your life. Just as food and water deserve proper storage and care, so does your ready pack. Just as you take care of rescue equipment, take care of your ready pack. Never leave your ready pack unattended. Review the contents often and maintain the contents required.

Hydration Water often is carried more comfortably on a belt around the waist or in a "hands-free" hydration system with a bladder or reservoir secured in the pack and a watering tube extending outside of the pack. These methods allow easy access so that water is consumed more often. Too often SAR personnel pack away water and drink only at breaks. This can be dangerous, especially at altitude and in hot environments. Water needs to be consumed continuously during a mission and, if the water is packed away, the searcher is less likely to stay hydrated.

At nearly 8.5 pounds per gallon, water is probably the heaviest material that will be carried. Carrying water properly—on the waist or tight against the back—more evenly distributes the weight, making it easier to carry.

Keep drinking water systems full. Water systems that are not full tend to shift in the pack, making travel more uncomfortable and difficult. However, water containers carried on the belt can shift and still be carried comfortably. If using hands-free hydration systems, always carry the bladder inside the pack, close to the searcher's back, aligned vertically with the spine to prevent spillage. An important consideration is the use of the cover to protect the water system. Bladders alone are not very durable and can rupture easily. This brings up another important point: always carry at least two different water sources in the unlikely event one does rupture.

Equipment Accessibility Several items included on the equipment list should be accessible to SAR personnel continuously, without having to unpack the ready pack. These items are termed "pocket items" and should be carried in an accessible pocket rather than in the pack itself. The decision to make a piece of equipment a pocket item is based on the item's frequency of use, size, and importance. Carrying some items in a pocket also allow more room in the pack or allow for a smaller pack.

Suggested pocket items include, but are not limited to: paper and pencil (not pen), compass, bandana or handkerchief, whistle (on lanyard attached to pack), tissue, watch (on wrist), water (on belt or tube/straw access), and a personal first aid kit. Some items may be considered pocket items, depending on the circumstances and situation. They include: flashlight (near dusk and at night), trail food (to munch on while traveling), sunglasses, sunscreen (where required), insect repellent (where required), knife, map, etc.

Research Contents The decision of what to purchase for inclusion in your ready pack should not be made hastily. Research all equipment thoroughly before purchasing anything. Ask experienced SAR personnel their opinions and find out what has worked for others in different conditions. Get details on the equipment in which you are interested and compare them to similar equipment for quality, durability, and applicability to the SAR field. Equipment suitable for a specific type of outdoor environment may be entirely unsuitable for SAR work (i.e., a ski jacket may get torn to pieces in SAR work, etc.).

Equipment doesn't necessarily have to be expensive to be ideal for SAR work. In many cases a military surplus garment or piece of equipment may be better than, or just as effective as, an expensive name-brand item. That said, consider purchases of SAR equipment as life-safety items. They are an investment and must protect and provide comfort against the elements. Most name-brand technical gear has a lifetime warranty and has stood the test of time.

Take your time and find out what is best for you and your needs before spending a great deal of money. You might be surprised how inexpensive it can be to save someone's life.

Mission Readiness Know what is in your ready pack and have it mission ready. Go through your pack and inventory the contents often. This keeps you familiar with the contents and helps identify problems before they make it into the field.

Keep your pack ready for the next mission by collecting and storing as much of the gear as possible together. Better yet, keep everything in the pack, ready to go, and simply check it often for completeness and serviceability. Food, water, and all perishables can be added at callout. A separate bag can be added to the core equipment to supplement the clothing portion as necessary in different seasons and for different environments.

> **INFO**
> The bottom line is: Know what you have and always have it ready to go.

> SARTips

Personal Body Management and Protective Equipment

Several items may be required in a wilderness area to minimize distractions and improve safety and comfort.

Insect Repellent

- A non-chemical approach to repelling insects includes wearing clothing made of slippery material such as silk and nylon. Additionally, avoid loose weave clothes that use materials such as cotton and wool when insects are a problem. Tying clothing at the wrists and ankles also aids in discouraging insects.

- Insect repellents that contain DEET, Indlone, Rutgers, and DMP have been effective, but beware of reactions and allergies. Stop using them if problems arise. Studies have shown that DEET is still the most protective repellent, although it's not necessary to use products that contain more than 35% DEET.

- Skin-So-Soft®, an Avon product, has been reported to reduce insect attacks and it smells much better than most other repellents.

- Avoid the use of perfumes and deodorant soaps before going into the field.

- Netting may be required to repel some insects such as gnats, fleas, black flies, horse flies, deer flies, and chiggers.

Sunscreen/Block

- Creams and balms may be of value in preventing chapped body parts; however, weigh any disadvantages regarding insects (due to sweet smell) before bathing in it.

- Sunscreen/block can save much discomfort in terms of pain from sunburn. At altitude the sun may not even feel hot, but its rays are burning your skin faster than at sea level. Look for blocks/screen with PABA or similar sun-blocking ingredients.

Eye Protection

- When working in brush (especially at night), it is advisable to wear protective goggles. These need not be heavy, and they should allow for ventilation around your eyes.
- When traveling in hot, sunny areas or at elevation, sunglasses should be worn to prevent eye injuries (snow blindness, etc.). Dark ski goggles that reflect 100% of UV light should be worn when traveling at high elevation in snow conditions.

Head Protection

- A helmet may need to be worn during rescue operations where injury is likely to the head. A hat that provides ear and neck protection is also important in cold environments.

Sleeping Systems

Sleeping during a SAR mission may be required on occasion, so information regarding what equipment is necessary is provided.

Ground Protection

- A pad placed between your body and the ground can serve two purposes: it can insulate you from the ground and provide a more comfortable sleeping surface. Both are good reasons to carry a lightweight sleeping pad.
- Ideally, insulating pads should be lightweight, soft, compact, waterproof, and efficient insulators. The traditional air mattress is relatively heavy, is not durable, and is least efficient among common sleeping pads because heat is lost through convection by the movement of the air inside the mattress.
- Urethane foam is soft and provides good insulation when dry. It is an open-cell structure and will absorb water (like a sponge), so a waterproof cover is generally used. Urethane foam is lighter than an air mattress, but bulkier.
- Ensolite or polyethylene is a closed-cell structure that does not provide as much padding as urethane; however, it does not absorb water, is more compact, and lighter than foam.

- A nylon cloth upon which to place your sleeping pad or tent provides an additional barrier between you and the ground, and will help to keep your tent, sleeping pad, sleeping bag, etc., clean and dry. Additionally, a ground cloth can be used as an improvisational item for things such as a shelter. It also reduces wear to other, more expensive items.
- Tree boughs or trash bags filled with leaves can be used, but they should only be considered an improvisational replacement for the real thing. A commercially made pad offers far more in terms of insulation and comfort.

Sleeping Bag

Full consideration must be given to the intended usage of a sleeping bag. Questions to ask include (Figure 9–2):

1. What type of camping will the bag be used for: backpacking, car camping, horse packing, or mountaineering?
2. What seasons will the bag be used?
3. What are the general warmth characteristics of the individual who will use the bag?

Insulating Material

The insulating material affects the cost, warmth, weight, and construction method. Selected specific materials are discussed in depth in Chapter 7 in the section on clothing.

Down Down is the fine insulating, fluffy feathers found under the stiffer feathers of ducks and geese. Its natural function as an insulator has made it the standard insulating material for lightweight sleeping bags. The primary reasons for its popularity are its light weight and compressibility for a given amount of insulation. Down is also soft, nontoxic, breathable, and resilient. On the negative side, down is expensive and loses its insulation when wet. In addition, down bags require special care in use and cleaning.

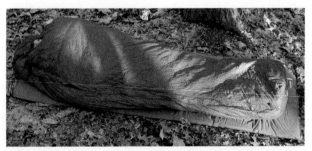

Figure 9–2 What type of camping will it be used for, in what seasons will it be used, and the general warmth characteristics of the individual using are all important questions to ask when choosing a sleeping bag.

Polyester Polyesters are synthetic fibers used as insulation in less expensive sleeping bags. Polyester has less loft, is heavier, and more bulky than down, but its fibers are water resistant, retain insulative properties when wet, and are relatively inexpensive. Many modified polyester fibers are on the market today including, but not limited to, PolarGuard™, Primaloft®, Dacron®, Hollofil®, and Quallofil®.

Construction Sleeping bags are compared generally by their quality of construction, their loft, and effective temperature range.

Quality of construction is determined primarily by the reputation of the manufacturer. A reputable manufacturer will stand behind its products, offering repair or replacement of damaged items.

Loft is generally used to specify the total thickness of a sleeping bag after it has had time to fluff up to its full thickness. Some manufacturers use it to specify the thickness of one wall. The criteria for determining loft should be determined for each product before a comparison is made so that the thickness of the actual insulating layer can be determined and compared.

Shapes and Sizes

- The rectangular bag is the roomiest. It is generally the least expensive construction, but is heavy and its roominess creates superfluous air space to heat. The additional material can make this style of bag too heavy, but the extra room makes it far more comfortable.
- The mummy bag is contoured to the body shape. It is the lightest, warmest, and most efficient design, but allows very little room for moving around inside. Mummy bags have a hood closure and the foot area is usually enlarged for comfort.
- The wedge shape is actually a tapered rectangle, with or without a hood.
- The modified mummy is barrel-shaped, and is widest at the midsection.

Construction Methods

The basic principle is to create a uniform loft throughout the bag to eliminate thin or cold spots.

1. Fiberfill is produced in battings and is sewn into sleeping bags in sheets, with some variations.
2. Down and some synthetic materials are subject to matting and shifting, so a method of baffling is necessary to control the filling to create a uniform loft.
3. The channel block (side-block baffle) is a longitudinal baffle in bags that extends the length of the bag on the side opposite the zipper to prevent down from shifting around the circumference of the bag.

4. The zipper baffle (draft tube) is an insulation-filled tube that extends the length of the bag on the inside of the zipper. Its purpose is to prevent heat loss through the zipper.
5. The use of heavy-duty nylon or non-corrosive synthetic zippers has eliminated much of the problems encountered with earlier metal zippers (snagging, breakage, freezing, and the danger of skin-to-metal contact in extreme cold). The full-length zipper is most popular and versatile, especially if it has a double tab to allow it to be opened from either end for ventilation.
6. The shells of nearly all sleeping bags are now made of nylon. It is strong, breathable, wind resistant, and light weight. Specifically:
   - Taffeta nylon is a flat weave fabric with a softer, more comfortable texture and a higher thread count than ripstop nylon.
   - Ripstop nylon has the same strength as taffeta, but has extra heavy threads every 3/16 inch to 1/4 inch that prevent tears from running, making ripstop more durable than taffeta. (See Figure 7-3, p. 90.)
   - Cotton shells are still used in some rectangular bags where weight and water considerations are not as important.

Baffling

Sleeping bag manufacturers want to construct sleeping bags to provide complete and uniform loft and insulation coverage to prevent thin or cold spots. Insulative materials, be it down or polyester fill, need to be managed in smaller tubes or "baffles" to maintain this uniform loft and coverage. There are a couple different types of construction used today in sleeping bags.

Quilted The least expensive is known as quilted, or "sewn-through" (**Figure 9–3**). This type of construction is the lowest quality. The outer layers of fabric are sewn together to create the baffles resulting in cold spots along the seams.

Box (Box Baffle or Square Box) Another fairly common type of construction is called the box baffle or square box (**Figure 9–4**). In this type of insulation, additional material is sewn between the outer layers to

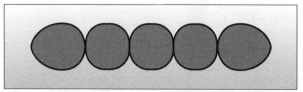

Figure 9–3 An example of quilted (sewn-through) baffle design in cross section.

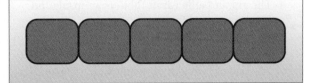
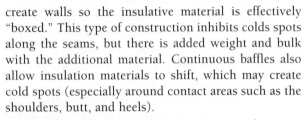

Figure 9–4 An example of box (box baffle or square box) baffle design in cross section.

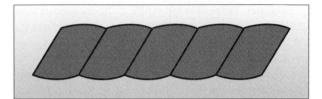

Figure 9–5 An example of shingle construction baffle design in cross section.

create walls so the insulative material is effectively "boxed." This type of construction inhibits colds spots along the seams, but there is added weight and bulk with the additional material. Continuous baffles also allow insulation materials to shift, which may create cold spots (especially around contact areas such as the shoulders, butt, and heels).

Shingle Construction The most common design in backpacking three- to four-season sleeping bags is the "shingle construction" (Figure 9–5). This particular design has slanted, overlapping layers of insulation that ensure no dead spots or areas with no insulation. Although a bit heavier and bulkier than recreational bags, it will provide essential protection from the elements.

Care of Sleeping Bags

Clean the bag when it gets dirty, but make sure to follow the manufacturer's instructions when doing so. Generally, do not wash sleeping bags in standard washing machines with central agitators, use detergents, or roughly handle a water-soaked bag. Generally, sleeping bags should be stored unstuffed, but again, it is important to follow the manufacturer's instructions for storage.

Ways to Sleep Warmer Inside a Sleeping Bag

- Sleep inside a shelter or tent (~10°F warmer)
- No tent? Improvise a windbreak.
- Do not set up camp in a ravine or valley bottom; it is warmer downwind just below peaks at higher elevations.
- Sleep in one layer of dry clothing in a good bag.
  - Protect the head, neck, shoulders, and wear a wool stocking hat.
  - Huddle with others for warmth.
  - Cold feet? Put on socks, booties.
  - Improve ground insulation.
  - Keep your sleeping bag dry
  - Use a vapor barrier in extreme cold.

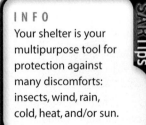

INFO
Your shelter is your multipurpose tool for protection against many discomforts: insects, wind, rain, cold, heat, and/or sun.

Shelters

Tarps are lightweight and versatile. Those made from coated nylon with a number of ties allow a variety of ways to rig a shelter. Plastic tarps are inexpensive, but are less durable and there is a tendency to leave torn plastic behind. Pitched properly, tarps can provide considerable water and wind protection. Their biggest disadvantage is their lack of complete insect protection.

Tents are generally heavier than tarps and relatively expensive, but provide the maximum in security. The features to be considered in selecting a tent include:

- In most applications warmth is a secondary consideration. However, where it is important (winter camping), tent warmth is a function of size, fabric, and design. Given the same design, a smaller tent will be warmer than a large one. A double-walled tent will be warmer because of the insulation value of the air space enclosed between the walls.
- Water repellency is provided either by using a waterproof tent fabric or a waterproof rain fly over a non-coated nylon tent. The waterproof fabric will not allow water vapor from breathing and insensible perspiration to pass through; the vapor condenses on the walls. In cold weather, the condensation freezes on the tent walls and "snows" on the occupants when the walls are touched or moved by the wind. The tent-rain fly combination is versatile and provides an insulation layer to reduce inside condensation and increase warmth. The disadvantage of this combination is the total weight involved.
- Weight is a function of fabric, size, and pole design. As much as 50% of a tent's weight can be concentrated in the pole system. Total weight must consider the basic tent, rain fly, poles, pegs, guy lines, and carrying sack.
- Size is usually determined by personal preference, based on the intended use of the tent. Backpacking tents are frequently tapered both in length and height, and have a simple pole system, all to reduce weight. At the other extreme, mountaineering expedition tents are generally much larger to allow for more comfortable living and gear storage

during extended stormy periods. Tunnel, dome, and wedge-shaped tents can provide up to 50% additional living space than A-frame tents with the same floor dimensions.

- One of the primary functions of a tent is insect protection. Most tents have a layer of mesh fabric sewn over the inside of each tent opening to provide insect protection while allowing for ventilation by tying back the main flaps of the tent.

- Considerations for tent fabrics include water repellency, breathability, wear resistance, weight, and wind resistance. The primary tent fabrics are cotton and nylon. The most popular fabric is ripstop or a similar weave nylon with a coated nylon rain fly.

- Pole design is a function of basic tent design. Some smaller tents are designed to use a pack frame or tree for support. Others use a single pole in the center or at the ends. A more stable A-frame design utilizes two poles at each end. The most complex design uses a system of exterior poles to which the tent is attached. However, the more complex the system, the more dependent is the system on each piece of the frame; the loss of one piece renders the whole frame useless. Single-piece poles are lighter than comparable multi-piece poles.

Food and Water

Because of the almost infinite variety of foods available, it can be very frustrating to plan a menu for SAR operations when you have to pack meals into the field. Your choices vary from simple add-hot-water meals to gourmet cooking, but one fact remains: most novices bring two to three times as much food as they need. While it may be impossible to starve over the three or four days of a SAR incident, food is necessary to maintain comfort and energy for demanding operations. If food is required, consider the weight and space the food will take before packing.

Table 9–1 shows a meal preparation strategy used by experienced outdoors people and SAR personnel. Realizing that large meals are not advocated during daily operations in the field and that light snacks will generally be used during SAR activities, dinner may be the only substantial meal of the day. One-pot meals are a quick and easy method of preparing a well-balanced dinner meal for the day. One-pot meals should be designed to consist of carbohydrates, protein, and seasonings/sauce. Carbohydrates and fats are important for quick and lasting energy. The process is simple and easy to prepare and helps to insure a more balanced meal.

Table 9–1	A "one-pot meal" is prepared by choosing one item from each of the three columns and combining/cooking them together.	
Carbohydrates	**Proteins**	**Seasonings/Sauces**
Minute rice	Canned tuna, shrimp, or meat	Tomato flakes/add water-type of powdered sauces
Instant potatoes	Chicken, salmon	Salt, pepper
Macaroni	Spam, corned beef	Onion or garlic salt
Spaghetti	Canned roast beef in gravy	Cloves or cinnamon
Noodles	Cheese	Gravy mixes
Top Ramen™	Meat or bacon bar	Cheese sauce mix
Kraft™ dinners	Bacon bits	Parsley flakes
Lipton™ dinners	Beef stick, pepperoni	Bouillon cubes
Tuna Helper®	Salami, thuringer	Sour cream sauce
Rice-a-Roni™	Freeze-dried meats	Vegetable flakes
Cup-a-Noodles®	Margarine, butter	Powdered milk
Dehydrated soups	Tuna casserole	Dried parsley, onion, and/or green pepper

Mess Kit and Utensils

A bowl, cup, and spoon are the only eating utensils needed. Meals are eaten one course at a time, so the same bowl may be used for an entire meal. Look for a one-quart heavy plastic bowl-shaped container with a handle and lid. Many shapes and sizes are available. This item is your cup, bowl, and plate.

Plastic bowls and cups will hold heat longer than metal and won't burn your lips when hot. Metal bowls and cups are easier to clean.

Aluminum cooking pots that stack inside each other make good use of space. A Teflon-coated frying pan is also handy, if you have the luxury of carrying one. Pack all cooking utensils in a cloth bag to prevent soot from rubbing off. Serving spoons, plastic spatula, and metal pot grips will complete the items needed.

Stoves

A good mountaineering/backcountry stove should have a low profile with a wide base for added stability. The top of the stove should be wide enough to provide a good base for a cooking pot. The main danger in stove operation is in overheating the fuel. For maximum safety, follow the manufacturer's operating instructions, and make sure to get a proper safety and operating briefing from the dealer.

Types of Stoves

A chemical fire (Sterno, Heat Tabs, Canned Heat) has a restricted heat output and is heavy for the amount of heat produced. They are adequate for heating a cup of tea or soup on the trail, but inadequate for cooking a full meal.

Alcohol stoves are simple to operate, lightweight, and easy starting. However, they have relatively low heat output and the fuel may be hard to purchase.

Other liquid fuel stoves usually burn white gasoline or kerosene, and some burn both. They have a high and controllable heat output, but require priming to start and special precautions in handling.

White gasoline is widely used and generally available, but is extremely volatile (Class I flammable liquid). It is especially dangerous when fumes are allowed to collect in an enclosed space, for example, when refueling a stove in a tent.

Coleman® fuel, or similar liquid fuels, can be used in stoves that burn white gasoline. It is less volatile and tends to burn cleaner and there is less stove clogging. In addition, Coleman® fuel is more widely available than white gasoline.

Kerosene is much less volatile than other liquid fuels; however, it requires a separate priming fuel (usually alcohol), has a distinctive and bothersome odor, and burns with a dirty, sooty residue, especially if the stove is not in top condition.

In extreme cold, precautions must be taken to avoid spilling any liquid fuel on the skin. Most types of liquid fuel do not freeze but will remain liquid down to very low temperatures. This extreme cold combined with the evaporative cooling effect can cause instant frostbite.

Gas cartridge stoves use liquefied gases (such as butane or propane) under pressure in sealed canisters. As the canister's pressure is released, the enclosed liquid boils, releasing the flammable gas. The lower the temperature and the less liquid in the canister, the lower the pressure and amount of gas produced. In comparison to other commercially available camp stove fuels, these liquefied gas cartridges are the most expensive per unit of heat. However, they do offer extreme convenience, simple stove valve operation, and they require no priming.

It is important to note that there are two ways manufacturers liquefy the fuels in these gas cartridges: high pressure and/or low temperature. The manufacturers of these types of products exclusively use pressure to liquefy their products, but temperature can also come into play when the canister is stored below the boiling point of its contents. If the contents are released at or just below its boiling point, very little or no flammable gas is produced. Since butane boils at 10°F and propane boils at −45°F, the ability of these canisters to produce flammable gases can be substantially reduced in cold temperatures. Propane is more efficient as a fuel because it works at lower temperatures. However, it also takes more pressure to liquefy because of its lower boiling point. So, the canisters in which it is contained must be stronger and, therefore, heavier—a distinct disadvantage when the canister must be carried.

A modern camping stove, like any other mechanical device, can malfunction. Often this happens at a very inappropriate time. The stove's chief enemy is the wind and the operator's impatience. When problems arise, take your time to identify possible causes before pouring on more fuel to preheat the generator.

Always carry the recommended tools and repair kit for your particular stove. Generally, your preventative maintenance and use of the proper fuels will help to reduce camp stove frustrations.

Water Bottles and Hydration Systems

Water containers come in many sizes and shapes, but the best have certain characteristics in common. They are light, durable, strong, and have a wide mouth.

Weight is always a factor, but keep in mind that the container must be able to withstand the rigors of SAR work. This means that it must be able to take a beating and not become ruptured, bent, or punctured. Plastic usually supplies this best, especially if it is a type of plas-

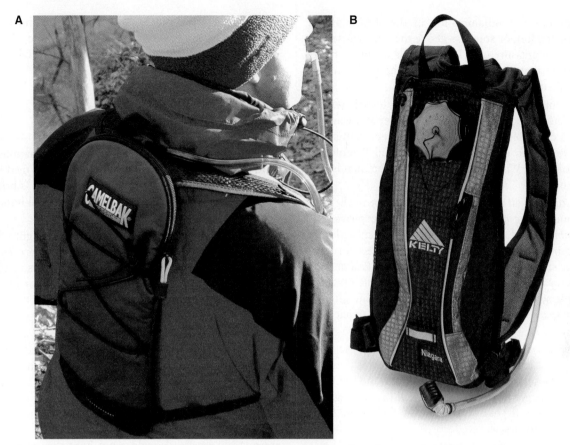

A

B

Figure 9–6 A hydration system can be integrated into varying sizes of packs or it can be worn alone. Either way, the easy access to water while moving is well suited for SAR field work. (A) Courtesy of T. P. Mier. (B) Kelty Niagara Hydration Pack courtesy of CMC Rescue, Inc.

tic that can withstand the contents freezing without breaking. Ask about this when purchasing one.

Some water carrying devices integrate with, or can be carried as, one's backpack (Figure 9–6). These allow the wearer to constantly drink from a tube that wraps over the shoulder and are sometimes referred to as "hydration systems." In their simplest form, they are made of two parts: a thin profile plastic bag of water—usually 2 liters or so—that can be carried comfortably on the back, and a tube (with a special "bite" valve on the end) from which water can be sucked while the device is being worn. The system can be integrated into varying sizes of packs or it can be worn alone. Either way, the easy access to water while moving is well suited for SAR field work. Note that because the tube is exposed to the environment, it may require special attention in very cold weather to prevent it from freezing.

Carrying one or two wide mouth bottles is also a good idea. They can be filled easily, flavorings and electrolyte powders can be added with less spillage, they lend themselves to easier cleaning, and snow is also easier to pack in for melting.

Boots

Tennis shoes and thin, leather-soled footgear are extremely hard on the feet in hilly and mountainous terrain. The foot bones and ligaments are not conditioned to the type of bending and stretching experienced by SAR personnel who wear these types of footgear and only occasionally get into the outdoors.

Boots should be adequate for their intended usage. They should provide good ankle support and have non-slip soles. The manufacturer's recommendations should be followed on methods and materials for waterproofing and cleaning.

Working in cliffs, and high-angle terrain requires tight fitting, stiff-soled boots. Hiking requires a lighter, more flexible boot.

Generally, avoid boots that reach higher than the ankle because ventilation to the feet may be hindered and ankle movement restricted. The use of a good pair of gaiters with lower cut boots may be better than high-topped boots.

Also, avoid boots with tight fitting "scree collars" because most of these collars ultimately cause a degree of tendonitis (an inflammation of the sheath of the Achilles' tendon, or soreness above the heel, caused by continuous pressure over long periods of time). Boots with backs that slope forward above the heel can also cause this injury.

Boots must fit properly. Boots that fit loosely will be better ventilated, will keep your feet drier and warmer, and will cause less "hot spots" and blisters than snug-fitting boots. To ensure a proper fit, Paul Petzoldt in his book, *The Wilderness Handbook* recommends the following:

> . . . *take off all socks, place the bare foot in the boot without lacing it, and push the foot as far forward as possible. Stand with full weight on the feet, with toes touching the end of the boot, and bend knees forward. There should be enough room between the heel and the back of the boot to insert a finger without pressure. People who wear larger sizes should allow slightly more space . . . from 5/8 inch for size seven to one inch for size 12.*

Now put on the socks that you will wear in the field, lace the boot comfortably, and stand. If there is pressure that stretches the boot outward, the boot is too tight and you need a larger width. Kick the toe of the boot against a solid surface. If your toes touch the end of the boot, you need a larger size.

Map and Compass

The specifics of what to look for, how to use a map and compass, and definitions of map and compass terms are covered in Chapter 10 (Navigation).

Walking Stick

A walking stick can be helpful when carrying a heavy pack over a long distance. It can help hold you up as well as offer assistance in probing those holes where snakes may lurk.

Chapter 13 (Tracking) discusses a common use of a walking stick for SAR: sign-cutting or tracking. A walking stick can do double duty and help substantially with tracking.

You can also improvise with a walking stick. It can serve as anything from a tent pole to a weapon or "motivator".

Weight is a factor and so is bulk, so avoid those logs that could as easily serve as a telephone pole and use one that is easily packed but can support your body weight.

Headlamp/Flashlight

A flashlight can be invaluable in certain situations in SAR work. SAR fieldwork usually demands a medium-brightness beam that is longer burning than it is bright. In most field situations, a little light for several hours is better than a bright light for a few minutes.

Don't become absolutely dependent on a light when working in the field. Many times, if you let your eyes adjust to the darkness enough ambient light exists to allow you to work quite safely. Save the flashlight for finding the toilet paper and other important uses. Don't waste it when you do not need it.

Always carry extra batteries and bulbs, and a second complete light source is not a bad idea. If you decide to carry more than one flashlight, it is recommended that the parts be interchangeable. Many different sizes and types of flashlights may be useful, but avoid large heavy "car battery" or "law enforcement" type lights. They are heavy, use many batteries, and are bulky to carry. Additionally, the white-hot light they give off is far better for starting fires or signaling the moon than it is for SAR work.

Hand lanterns are fine for most outdoor work, but a headlamp can be invaluable for night SAR work. It keeps your hands free to pursue other interests and it always points where you are looking. Bright, white light emitting diodes (LED) devices are now available that can remain lit for hundreds of hours using just one or two small batteries. Some of these are ultra small and can be used as a headlamp (**Figure 9–7**).

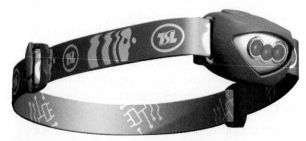

Figure 9–7 The TSL Noxys LED headlamp is an example of a long-lasting, convenient light source for SAR work. Photo courtesy of Pigeon Mountain Industries (PMI), Inc.

Tools and Equipment

During SAR operations, a few tools can be invaluable when attempting to repair essential equipment, improvise, or just make yourself more comfortable. Three items in particular have been recognized as essential in SAR work.

Knife

Criteria for a knife are simple, but rarely followed for some reason. A knife for use in field SAR work should simply have the following: two blades of different sizes, neither of which is over 3 inches long, one sharp blade, and multipurpose applications. An all-purpose "Swiss Army" or "multipurpose" type of utility tool is recommended (Figure 9–8).

Repair/Sewing Kit

A repair kit consisting of wire, pliers, needle, thread, etc., is handy for minor repairs like torn clothing, broken pack parts, etc. But, its potential weight and bulk could make it unsuitable for light "24-hour" ready packs.

General "Hell Box"

This is simply a small bag of "possible items." These include anything that might come in handy for comfort, repairs, and emergencies. Tape, screwdriver, screws,

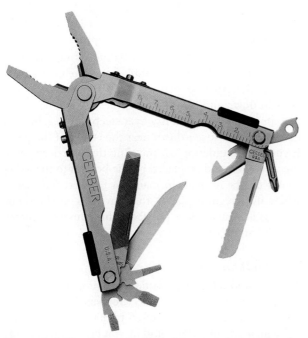

Figure 9–8 The Gerber Multiplier® is a good example of a multi-use tool for SAR work. Photo courtesy of Pigeon Mountain Industries (PMI), Inc.

wire, pliers, clevis pins, stove parts, flashlight/headlamp parts, string, cord, horseshoe nails, etc., are all possibilities. The lighter you want to pack, the smaller the "box." As a matter of fact, a bag may actually work better. A small nylon bag, or, better yet, a sealable plastic bag, can be carried in a pocket (if small enough) or crammed into a small spot in your pack.

Hygiene and Sanitation

Toilet paper, toothbrush, toothpaste, biodegradable soap, sanitary napkins or tampons (with paper, not plastic, inserters), and shaving equipment (razor, blades, small mirror, soap) are all examples of items that most of us consider necessities. However, many of these can be done without or improvised from other pack contents. Decide for yourself what item is actually a necessity and what is merely a comfort, and pack accordingly.

Some hygiene items are more important than others. For instance, toilet paper is so light and useful that no one should be without it in the wilderness. Anyone who has ever had to do without it knows how important it is. Packing it in a sealable plastic bag will keep the paper dry.

We are taught that both toothpaste and toothbrush are important for oral hygiene, but what is really the priority is getting the mouth clean on a regular basis. Simply rinsing the mouth frequently with clean water and scrubbing the teeth with a towel, on occasion, can serve the purpose.

Packs

Selection and use of a pack is a function of the following variables:

- Your intended use and needs
- The individual characteristics of the various types of packs
- Your body structure
- The combined weight and space (cubic inches) of all the items that you intend to put inside.

A specific list of needed equipment for search and rescue is detailed in Appendix 6 (SAR Tech II equipment list).

To help decide how big a pack you need, make a pile of the equipment that you intend to carry. Separate the items into different piles: items that will go into the pack itself, items that will be attached to the outside of the pack, and item for your pockets. For size comparison, the average grocery paper bag will hold about 1400 cubic inches.

Soft, body-hugging packs that do not extend far from the body are more appropriate for most SAR fieldwork, but they may not be as comfortable over long distances as packs that use external frames. The soft, internally framed packs are easier to carry when you are climbing or covering difficult terrain, and they do not stick out and cause snagging problems with trees and brush. Externally-framed packs allow ventilation under them and keep the back more comfortable when properly packed. It also helps, in general, to minimize the number of items that are hung on the exterior of the pack.

Types of Packs

Belt, waist, and fanny packs are small bags designed to wear as a belt around the waist.

- Capacity: 100 to 300 cubic inches, 3 to 10 pounds
- Uses: lunches, the essentials, cameras, and personal gear.

Daypacks are small packs designed to hang from the shoulders.

- Capacity: 700 to 1000 cubic inches, 20 to 25 pounds
- Uses: general day-hiking equipment, water bottle, emergency gear
- Options include:
  - A waistband helps prevent the pack from shifting on the back.
  - Vertical or horizontal partitions provide more efficient loading and access.
  - For the larger daypacks, semi-rigid aluminum or fiberglass frames in the form of sewn-in stays helps distribute the load between the shoulders and hips.

Overnight packs are a further development and refinement of the daypack to a more comfortable, larger capacity pack.

- Capacity: up to 5500 cubic inches, up to 60 pounds depending on the strength of the user.
- Uses: two- to three-day trips.
- Characteristics:
  - The body pack is designed to conform directly to the user's back, thus using the user's back for support. The efficiency of this design is a function primarily of the method of packing equipment into the bag.
  - The internal frame pack provides support for the large bag by the use of adjustable metal or synthetic rods or slats sewn into the bag. A padded waist belt increases comfort and distributes part of the weight to the hips.

Internal frame packs are better suited for activities requiring good balance and freedom of movement (**Figure 9-9**). They fit close to the back, provide for a lower center of gravity, and are flexible. Rigid (external) pack frames with fitted bags provide the most comfortable and convenient method of carrying large loads on extended trips (Figure 9-9).

- Capacity: up to 6000 cubic inches, weight limited only by user's strength
- Uses: extended trips of several days, heavy or bulky loads
- Options:
  - Waist or hip suspension systems help distribute weight between hips and shoulders.
  - Most bags have multiple outside pockets that provide convenience in organizing and finding equipment easily.
  - Bags may be a single compartment or may be divided into various arrays of zippered compartments.
  - Some bags are waterproof; others provide an optional waterproof covering.

Pack a soft pack for comfort with softer items placed near your back. Avoid overloading either by weight or bulk. Pack the frame/bag with heavy items high and near the back, least needed items at the bottom, and frequently used items in the outside pockets. Waterproof all items individually in plastic bags. Although most pack fabrics are "waterproof," water can enter the pack through unwaterproofed seams or when it is opened. Blowing sand or snow can be forced right through zippers.

How to pack your pack can be just as important as what to pack. On smooth trail, heavy items are kept high in the pack so that much of the weight comes straight down and is balanced. If the trail is rough, or if you are going cross-country over steep inclines, heavier gear should be lower down near the center of the pack. If you are "bouldering" or traveling through deep snow, the weight should be placed on the bottom to the lower center of gravity to help maintain balance. No matter where the weight is placed, the heavier items should be as close to your back as possible. This conserves energy and aids with balance.

Making It Fit

To be comfortable, a pack must fit properly. Just like boots, most packs made today are available in various sizes. Pack manufacturers often publish tables that detail which size of pack would fit you best. To determine whether or not a pack is a good fit, a good rule of thumb to follow is to get it sized at the store.

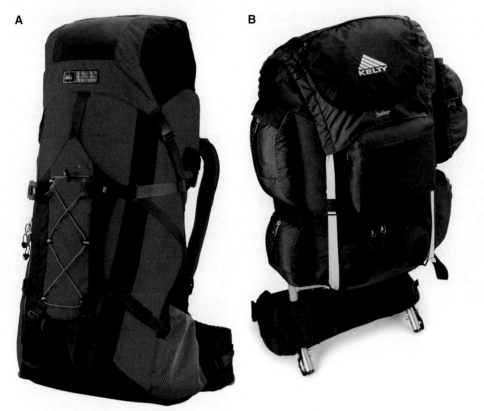

Figure 9–9 An example of a large internal (A) and a large external (B) frame pack. (A) Courtesy of REI. (B) Courtesy of Kelty.

With the pack loaded to capacity and the hip belt placed where you want it (make sure it is snug), the shoulder straps should be high enough so that you can drop a shoulder down without the strap falling off to that side. The straps should be aligned perpendicular to the shoulders with only a small portion of the weight of the pack resting on the shoulders.

Many packs today are designed with a variety of adjustable suspension features to assure a good personal fit. Don't let the variety of buckles, straps, sliders and pins overwhelm you. Load the adjustable pack to maximum weight, put the pack on, and adjust the shoulder and lift straps until the weight moves off your shoulder and onto your hips. Most of the weight should be on your hips. Adjustments should be made while wearing the pack, so at least for the first time wearing it you may need assistance from another person.

Packs without hip belts contain few, if any, adjustments. Basically you will be carrying all of the weight on your shoulders. For SAR work, except in the most accommodating situations, get a pack with a hip belt that has multiple adjustments, or fits you perfectly.

What to Look for in a Frame Pack

Frame Construction Most pack frames are constructed with either welds or coupling devices. In either case, you should only be concerned that the frame hold up to the weight and stress of its intended use. Evaluate how it takes diagonal stress (the toughest stress that a pack will endure) by putting one leg of the frame on the floor, and apply weight on top. Increase the pressure until you have a fair idea of the amount of stress the frame will take. U-shaped frame designs and most H-shaped frames will show no weakness against this test (and stress).

Shoulder Straps Shoulder straps should be padded, adjustable, and wide enough for comfort.

Stitching Look for nylon or cotton wrap nylon thread in the stitching. Stitching should be small (the smaller the length of stich, the better), straight, and even. Check the seams on the pack bottom and on the pockets that there are no thread breaks and no bunching of fabric.

Reinforcing Check for extra reinforcing material, extra (double rows) stitching at stress points, for example, where the bag fastens to frame, at zipper endings, corners, etc.

Hip Belt A two-piece hip belt will hold the frame a little too tight to your back. A one piece belt will allow the frame to float a bit more on your hips as you walk.

Back Bands These help distribute the weight of the pack evenly across your back, and will keep the frame and bag far enough from your back so that nothing pokes you while you are moving. One-piece back bands are probably the best; narrow bands will need to be adjusted to the spot(s) affording the most comfort.

Pack Fastenings The bag should have four or more points of contact with the frame on each side. All grommets and tabs should be reinforced. Look for how easy the bag can be removed and reattached.

Waterproofing Most packs claim to be "waterproofed" or "water repellent." Don't believe it! Obtain a rain cover designed to fit the pack itself, pack your gear in waterproof plastic bags, and then place the smaller bags in the pack.

Storm Flap Make sure that the storm flap will cover the top of the pack when it is fully loaded.

Outside Pockets While handy for things you need to access often, one shortfall is that pockets will tend to catch on branches and bush. Look carefully at the placement of pockets and other external features. Remember, SAR work is mostly "off trail." Consider internal smaller compartments that are accessible by zippers or Velcro®.

Zippers Zippers should be heavy-duty nylon. Metal zippers will freeze stuck during cold weather operations.

Compartments Many variables and options are offered. Multiple compartments will help keep your pack organized, but may limit the positioning of large heavy items.

Lash Points Look for multiple options. You will find it handy to be able to strap some gear and equipment on the outside (e.g., skis, ice axe, crampons, foam pads, tent, marmot cup, etc.).

Rain Cover A rain cover is optional on some packs and can be easily improvised; however, a rain cover that fits your pack perfectly is worth its weight in gold.

References

Auerbach, P.S. (2003). *Medicine for the Outdoors*, 4th ed. Guilford, CT: The Lyons Press.

Auerbach, P.S., ed. (2001). *Wilderness Medicine*, 4th ed. St. Louis, MO: Mosby, Inc.

Cox, M., & Fulsass, K., eds. (2003). *Mountaineering: Freedom of the Hills*, 7th ed. New York, NY: Mountaineers Books.

Farmer, K. (1976). *Woman in the Woods*. New York, NY: Stackpole Books.

Getchell, A. (1995). *The Essential Outdoor Gear Manual: Equipment Care and Repair for Outdoorspeople*. New York, NY: International Marine/Ragged Mountain Press.

Gilpatrick, G. (1999). *Building Outdoor Gear*. Bangor, ME: Gil Gilpatrick.

Johnson, M. (2003). *The Ultimate Desert Handbook: A Manual for Desert Hikers, Campers, and Travelers*. New York, NY: Ragged Mountain Press/McGraw Hill.

Manning, H. (1986). *Backpacking: One Step at a Time*, 4th ed. New York, NY: Vintage Books.

McManners, H. (1998). *The Complete Wilderness Training Book*. New York, NY: DK Publishing.

Petzoldt, P. (1974). *The Wilderness Handbook*. New York, NY: W.W. Norton & Company, Inc.

Rawlins, C., & Fletcher, C. (2002). *The Complete Walker IV*, revised ed. New York, NY: Alfred A. Knopf, Inc.

Schuh, D.R. (1979). *Modern Survival: Outdoor Gear and Savvy to Bring You Back Alive*. New York, NY: David McKay Company.

Chapter 10

Navigation

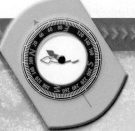

Objectives

Upon completion of this chapter and any course activities, the student will be able to meet the following objectives:

Define the following terms or concepts:
    Determining distances. (p. 161)
    Contour lines. (p. 144)
    True north. (p. 151)
    Grid north and magnetic north. (p. 145)

Demonstrate the use of the UTM (Universal Transverse Mercator) Grid System to determine the coordinates for a given point. (p. 146-148)

Describe the procedures used to obtain a back azimuth. (p. 158-160)

Describe how to take bearing in the field and transfer it correctly to the map, and obtain a bearing on the map and transfer it correctly to the field. (p. 164-165)

Describe techniques used to navigate during daylight hours while wearing a 24-hour pack. (p. 151-165)

List three advantages and three limitations of GPS (Global Positioning System) units as employed during search operations. (p. 166-168)

Global Mapping of Points

Many approaches to plotting points on the Earth exist, each with their advantages and disadvantages, depending on one's needs and perspective.

Map-Related Definitions

- **Agonic Line** – An imaginary line on the Earth's surface connecting points where the magnetic declination is zero as of a given date.
- **Contour** – Imaginary line on the ground, all points of which are at the same elevation above or below a specified datum.
- **Contour Interval** – Difference in elevation between two adjacent contours.
- **Coordinates** – Linear and (or) angular quantities that designate the position of a point in relation to a given reference frame.
- **Datum** – A reference system for computing or correlating the results of surveys. There are two principal types of datums: vertical and horizontal. The vertical datum is a level surface to which heights are referred and the horizontal datum is used as a reference for position. Several datums exist including the North American Datum of 1983 (NAD 83), which is now a three-dimentional datum (horizontal and vertical) thanks to GPS.
- **Grid** – Network of uniformly spaced parallel lines intersecting at right angles. When superimposed on a map, it usually carries the name of the projection used for the map, that is, Lambert grid, UTM grid, etc.
- **Isogonic Line** – Line joining points on the Earth's surface having equal magnetic declination as of a given date.
- **Latitude** – Angular distance, in degrees, minutes and seconds, of a point north or south of the equator.

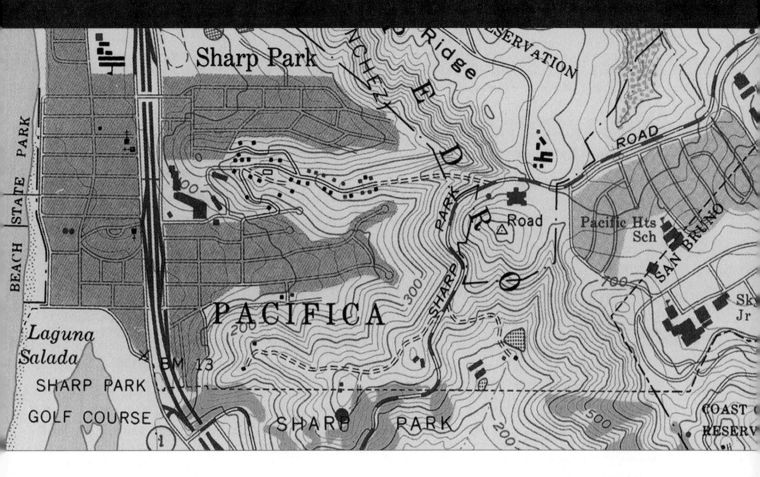

- **Longitude** – Angular distance, in degrees, minutes and seconds, of a point east or west of the Greenwich meridian.

- **Magnetic Declination** – The angular difference between magnetic north and true (geographic) north at the point of observation; it is not constant but varies with time because of the "wandering" of the magnetic north pole.

- **Meridian** – Great circle on the surface of the Earth that passes through the geographical poles and any given point on the Earth's surface. All points on a given meridian have the same longitude.

- **Parallel of Latitude** – A circle, or approximation of a circle, on the surface of the Earth, parallel to the equator, and connecting points of equal latitude.

- **Prime Meridian** – Meridian of longitude 0 degrees, used as the origin for measurements of longitude. The meridian of Greenwich, England, is the internationally accepted prime meridian.

- **Quadrangle (Quad)** – Four-sided area, bounded by parallels of latitude (dimensions are not necessarily the same in both directions).

- **Relief** – Elevations and depressions of the land or sea bottom.

- **Section** – Unit of subdivision of a township, normally a quadrangle one mile square with boundaries conforming to meridians and parallels within established limits, and containing 640 acres as nearly as practical.

- **Scale** – Relationship existing between a distance on a map, chart, or photograph and the corresponding distance on the Earth.

- **Topography** – Configuration (geographic relief) of the land surface; the graphic delineation or portrayal of that configuration in map form, as by contour lines.

- **Township** – Unit of survey of the public lands of the United States, normally a quadrangle approximately six miles on a side with boundaries conforming to meridians and parallels within established limits, containing 36 sections.

- **Variation** – Another term for "declination."

Geographic Mapping

The geographic approach to plotting points on the globe is, by far, the method with which humans are most familiar. This approach uses addresses, specific known geographic locations, or other such places as descriptive points.

In the geographic system, references are made to a specific place such as, "456 Main Street," "Kelly's Diner," or "Swan Lake." References can also be relative to such known points (i.e., 1 mile south of Swan Lake). These references can be measured in travel distances (4 miles west of Swan Lake) or in map distances (1 inch east of Kelly's Diner on the map). As long as everyone using the system understands the reference, the system works. Maps may not even be necessary with this system if all are familiar with the area and specific landmark names.

The geographic system requires little or no training, and is easily learned. Even though this system can be time consuming when coordinates are to be transmitted via radio, it seems best suited for novices. During SAR situations, the geographic approach works best as a backup to other more sophisticated mapping systems.

Geographic Coordinate System: Latitude and Longitude

One way to identify points on the curved surface of the Earth is with a system of reference lines called parallels of latitude and meridians of longitude. On some maps, the meridians and parallels appear as straight lines. On most modern maps, however, the meridians and parallels appear as curved lines. These differences are due to the mathematical treatment required to portray a curved surface on a flat surface so that important properties of the map (such as distance) are shown with minimum distortion. The system used to portray a part of the round Earth on a flat surface is called a map projection.

To simplify the use of maps and to avoid the inconvenience of pinpointing locations on curved reference lines, map makers superimpose on the map a rectangular grid consisting of two sets of straight, parallel lines, uniformly spaced, each set perpendicular to the other. This grid is designed so that any point on the map can be designated so by its latitude and longitude or by its grid coordinates (see UTM below), and a reference in one system can be converted into a reference in another system. Such grids are usually identified by the name of the particular projection for which they are designed.

The geographic coordinate system (latitude and longitude) uses a grid system that covers the entire globe and uses lines of longitude (meridians), which run north-south, and latitude lines (parallels), which run east-west (**Figure 10–1**). Quite a bit of skill is required to accurately describe a point in the field with this system, but it gets much easier with practice. This system is not nearly as effective for ground personnel as it is for those that do not require as much accuracy (i.e., aircraft, boats, etc.), but works fairly well for all-around, general use, especially when coordinate information must be exchanged between air and ground forces, or between international units.

In the late 1800s, geographers met and decided that a line from pole to pole, forming a huge half-circle passing through Greenwich, England, would be called the prime meridian. From this longitudinal line, considered zero, the angular distance, east or west, to any point on the Earth's surface is measured by an angle in degrees up to 180 in either direction. At this 180-degree mark, called the International Date Line, another meridian is formed that connects with the prime meridian.

Latitude starts at the equator, considered zero, with a big circle that encompasses the entire globe midway between both poles. The angular distance of any point on earth, north or south of the equator, is measured in degrees with 90 being the maximum at each pole. Lines of latitude are parallel to the equator and are referred to as parallels.

One degree equals 60 minutes and 1 minute equals 60 seconds. Plotting a point to within 1 navigational second is accurate to within approximately 1000 square feet. This is very accurate as mapping methods go, but it is very difficult to define 1 second (1.3 mm) on a 7.5-minute map. Fifteen-second accuracy is much more realistic.

Universal Transverse Mercator System (UTM)

The National Imagery and Mapping Agency (NIMA; formerly, Defense Mapping Agency) adopted a special grid for military use throughout the world called the Universal Transverse Mercator (UTM) grid. In this grid, the world is divided into 60 north-south zones, each covering a strip 6° wide in longitude. These zones are numbered consecutively beginning with Zone 1, located between 180° and 174° west longitude, and progressing eastward to Zone 60,

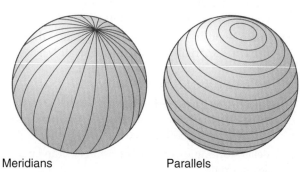

Meridians   Parallels

Figure 10–1 Examples of parallels (latitude) and meridians (longitude). (Courtesy of the United States Geological Survey.)

between 174° and 180° east longitude. Thus, the conterminous 48 United States are covered by 10 zones, from Zone 10 on the west coast through Zone 19 in New England (Figure 10–2). In each zone, coordinates are measured north and east in meters (where one meter equals 39.37 inches, or slightly more than 1 yard). The northing values are measured continuously from zero at the equator, in a northerly direction. To avoid negative numbers for locations south of the Equator, the designing cartographers assigned the Equator an arbitrary false northing value of 10,000,000 meters. A central meridian through the middle of each 6° zone is assigned an easting value of 500,000 meters. Grid values to the west of this central meridian are less than 500,000, and to the east, more than 500,000 meters.

The UTM grid is shown on all quadrangle maps prepared by the U.S. Geological Survey (USGS). On 7.5-minute quadrangle maps (1:24,000 and 1:25,000 scale) and 15-minute quadrangle maps (1:50,000, 1:62,500, and standard-edition 1:63,360 scales), the UTM grid lines are indicated at intervals of 1,000 meters, either by blue ticks in the margins of the map or with full grid lines. The 1,000-meter value of the ticks is shown for every tick or grid line. In addition, the actual meter value is shown for ticks nearest the southeast and northwest corners of the map. If the map does not already have the grid lines on the map, the lines can be hand-drawn by connecting the tick marks.

On the 7-1/2 minute map, each tick is represented by 4 numbers. The first two numbers are in superscript (e.g., ^{49}98). The numerals in superscript represent the 1,000,000- and 100,000-meter grids. The last two numerals represent the 10,000- and 1000-meter grids. Thus, using the northing (that is, the left and

right margins), ^{49}98 represents 4,998,000 meters north of the equator. Computer programs exist that can convert these figures into latitude and longitude, and most GPS units (see page 166) can easily switch between UTM and latitude/longitude.

To use the UTM grid, you can place a transparent grid overlay ("interpolator") on the map to subdivide the grid, or you can draw lines on the map connecting corresponding ticks on opposite edges (Figure 10–3). The distances can be measured in meters at the map scale between any map point and the nearest grid lines to the south and west. The northing of the point is the value of the nearest grid line south of it plus its distance north of that line; its easting is the value of the nearest grid line west of it plus its distance east of that line (Figure 10–4).

In use, the numerals in superscript are most often ignored when describing points on a UTM grid. Thus, a point falling midway between ^{3}61 and ^{3}62 (easting) and ^{49}97 and ^{49}98 (northing) would be described as 61500/97500. The use of all 10 digits to describe a UTM point describes a point to within 1 meter and is called "10-digit accuracy." In actual use, the right-most (fifth) digits in the description of the easting and northing are infrequently used because describing a point to within 100 square meters (10 m × 10 m) is usually sufficient for land navigation. This level of accuracy requires the use of only 8 digits. So, the same point may more realistically be described as 6150/9750 ("8-digit accuracy"). Measurements in this system are always made from the

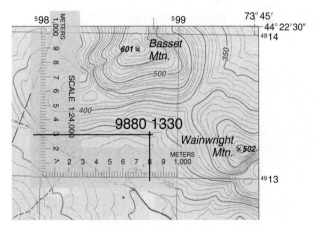

Figure 10–3 Finding a UTM point using an interpolator. To plot a point at coordinates of 9880/1330, the easting (9880) is first located by finding the blue tick marked with the upper case 98 on the bottom or top margin of the map then measuring an additional 8/10ths of the way (800 meters) to the tick line at 99. The northing is located by finding the blue tick marked with the upper case 13 on the right or left margin of the map then measuring an additional 300 meters north (approximately ⅓ of the way to the tick line at upper case 14).

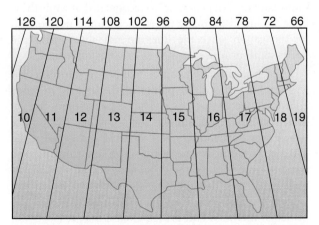

Figure 10–2 The Universal Transverse Mercator grid that covers the conterminous 48 United States comprises 10 zones, from Zone 10 on the west coast through Zone 19 in New England. (Courtesy United States Geological Survey.)

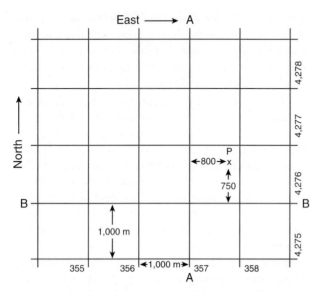

Figure 10–4 In Zone 19, the grid value of line A-A is 357,000 meters east. The grid value of line B-B is 4,276,000 meters north. Point P is 800 meters east and 750 meters north of the grid lines. Therefore, the grid coordinates of point P are east 357,800 and north 4,276,750. Ignoring the superscript numerals, the UTM point would be read, "Zone 19, 57800 76750," and is theoretically within one square meter accuracy. (Courtesy United States Geological Survey.)

left margin to the point, then from the bottom margin to the point (Read-Right-Up).

The Uniform Mapping System (UMS)

The Uniform Map System (UMS) was devised in Washington State in the mid 1960s and was widely used prior to the proliferation of inexpensive, handheld GPS devices. The system was designed to help air and ground operations in communicating location information accurately and quickly to other operating units. However, UTM and the geographic coordinate system have almost completely supplanted UMS everywhere it was used.

UMS is a system that uses letters and numbers to describe points, and is tied into Sectional Aeronautical Charts (1:500,000) that are broken down into a grid and used by the Civil Air Patrol and U.S. Air Force. UMS is also keyed into 15-minute topographical (topo) maps (15° latitude by 15° longitude; 1:62,500 scale) that have recently been abandoned by the USGS.

Because of the maps on which the system is based, the UMS permits the exchange of location points between ground SAR teams and aircraft, and is also considered, particularly by those who do not use it often, to be difficult to teach and apply in the field. Some claim that the problem may be a consequence of attempting to adapt an air search system to ground SAR operations. Others swear by its effectiveness.

An example of a UMS designated point is, *SFO 123 B 4567*, where: "SFO" designates the three-letter name of the Sectional Aeronautical Map within which the described point lies, "123" is the 15-minute quad (15 minute latitude by 15 minute longitude quadrant) within the SFO map that is indicated on the Section Map; "B" represents the upper right quadrant of the 15-minute quad (A is upper left, C is lower left, and D is lower right [all 7.5-minute quads]); "4567" represents measurements made from the corner of the 7.5-minute quad (A, B, C, or D corner, as indicated), horizontally first, then vertically (Read-Right-Up); "45" is 4.5 miles horizontally from the upper right corner (B), and 6.7 miles vertically from that point. The entire designation describes an area 1/10th of a square mile.

Township and Range: U.S. Public Land Survey

In 1785, the United States Public Land Survey (USPLS) was started with the territories northwest of the Ohio River as a test area. According to the plan, also known as the "Public Land System," land was to be divided into townships six miles square with boundaries running north, south, east, and west, and townships were to be subdivided into 36 numbered sections of one square mile (640 acres) each (**Figure 10–5**). Principal meridians and baselines were established as a reference system for the township surveys.

The thought was that all areas in the United States would be surveyed using this system, thereby setting a national mapping standard. The surveys were not entirely completed and, thus, the system is not applicable to many parts of the United States. For this reason, not all USGS maps have township and range lines on them. It is also important for SAR personnel to recognize that while these lines are found on many maps, they should not be used for navigation since the lines do not always run true north-south or true east-west as originally intended.

In each area that was to be mapped, a starting point was established and all points in the area were referenced relative to that point. The reference point for the Washington-Oregon survey, for example, was established near Portland, Oregon, in 1851 and is called the Willamette Stone. A true north-south line runs through the stone and is called the Willamette Meridian. An east-west line runs through the stone and is called the Willamette Baseline. These are also referred to as the principal meridian and principal base line, respectively. Although the boundaries of townships and section were originally intended to be aligned with the true cardinal directions, in reality, they are far from it. Thus, they should not be used for navigation.

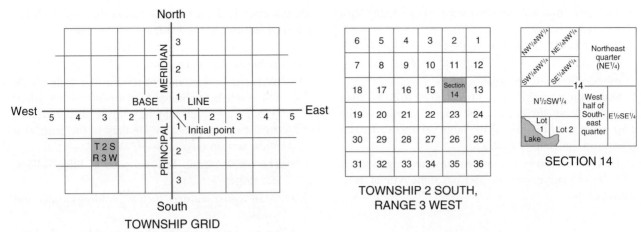

Figure 10–5 General diagram of the U.S. rectangular system of surveys. (Courtesy United States Geological Survey.)

A specific point on the map is described by first identifying the township in which it falls. The township number is described as either north or south of the principal base line and east or west of the principal meridian. For example, the township in **Figure 10–6** is two townships (tiers) south of the principal base line and three columns (ranges) from the principal meridian. Thus, the township is described as "Township 2 South, Range 3 West" or "T 2 S, R 3 W."

A point in a township could be further described by its section number. Sections are numbered consecutively, starting at the northeast corner and ending in the southeast corner of the township. Section 31 is at the lower left of the township, and section 6 is at the upper left (Figure 10–6). Indicating the section in which a point is located plots it to one square mile accuracy. A point can be more accurately described by indicating that corner (1/4) of the section where the point is located. Describing a point as being within the NW corner of a section describes a point within 166 acres of accuracy. Describing a point as being in the NW corner of the SE corner of a section describes a point within about 40 acres of accuracy. A description of a point within 40 acres of accuracy would look like: NE/4, SE/4, Section 2, T 2 S, R 3 W.

SDMRT System

The San Diego Mountain Rescue Team (SDMRT) uses a system to describe a point on a map that is simple, fast, and easy to learn. Unlike the other absolute navigation systems, the SDMRT system can work on any map, regardless of the terrain or area it describes. Because this system is useless without a map, it cannot be strictly considered a method of absolute navigation. However, it is so simple and useful in the "real" world that it deserves more than just a mere mention.

The first step in the SDMRT system includes identifying the map to be used by scale (15- or 7.5-minute) and quadrant name. Second, a measuring device (ruler) is required to measure the point from the nearest borders. The coordinates are read by simply indicating the distance, in inches, from the left map margin as well as

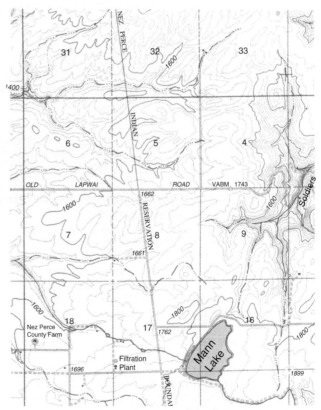

Figure 10–6 Examples of red township and range boundaries on a map. (Courtesy United States Geological Survey.)

the distance from the bottom margin (Read Right Up). One example is:

> Point A is 12-1/2 inches from the left and 4-3/8 inches from the bottom of the 7.5-minute series, Northampton Quadrangle topo map.

Make sure any measurements are taken from the map margin and not the edge of the map. The edge of the map is not used because of the large variances that can exist from one map to another.

This system can be used on any map as long as it has a border or margin, and the user has some type of measuring device.

Maps

A map is a pictorial representation of the Earth's surface drawn to scale and reproduced on a flat piece of paper. In SAR, reading a map allows SAR personnel to associ-ate the graphic details appearing on the map with the physical features in the field, and vice versa.

As a minimum, maps for land navigation should provide the following information:

- An accurate depiction of terrain in a scale that is achievable by walking (or flying or boating, whatever the approach may be). "Scale" is the ratio of the area represented by the map to the same area in the terrain (e.g., 1 to 24,000).
- The major terrain features such as hills, valleys, and ridges
- "Man-made" features such as buildings, trails, and roads
- An accurate depiction of measurable relief, elevation, and contour (lay of the land)
- The location of water and water courses (important information for SAR personnel and search planning)

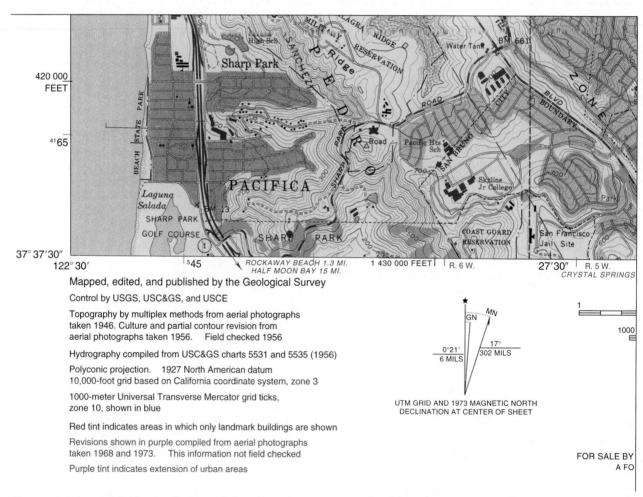

Figure 10–7 Lower left margin of a 7.5-minute topographic map at a scale of 1:24,000 (San Francisco South, California, quadrangle). (Courtesy United States Geological Survey.)

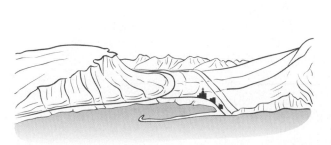

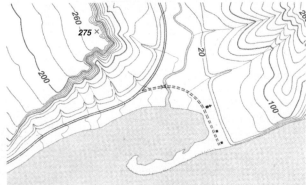

Figure 10–8 The terrain on the left is depicted by the topographical map on the right. (Courtesy United States Geological Survey.)

Topographical Maps

Topographical (topo) maps portray the shape and elevation of the terrain while showing a graphic representation of selected man-made and natural features on a part of the Earth's surface plotted to a definite scale.

The USGS publishes topo maps in a variety of scales; the most popular for land SAR is the 1:24,000 or 7.5-minute map (**Figure 10–7**). These maps have quadrangle dimensions of 7.5 minutes in latitude and longitude, the bounding parallels and meridians being integral multiples of 7.5 minutes. The series includes the few maps whose boundary lines are offset or extended to cover islands, irregular coastal features, or areas needed to complete mapping to political boundaries.

USGS topo maps are supposed to be updated every 5 to 10 years, but in reality it is often longer. Because of this, they accurately depict terrain and relief (elevation and slope), but the man-made features in the terrain may occasionally differ from what the map depicts due to the extended length of time between map updates (**Figure 10–8**). The 7.5-minute series maps are the most commonly used maps in ground SAR work because of the appropriateness of scale and wide availability. They are also available as digital files on CD-ROM computer disks. This electronic version has become very popular with the wide use and availability of laptop computers.

The top of a USGS topo map is always true (geographic) north. Thus, the vertical lines of longitude on the map point north and south, and the horizontal lines of latitude point east and west.

The space outside the margin line (called the "margin") on USGS topographical maps identifies and explains the map. The marginal information corresponds somewhat to the table of contents and introduction of a book; it tells briefly how the map was made, where the quadrangle is located, what organizations are responsible for the contents, and gives other information to make the map more useful.

PENINSULA QUADRANGLE
OHIO—SUMMIT CO.
7.5 MINUTE SERIES (TOPOGRAPHIC)

Figure 10–9 Quadrangle name found in the upper right margin of a USGS topographical map. (Courtesy United States Geological Survey.)

Each map is identified in the upper right margin by its quadrangle name, state, or states in which it is located, series, and type (**Figure 10–9**). It is usually named after a prominent, immovable place or landmark within the mapped area. If the quadrangle includes areas of more than one state, the state names are shown in the title in the order of decreasing area. The "series" refers to the area mapped in terms of minutes or degrees; "type" is either topographic or planimetric (no topographic features). If a new 7.5-minute map covers a part of a published 15-minute quadrangle, a note is added giving the position of the 7.5-minute quadrangle.

The title block in the lower right margin shows the quadrangle name, state name, and the geographic index number (**Figure 10–10**). For a 7.5-minute map, the margin also gives the position in relation to the 15-minute map, if applicable, and the year the map was published. The geographic index number is the geographic position of the corner of the map nearest the Greenwich meridian and the equator, followed by the series, such as "7.5-minute." Just to the left of the title block is a diagram of the location of the quadrangle within the state.

Adjoining quadrangle names are shown so that map users may know that topographic data are available for these adjacent areas (**Figure 10–11**).

Geographic coordinates are shown at all four map margin corners and along the margin lines at 2.5-minute intervals for 7.5-minute maps (**Figure 10–12**). Coordinates

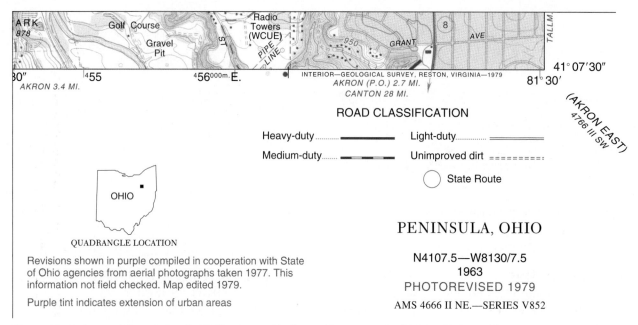

ROAD CLASSIFICATION

Heavy-duty..............━━━━━   Light-duty.............══════

Medium-duty........▬▬▬   Unimproved dirt ═════════

◯ State Route

PENINSULA, OHIO

N4107.5—W8130/7.5
1963
PHOTOREVISED 1979

AMS 4666 II NE.—SERIES V852

OHIO

QUADRANGLE LOCATION

Revisions shown in purple compiled in cooperation with State of Ohio agencies from aerial photographs taken 1977. This information not field checked. Map edited 1979.

Purple tint indicates extension of urban areas

Figure 10–10 Lower right margin of a USGS topographical map. (Courtesy United States Geological Survey.)

for both the state (each state has its own zone grid based on various projections) and UTM grid systems are shown near the map margin corners.

The credit legend is located in the lower left margin (see Figure 10–7). Because of the almost infinite number of possible combinations of data, credit legends cannot be rigid. However, they usually include the name of the mapping agency, the name of the editing and publishing agency, name of the agency that furnished the geodetic (the science that deals with the measurement and mathematical description of the size and shape of the earth) control, method by which the mapping was performed,

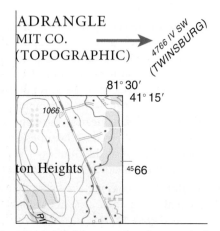

Figure 10–11 Adjoining quadrangle name indicated by blue arrow. This example shows the upper right map margin.

credit note for hydrographic (the science that deals with measurement and description of the physical features of the Earth's oceans, seas, and other waterways) information, and informative and explanatory notes.

The magnetic declination for the year of field survey or revision is determined to the nearest 0.5 degree from the latest isogonic chart. It is shown by a diagram centered between the credit legend and bar scale (**Figure 10–13**). The declination diagram indicates the angular relationship between true north, grid north, and magnetic north.

The center of the lower margin contains the following information, arranged in the order indicated:

1. Publication scales expressed as a ratio
2. Bar scales in metric and imperial units
3. Contour-interval statement. If the map contains supplementary contours, a statement to the effect is added. When the maximum elevation on the quadrangle is less than the specified contour interval, a note stating, "entire area below 5 feet" is used in place of the standard contour interval.
4. Vertical datum: The statement, "Datum is mean sea level" is on standard survey topographical maps printed prior to 1975. On maps published since, the statement is "National Geodetic Vertical Datum of 1929."
5. Depth-curve sounding statement, where applicable
6. Shoreline and tide-range statements, shown on maps that include tidal shoreline

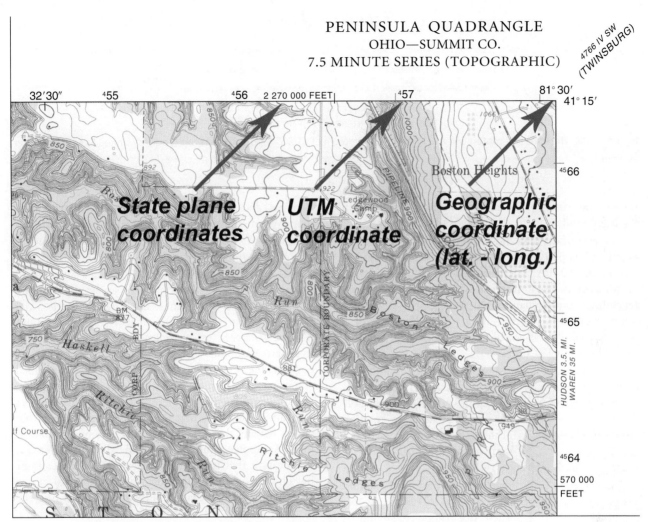

PENINSULA QUADRANGLE
OHIO—SUMMIT CO.
7.5 MINUTE SERIES (TOPOGRAPHIC)

4766 IV SW
(TWINSBURG)

Figure 10–12 UTM coordinates, state plane coordinates, and geographic coordinates (latitude and longitude) at the map margin corners of a 7.5-minute topographical map. (Courtesy United States Geological Survey.)

7. Map accuracy statements. The standard statement is, "This map complies with national map accuracy standards."

The Bar Scales (distance determination) are located at the bottom center margin of the map (**Figure 10–14**). Distance can be determined by measuring the distance on the map with a piece of paper, piece of string, or a ruler, then comparing the measured distance to the Bar Scale, which is in meters, miles, and feet. The Metric System (meters) is the measurement of choice for SAR.

A legend explaining the various road symbols that are shown on the map is placed in the lower right margin (**Figure 10–15**). This legend is tailored for each map to include only the classes of roads and route markers that are

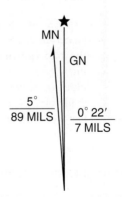

UTM GRID AND 1979 MAGNETIC NORTH
DECLINATION AT CENTER OF SHEET

Figure 10–13 Magnetic declination diagram on a USGS topo map, found in the bottom margin of the map.

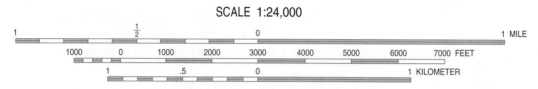

SCALE 1:24,000

CONTOUR INTERVAL 40 FEET
DOTTED LINES REPRESENT 20-FOOT CONTOURS

Figure 10–14 The scale and contour interval in the bottom margin of a USGS topographical map. (Courtesy United States Geological Survey.)

shown in the body of the map. Trails are not included in the legend unless there are no roads on the map.

The year of the data shown on the map is printed beneath and as part of the title in the lower right margin (see Figure 10–10). The latest date of field completion or revision is used. It remains unchanged in future reprintings, but is changed when the map is revised. If minor cartographic corrections are made for a reprint, a note in small type is added under the year (i.e., "1957, Minor Revision 1973").

Road destinations are shown in the map margin for convenience in determining the distance to the next town or important road junction beyond the map border, and to facilitate orientation of the map with respect to well-known features.

The USGS has a free pamphlet that has every map symbol found on a topo map (Figure 10–16). These free pamphlets should be available where topo maps are sold, or are free from the USGS by writing, calling, or by visiting their web site.

Colors on the Map

Generally there are six colors on the map. Brown denotes contour lines, green is for vegetation, blue for water, black for man-made objects, red for man-made features such as roads and built-

up areas, and purple for new changes or updates on the map. When contour lines are showing elevation on glaciers or snow-capped mountains, these lines are blue.

Contour lines represent relative elevation (Figure 10–17). Each contour line on the map connects all points at the same elevation above sea level. There are three types of contour lines: Index, Intermediate, and Supplementary. Every fifth line is darker and has a number superimposed on it, indicating the elevation along that particular line. This darker contour is an "index" contour line. The lighter brown contour lines are called "intermediate" contour lines, and they fall between index lines and are not numbered. Supplementary contour lines are dashed lines that may be used when the terrain is very flat and there are large distances between contour lines. A supplementary contour line shows a difference in elevation that is half of the elevation of the contour lines between which it falls. The contour interval can be found in the bottom margin of the map, usually near the distance scale. When successive contour lines are close together, the terrain is steep. Contour lines that touch indicate a cliff. Widely spaced contour lines indicate a gently sloping or flat terrain.

Terrain Features

All terrain features evolve from a complex landmass known as a "ridgeline" (Figure 10–18). This ridgeline should not be confused with, and is not a synonym for, a "ridge," which is an individual terrain feature. A ridgeline is a line of high ground, usually with variations in elevation along its top and low ground on all sides, which is the source of many terrain features. A "ridge" is simply one of the terrain features that may arise from a ridgeline.

A total of ten natural or man-made terrain features may arise from a ridgeline, each with unique and notable characteristics. These features fall into two categories: major and minor (Figure 10–19).

Major Terrain Features

Hill: A hill is an area of high ground. From a hilltop, the ground slopes down in all directions. A hill is shown on the map by contour lines forming concentric circles

ROAD CLASSIFICATION

Primary highway, all weather, hard surface .... ▬▬▬

Light-duty road, all weather, improved surface .... ═══

Secondary highway, all weather, hard surface .... ▬▬▬

Unimproved road, fair or dry weather .... ========

⬭ Interstate Route   ⬠ U.S. Route   ◯ State Route

Figure 10–15 Legend showing various road symbols.

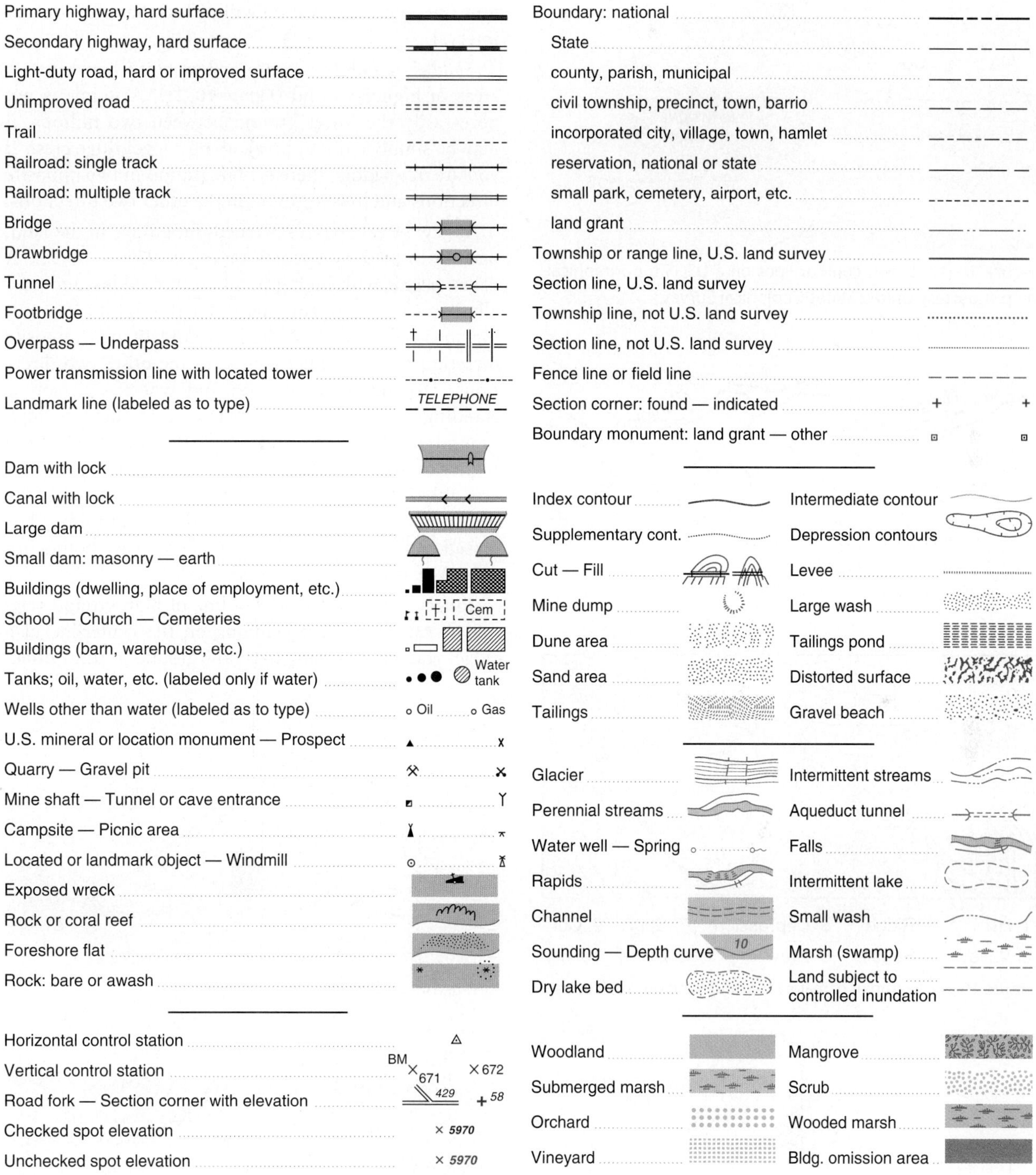

Primary highway, hard surface		Boundary: national	
Secondary highway, hard surface		State	
Light-duty road, hard or improved surface		county, parish, municipal	
Unimproved road		civil township, precinct, town, barrio	
Trail		incorporated city, village, town, hamlet	
Railroad: single track		reservation, national or state	
Railroad: multiple track		small park, cemetery, airport, etc.	
Bridge		land grant	
Drawbridge		Township or range line, U.S. land survey	
Tunnel		Section line, U.S. land survey	
Footbridge		Township line, not U.S. land survey	
Overpass — Underpass		Section line, not U.S. land survey	
Power transmission line with located tower		Fence line or field line	
Landmark line (labeled as to type)	TELEPHONE	Section corner: found — indicated	
		Boundary monument: land grant — other	

Dam with lock		Index contour	Intermediate contour
Canal with lock		Supplementary cont.	Depression contours
Large dam		Cut — Fill	Levee
Small dam: masonry — earth		Mine dump	Large wash
Buildings (dwelling, place of employment, etc.)		Dune area	Tailings pond
School — Church — Cemeteries	Cem	Sand area	Distorted surface
Buildings (barn, warehouse, etc.)		Tailings	Gravel beach
Tanks; oil, water, etc. (labeled only if water)	Water tank		
Wells other than water (labeled as to type)	o Oil o Gas	Glacier	Intermittent streams
U.S. mineral or location monument — Prospect	▲ x	Perennial streams	Aqueduct tunnel
Quarry — Gravel pit	⚒ x	Water well — Spring o o~	Falls
Mine shaft — Tunnel or cave entrance	▫ Y	Rapids	Intermittent lake
Campsite — Picnic area	🏕 ⚞	Channel	Small wash
Located or landmark object — Windmill	⊙ ⚐	Sounding — Depth curve 10	Marsh (swamp)
Exposed wreck		Dry lake bed	Land subject to controlled inundation
Rock or coral reef			
Foreshore flat		Woodland	Mangrove
Rock: bare or awash		Submerged marsh	Scrub
		Orchard	Wooded marsh
Horizontal control station	△	Vineyard	Bldg. omission area
Vertical control station	BM ×671 ×672		
Road fork — Section corner with elevation	429 +58		
Checked spot elevation	× 5970		
Unchecked spot elevation	× 5970		

Figure 10–16 Topographical map legend available from USGS.

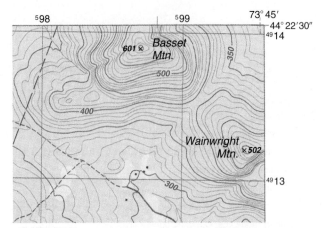

Figure 10–17 Brown contour lines on a USGS topographical map. (Courtesy United States Geological Survey.)

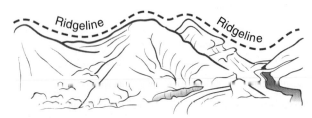

Figure 10–18 A ridgeline.

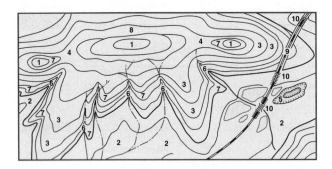

| 1. Hill | 3. Ridge | 5. Depression | 7. Spur | 9. Cut |
| 2. Valley | 4. Saddle | 6. Draw | 8. Cliff | 10. Fill |

Figure 10–19 Examples of major (1–5) and minor (6–10) features.

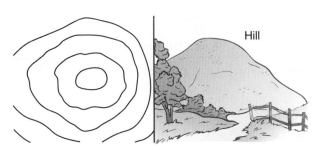

Figure 10–20 Hill.

(Figure 10–20). The inside of the smallest closed circle is the hilltop. It is important to note that it is rare to have a completely flat hilltop. It is very possible that the hill will rise slightly in elevation beyond the very top contour line, but the elevation will be less than the contour interval.

Saddle: A saddle is a dip or low point between two areas of higher ground (Figure 10–21). A saddle is not necessarily the lower ground between two hilltops; it may be simply a dip or break along a level ridge crest. If you are in a saddle, there is high ground in two opposite directions and lower ground in the other two directions.

Valley: A valley is a stretched-out groove in the land, usually formed by streams or rivers (Figure 10–22). A valley begins with high ground on three sides, and usually has a course of running water through it. If standing in a valley, there is high ground in two opposite direction and a gradual incline in the other two directions. Depending on its size and where a person is standing, it may not be obvious that there is high ground in the third direction, but water flows from higher to lower ground. Contour lines forming a valley are either U shaped or V shaped. To determine the direction water is flowing, look at the contour lines. The closed end of a contour line (U or V) always points upstream or toward high ground.

Ridge: A ridge is a sloping line of high ground (Figure 10–23). If you are standing on the centerline of a ridge, you will normally have low ground in three direc-

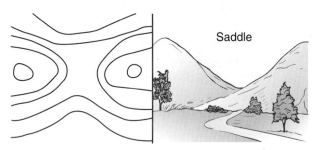

Figure 10–21 Saddle.

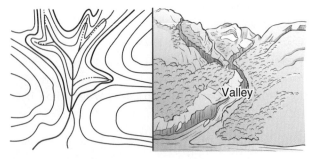

Figure 10–22 Valley.

tions and high ground in one direction with varying degrees of slope. If you cross a ridge at right angles, you will climb steeply to the crest and then descend steeply to the base. When you move along the path of the ridge, depending on the geographic location, there may be either an almost unnoticeable slope or a very obvious incline. Contour lines forming a ridge tend to be U-shaped or V-shaped. The closed end of the contour line points away from high ground.

Depression: A depression is a low point in the ground (Figure 10–24). It could be described as an area of low ground surrounded by higher ground in all directions, or simply a hole in the ground. Usually only depressions that are equal to or greater than the contour interval will be shown. On maps, depressions are represented by closed contour lines that have tick marks pointing toward low ground.

Minor Terrain Features

Draw: A draw is a less developed water course than a valley (Figure 10–25). In a draw, there is essentially no level ground and, therefore, little or no maneuver room within its confines. If you are standing in a draw, the ground slopes upward in three directions and downward in the other direction. A draw could be considered the initial formation of a valley. The contour lines depicting a draw are U-shaped and V-shaped, both pointing toward high ground.

Spur: A spur is a short, continuous sloping line of higher ground, normally jutting out from the side of a

ridge (Figure 10–26). A spur is often formed by two roughly parallel streams cutting draws down the side of a ridge. The ground will slope down in three directions and up in one. Contour lines on a map depicted a spur with the U or V pointing away from high ground.

Cliff: A cliff is a vertical or near vertical feature; it is an abrupt change of elevation. When a slope is so steep that the contour lines converge into one "carrying" contour or contours, this last contour line has tick marks pointing toward low ground (Figure 10–27). Cliffs are also shown by contour lines very close together and, in some instances, touching each other.

Cut/Fill: A cut is a man-made feature resulting from cutting through raised ground, usually to form a level

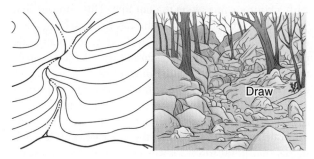

Figure 10–25 Draw.

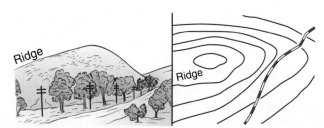

Figure 10–23 Ridge.

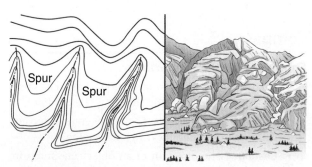

Figure 10–26 Spur.

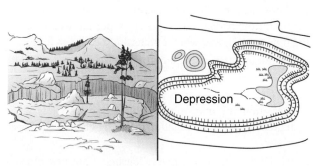

Figure 10–24 Depression.

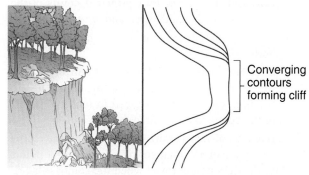

Figure 10–27 Cliff.

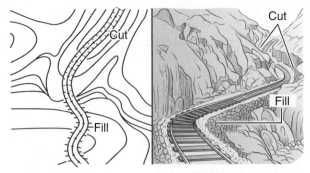

Figure 10–28 Cut/fill.

bed for a road or railroad track. Cuts are shown on a map when they are at least 10-feet high, and they are drawn with a contour line along the cut line. This contour line extends the length of the cut and has tick marks that extend from the cut line to the roadbed, if the map scale permits this level of detail (Figure 10–28). A fill is a man-made feature resulting from filling a low area, usually to form a level bed for a railroad track. Fills are shown on a map when they are at least 10-feet high, and they are drawn with a contour line along the fill line. This contour line extends the length of the filled area and has tick marks that point toward lower ground. If the map scale permits, the length of the fill tick marks are drawn to scale and extend from the base line of the fill symbol.

Compass

Compass-Related Definitions

- **Azimuth** – For land navigation, has the same meaning as "bearing" or "heading" (see below).
- **Back Azimuth** – Refers to 180 degrees opposite from one's azimuth, bearing, or heading.
- **Bearing** – The direction of an object measured in degrees from north. Azimuth and bearing are often used interchangeably. The term "heading" is also often used in lieu of azimuth or bearing.
- **Cardinal Points** – The four principal points of the compass: north, south, east, and west.
- **Course** – Plan of travel using a compass, map, or both.
- **Direction** – The relative location of one terrain feature to another; similar to bearing, azimuth, and heading, but usually described in terms of points of the compass rather than degrees.
- **Direction-of-Travel Arrow** – The arrow or line on the base plate of an Orienteering Compass that points in the direction of travel when the compass is oriented.

- **Grid North** – The north established by the vertical UTM grid lines on the map. In the declination diagram of a USGS topographical map, grid north is usually indicated by the letters "GN" and the grid north line has no arrow on it.
- **Heading** – For land navigation, has the same meaning as "bearing" (see above).
- **Intercardinal Points** – The four points of the compass between the four Cardinal Points: northeast, southeast, northwest, and southwest.
- **Landmark** – A feature in the landscape which can be readily recognized – anything from a prominent tree or rock, to a building or lake.
- **Magnetic North** – The direction to which the compass points. In the declination diagram of a USGS topographical map, magnetic north is usually indicated by the letters "MN" and the magnetic north line has an arrow on it.
- **Orientation** – The process of determining one's location in the field with the help of landscape features, map, or compass, or with all three combined.
- **Orienteering Compass** – A compass especially designed to simplify the process of finding one's way with map and compass. It usually has a compass housing mounted on a rectangular base plate in such a way that it can be turned easily.
- **Protractor** – Instrument for measuring angles, usually in degrees.
- **True North** – A line from any position on the Earth's surface to the North Pole. All lines of longitude are true north lines. In the declination diagram of a USGS topographical map, true north is usually indicated by a star.
- **Tune-in or Set** – Terms coined to mean to adjust the compass bezel to a certain number or degree heading as indicated on the 360-degree dial.

There are generally two different styles of compasses: Orienteering (clear base plate) and Lensatic (military). Although either style will work in the right hands, the Orienteering style of compass is the preferred compass for SAR. Regardless of the style, all compasses have the similar basic features (Figure 10–29). Knowing the proper names for the parts of a compass is important when learning how to use it and when purchasing a compass for SAR.

Characteristics of a quality compass for use in SAR include the following:

Base Plate or Base – Clear, rectangular, and with various measurement markings and UMT scales. It is also beneficial to have a small magnifying glass in the base plate.

Bezel, Dial, Ring or Compass Housing – Marked clockwise in 360 degrees, in 2-degree increments.

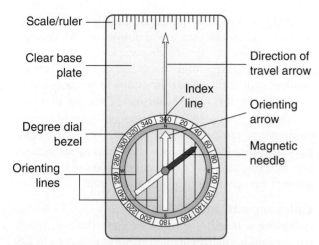

Figure 10–29 Parts of a base plate-type, Orienteering Compass. Note that a sighting compass would be similar but would extend the direction of travel arrow onto a mirror that could be used to sight a distant object much like a gun sight.

Bearing/Orienting Lines – Parallel lines within the bottom, center of the dial. These orienting lines will be used with the map to obtain headings. Most compasses also have an outline of a compass needle, called an Orienting Arrow, also within the dial, or possibly two marks near the north end of the capsule. These items are used to align the magnetic needle with the orienting arrow so that an azimuth (bearing) can be followed.

Magnetic Needle – For most compasses, the red or colored end points toward magnetic north. The magnetic end of the needle may be indicated by a small luminous dot at the point of the needle. In a quality compass, the magnetic needle usually pivots on a jeweled bearing for smooth action. To help the needle move smoothly and settle quickly, the dial is filled with a non-freezing liquid.

Direction of Travel Arrow – On most compasses, this is an arrow inscribed in the base plate of the compass, the base of which forms the index or lubber line. In higher quality compasses, this Direction of Travel Arrow might be something as small as a small luminous mark near the front end of the compass. The Direction of Travel Arrow must be pointing in the desired direction of travel while navigating.

Index Line or Lubber Line – Location where the degree reading (azimuth) is read, usually at the bottom of the Direction of Travel Arrow. The Index Line is also called the Index Mark.

Sighting Mirror – A mirror that is usually on the hinged cover of the compass, which has a fine line that runs from the top (near a rifle-like sight) to its bottom,

within the center of the mirror. This center line can also be an extension of the Direction of Travel Arrow. Not all compasses will have a sighting mirror. However, a higher quality compass with a sighting mirror is recommended for SAR. This feature on your compass will help make more accurate sightings, plus the mirror might also be used for signaling during an emergency.

The other category of compass is the Lensatic Compass. This is a good quality compass that is mostly used by the military. The Lensatic Compass is useful to those who already know how to use it; however, it may be difficult to use accurately, especially for a beginner.

There are many other kinds of compasses on the market, including some electronic varieties. These compasses have no moving parts, but the electronic units rely completely on batteries to function properly—a significant shortcoming. SAR personnel must first learn to use an Orienteering type compass before learning other navigational devices such GPS (see below) and other types of compasses.

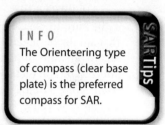

INFO
The Orienteering type of compass (clear base plate) is the preferred compass for SAR.

Navigating With a Compass

When first learning how to use a compass, it is important to remember good compass posture. To hold the compass for use, stand still with your arms comfortably at your sides, elbows bent so that both hands can hold the compass directly in front of your body. For most people, this position will have the compass at either chest-level or belt-level. The next step is to ensure that the direction of travel arrow is pointing in the same direction as your toes. To get where you want to go, your toes must always be pointing in the same direction as the direction of travel arrow on the compass. Hereafter, when you move the compass to a specific heading, move your entire body as a solid extension of the compass. Make absolutely sure that you hold the compass level so that the needle may move freely to settle on a direction.

For practice, try facing in the direction of 160 degrees. This is a three-step process:

1. First, turn your compass bezel (dial ring) so that 160 degrees is on the Index Line.
2. Second, use good compass posture. Hold the compass level with the direction of travel arrow pointing in the same direction as your toes.
3. Third, turn your entire body and compass (as one unit) until the magnetic end of the floating needle is directly aligned over the pointed end of the Orienteering Arrow painted on the bottom, center of the bezel.

The magnetic needle will still point to magnetic north, but you will now be facing a magnetic heading of 160 degrees.

To determine the bearing of a distant object (e.g., radio tower, mountain peak, etc.) from you, do the following:

1. First, use good compass posture. Hold the compass level with the direction of travel arrow pointing the same direction as your toes and turn your body until you are facing the distant object.

2. Second, turn your compass dial until the pointed end of the Orienting Arrow in the bottom center of the bezel is perfectly aligned under the pointed end of the magnetic needle.

3. Third, read the heading (number on the dial ring) at the index line at the base of the direction of travel arrow.

Be sure to check for anything near you, or on you, that might be metallic. Depending on how close you are to metallic items, the magnetic needle could be affected by the metal object(s). Keep these items away from your compass when it is use: belt buckles, watches, jewelry, brass-colored objects (many have steel in them), eyeglasses, automobiles, frame packs, utensils, ink pens, whistles, radios, vehicles, and anything else metallic. Note that power and telephone lines (anything conducting or producing electric current) can also cause deviation. Also, be aware that there are certain areas of the United States that have a high mineral content in the ground that can affect your compass. One such area located in Arkansas is appropriately named Magnet Cove.

When using a compass with a sighting mirror, use the same procedures, but the compass will have to be brought up to eye level to view distant objects using the sight. In doing so, it is still best to use both hands and keep the compass level. Most sighting mirrors have a fine line down the center that will help you align with the distant object. The mirror casing will also have a "gun site" at the top of the mirror casing, which makes it easier to sight the distant object. When the sight, direction of travel arrow, your toes, and the image of the index line are all aligned, any object viewed through the sight is directly on the heading set on the compass.

Cardinal Directions are those directions that correspond to bearings that are multiples of 90 degrees. North is either "0" or 360 degrees, east is 90 degrees, south is 180 degrees, and west is 270 degrees. If you are familiar with the cardinal directions in relationship to your position, it is easier to estimate direction of travel.

When in the field, SAR personnel should always know where north is located, with or without a compass. This provides a constant awareness of one's direction of travel and may come in handy should improvisational navigation be required at any time.

Following a Heading

Following a lengthy compass heading through rough terrain can be challenging and requires practice. To follow a heading over some distance do the following:

Once you have selected a heading, with the direction of travel arrow and your toes facing the direction that you wish to travel, sight an object in the distance. The object, such as a distinctive tree, rock, or other unique feature, must be something that is attainable, immovable, and visible. Once you have confirmed your object in the distance, close your eyes for just a few seconds. Then, open your eyes to reconfirm that you can easily find your object again. Reconfirm your heading to that object and lower your compass. Now, simply walk to the object. The route you take to the object is irrelevant. You can meander as much as you like as long as you can always see your target object. Once you arrive at your object, repeat the process with another distant object. Continue to repeat the process until you reach your destination. Generally, the further away the sighted object is, the more accurate the heading will be over a long distance. The closer the sighted object is, the less accurate the heading will be over a long distance.

Traveling a long distance on a compass bearing can be challenging but gets easier with practice. The real challenge is searching well while moving between objects and navigating around obstacles and over rough terrain. Thus, in SAR, competent navigation becomes a critical and necessary secondary skill without which your primary purpose (searching) could not be accomplished. Navigation with a map and compass must become so easy and natural to SAR personnel that they can safely focus on other issues—like finding the lost subject.

Using Map and Compass Together

When using an Orienteering Compass with a map, the compass is used primarily as a protractor and ruler. The 360-degree dial, in association with the orienting lines in the base of the bezel, serve as the protractor and the straight sides of the rectangular base plate serve as a straight edge. When using the compass as a protractor, the magnetic needle can be completely ignored.

To determine the heading from one point to another on the map, place the compass on the map so that one edge of the base plate touches both the starting point and the destination, with the direction-of-travel arrow pointing in the direction of the destination. Then, turn the dial ring until the orienting arrow, with the arrow pointing north, is parallel to the nearest north-south meridian. The heading from the starting point to the destination is now indicated on the dial ring at the index line.

The scales on the bottom margin of the map can be used to measure distance on the map. On a 1:24,000 scale map, one inch on the map equals 24,000 inches (or 2000 feet) in the terrain. To get the distance in feet in the terrain, measure the inches on the map and multiply by 2000. The bar scale can also be used directly by marking on the edge of a piece of paper the distance between two points on the map. Then, measure it against the bar scale in the bottom margin of the map (Figures 10–30 and 10–31). The base plate on the compass or the compass lanyard, in lieu of the paper, also works well.

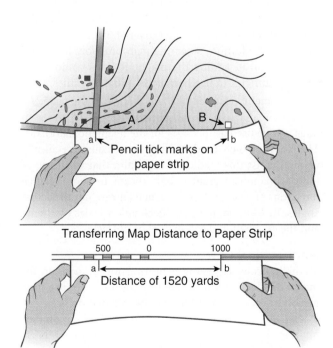

Figure 10–30 Measuring straight line map distances. Use a ruler, piece of paper, lanyard, or ruler edge of a compass, to indicate distance, then compare it to the map scale.

Adjusting for Magnetic Declination

The angle between the direction the magnetic needle points (magnetic north) and true north is called "declination." Due to the geology of the Earth, the magnetic needle on a compass only points to the north pole (true north) when the compass is along a line in the United States that (as of 2004) generally runs from just east of New Orleans, through the middle of Alabama and the eastern tip of Arkansas, through eastern Iowa and eastern Missouri, through eastern Minnesota and western Wisconsin, and up to the magnetic north pole just north of Hudson Bay. This line along which a compass needle points to both true north and magnetic north is called the "Agonic" line (Figure 10–32). East of this line, a compass needle will point west of true north (west or negative declination),

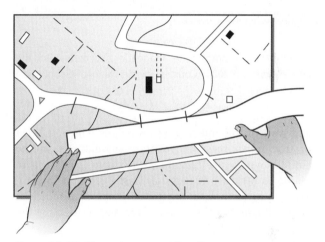

Figure 10–31 Measuring curved line distances.

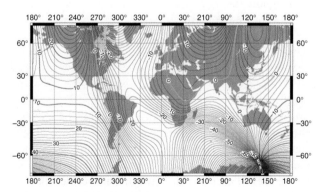

Units (Declination): degrees
Contour Interval: 2 degrees
Map Projection: Mercator

Figure 10–32 Approximate magnetic declination around the Earth. The green lines are agonic lines on which declination is zero. (Courtesy of the National Geophysical Data Center.)

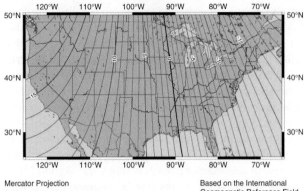

Magnetic Declination for the U.S. 2004

Mercator Projection

Contours of Declination of the Earth's magnetic field. Contours are expressed in degrees.
Contour Interval: 1 Degree (Positive declinations in blue, negative in red)

Produced by NOAA's National Geophysical Data Center (NGDC), Boulder, Colorado

Based on the International Geomagnetic Reference Field (IGRF), Epoch 2000 updated to December 31, 2004

The IGRF is developed by the International Association of Geomagnetism and Aeronomy (IAGA). Division V

http://www.ngdc.noaa.gov

Figure 10–33 Approximate magnetic declination in the United States in 2004. (Courtesy of the National Geophysical Data Center.)

and west of this line a compass needle will point east of true north (east or positive declination). In the United States, declination varies from 20° west in Maine to 30° east in parts of Alaska. The declination diagram in the bottom margin of a topo map indicates the declination in the center of the map at the time the map was printed (**Figure 10–33**).

If you know the magnetic declination of the area in which you will be navigating, you have four options:

1. Ignore it.
2. Adjust for it on the compass.
3. Adjust for it by drawing magnetic meridians (north-south lines) on the map.
4. Adjust for it mathematically.

Ignore It

In some situations, magnetic declination can be ignored altogether. When using a compass without a map, all references should be made to magnetic north and so declination is irrelevant. If you are operating on the agonic line (see above) where the angle between magnetic declination and true north is zero, magnetic declination can be ignored even when using a map and compass together. The same philosophy may be applied when the compass being used has 2-degree increments on the dial ring and you are operating in an area with a declination of less than 1 degree. The level of accuracy at which you are navigating makes adjusting for small declinations unnecessary. The inverse is also true: If your compass is extremely accu-

rate and has 0.5-degree increments on the dial, and you will be using the compass with a map, corrections should be made for even the smallest magnetic declination.

Adjust the Compass

Some compasses have a small screw on them that allow the user to adjust the compass for declination. This is a simple and easy method of adjusting for declination that is often used in SAR. What adjusting the compass does is offset the orienting arrow and the index line in the base of the bezel just enough to compensate for declination when the compass is used as a protractor with a map. Once adjusted, the orienting arrow in the bezel is no longer parallel to the orienting lines. A scale marked in the bezel allows the index line to be offset in relation to the orienting lines for the precise amount and direction of magnetic declination.

Make sure to check the adjustment on the compass each time it is used with a map.

Draw Magnetic Meridians on the Map

Another way to account for magnetic declination is to prepare the map by adding magnetic north lines to it. If magnetic north-south lines are drawn on the map, the magnetic needle on a compass will point to the north end of the lines drawn on the map. Adding these lines requires a protractor, long straight edge, and the angle of declination. On computer generated topo maps, the lines can be added with a click of the mouse. Because of the difficulty in accomplishing this manually, especially with multiple maps, this method is not recommended for SAR. In addition, since the map probably has UTM grid lines on it, adding the magnetic lines could make the map difficult to use because of too many lines.

If this method is used, the actual angle in the magnetic declination diagram in the bottom margin of the map must not be used as the basis for the magnetic meridians. The USGS, which produces the topo maps, specifically warns against this method. They claim that the angle of the declination diagram is only meant to show relative directions of true, grid, and magnetic north, not the actual angles. In addition, magnetic declination varies over time and the declination diagram may be obsolete.

Mathematical Correction

Mathematically adjusting a bearing to compensate for magnetic declination is another option. To use this method, you must first know if the declination is east or west. Determine this by inspecting the declination diagram in the bottom margin of your map. If the "MN" is to the left of the star in the diagram, the declination is west. If the "MN" is to the right of the star in the diagram, the declination is east. Next, you must determine if you are going from the map to the compass (e.g., plotting a bearing based on the true north lines on the map, then using the bearing to navigate with a compass) or going from the compass to the map (e.g., taking a bearing with a compass then plotting it on the map). This combination gives you four options for mathematically correcting for magnetic declination, and each of the four options has a rule for correcting for declination (**Table 10-1**). Since most SAR personnel are unlikely to use both easterly and westerly declinations—they mostly stay on one side of the agonic line or the other—the rules necessary to mathematically correct for declination are usually reduced to two.

The simplicity of the rules makes remembering them easy, but the similarity between the options also makes it likely that they will be confused with each other. Worse, using the wrong set of rules (adding when you should have subtracted) will actually double the error of declination. So, it is recommended that a small note be added to one's map case or compass that includes the two rules most likely to be used, or just copy Table 10-1, reduce it in size, cut it out, and attach it to your map case or compass. This will preclude the need to remember the various rules and reduce the chances of error.

Declination Correction Examples
Here are two examples of using the magnetic declination adjustment rules to correct the magnetic declination:

Example 1: In the bottom margin of your map, you note that the declination diagram indicates that the magnetic declination is 4 degrees east. You plot a course on the map from point A to point B using true north and determine that the bearing is 100 degrees (true). What is the bearing you would follow in the field to travel from point A to point B? Using the magnetic declination adjustment rules found in Table 10–1, you determine that the declination is east and you are going from the map to the compass. So, the rule that applies is to "subtract declination." Since the map course was 100 degrees, and the declination is 4 degrees east, the magnetic course to follow in the field is a bearing of 96 degrees (100 − 4).

Example 2: The declination diagram indicates that the magnetic declination is 9 degrees west. You follow a compass heading of 355 degrees (magnetic) to travel from a church to a distant peak. Arriving at the peak, you note that there are many similar peaks in the area and you want to determine which one on the map you are on. So, you want to draw a line on the map that indicates the route you just traveled. Using the magnetic declination adjustment rules found in Table 10–1, you determine that the declination is west and you are going from the compass to the map. So, the rule that applies is to "subtract declination." The corrected bearing for the map would be 346 degrees (355 − 9). Using your compass as a protractor, enter 346 degrees at the index line of the compass. With the direction of travel arrow pointing from the church to the peak on the map and the edge of the compass base plate next to the church, turn the entire compass (base plate and all) until the orienting lines in the compass bezel are aligned with the true north lines on the map. Draw a line from the church along the edge of the compass base plate. The peak on which you stand is on that line.

When adjusting for declination, it is very important that it be compensated for properly (according to one of the accepted methods described above) and only ONCE. Accounting for declination twice is just as bad as accounting for it improperly. Be very careful and practice often.

OPERATIONS
"Orient" your map by turning it so that north on the map points to north in the landscape.

SARTips

Using the Map and Compass in the Field
An important step in using a map as a guide in the field is to "orient" it. Orienting the map means to turn it so that north on the map points to north in the landscape. Once this is done, the terrain and man-made features on the map should align with the same features in the field. To do this, inspect the map and the surrounding landscape and, using a compass to help determine when you are facing north, turn your body while holding the map until the compass, map, and landscape all match. This can also be done while turning the map and compass on the ground (**Figure 10–34**).

Table 10–1	To correct for magnetic declination, determine if declination is east or west, and then establish if you are going from map to compass or compass to map.	
	East Declination	**West Declination**
Map to Compass:	Subtract declination	Add declination
Compass to Map:	Add declination	Subtract declination

Map Orientation With Compass

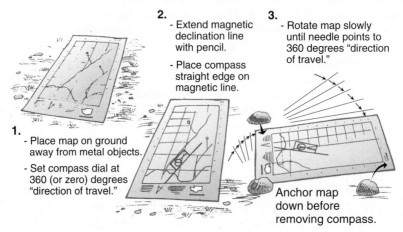

2.
- Extend magnetic declination line with pencil.
- Place compass straight edge on magnetic line.

3.
- Rotate map slowly until needle points to 360 degrees "direction of travel."

1.
- Place map on ground away from metal objects.
- Set compass dial at 360 (or zero) degrees "direction of travel."

Anchor map down before removing compass.

Figure 10–34 Orienting the map to the surrounding landscape using a compass.

It also may be useful to determine your exact location on the map. Either of two approaches should work to determine your location, depending on your situation: observation and resection (triangulation).

In the observation or inspection method, simply visually identify features or landmarks in the landscape by looking around. Then, slowly turn the map around until the features on the map actually match the features within sight of where you are standing (Figure 10–35).

In the resection method a compass is required. But, it starts the same way: Look around and identify features or landmarks in the landscape around you. Then, determine the bearing from your location to the feature/landmark you see (Figure 10–36). Let's assume that the bearing is

70 degrees (magnetic) to a radio tower on a nearby mountain peak and try an example.

Leave the heading of 70 degrees on your compass and place the compass (now used as a protractor and ignoring the magnetic needle) on the map with the edge of the base plate immediately next to the distant object (tower on mountain). While keeping the edge of the base plate on the map next to the tower, pivot the edge of the compass around the tower until the Orienteering lines in the bottom of the bezel are aligned with the north-south grid lines on the map. When using this method, the Orienting arrow on the compass should always be pointing to the top (north) of the map. Once everything is aligned, draw a line with the edge of the compass through the distant

Point Position from Observation

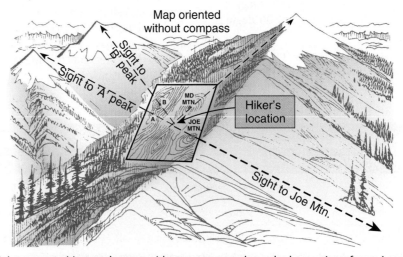

Map oriented without compass

Sight to "B" peak

Sight to "A" peak

MD MTN

B

A

JOE MTN

Hiker's location

Sight to Joe Mtn.

Figure 10–35 Determining your position on the map without a compass through observation of prominent features or landmarks in the terrain.

Point Position
from Oriented Map and Compass Bearings

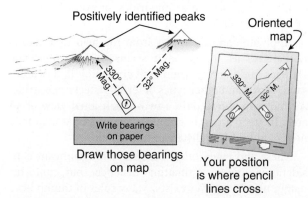

Figure 10–36 Determine your position using a compass and map together (resection). Using three prominent points can add accuracy to the position.

object (the tower in this example). Your location is somewhere on this line. To narrow down your location on this line, select another distant object that is approximately 90 degrees from the first object you chose. For our example, let's assume you also see a water tower at a bearing of 160 degrees. Follow the same procedure as you did with the first distant object and draw a second line on the map. The intersection of the two lines is very close to your location on the map.

Other Compass Skills

Traveling at night with a compass presents many of the same problems as traveling through dense underbrush. Using a flashlight properly with a compass at night can

simplify things substantially, and using a flashlight improperly at night can hinder the most skilled navigator. A dim wide-beamed light can be held underneath the base of the compass, pointed primarily in the direction of travel, to allow some light for reading the compass at night. However, care must be taken not to shine the light in anyone's eyes. When the needle is aligned with the Orienteering Arrow, the light can be directed in the direction of travel where an object can be sighted. Some compasses also have a small light integrated into the compass. The light is small and just the right size to easily see the heading while not disturbing night vision.

Traveling around obstacles is often necessary in the field when using a compass for navigation. The easiest way to travel around an obstacle, such as a lake, pond, cliff, or other hazard, is to sight an object beyond the obstacle and then travel to that object by the easiest route possible. This approach, however, is limited to those obstacles that can be seen over or through. When obstacles cannot be seen over or through, a completely new course may be required, or a method similar to the one in Figure 10–37 can be used.

Measuring Distance by Stride: "Tally"

A method of estimating distance in the field may be required for some situations in SAR. Distance can be estimated by knowing the length of one's stride and multiplying it by the number of strides walked.

Being able to estimate distance traveled in the field can be of value in several situations that often arise in SAR. For instance, estimating distance can be of value

Navigating Accurately Around Obstacles

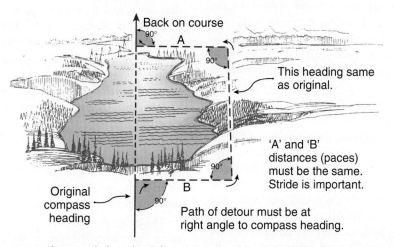

Figure 10–37 Navigating accurately around obstacles. Take a 90° turn right or left of obstacle. Count paces until clear of obstacle (B). Resume original bearing until past obstacle. Take 90° turn opposite of first turn and walk exact distance as you did to clear the obstacle (A). Continue on original bearing.

when a mapped object or area is a known distance from a starting point (measured from a map) and searchers want to know when, in their travels, to start looking for the object or area. Also, being able to estimate how far a clue was found from the start of a search might be valuable during debriefing.

The English term "mile" is derived from a Roman term meaning "1000 Roman Paces" or double steps. The Romans considered the pace to be five times the length of a Roman legionnaire's foot and, thus, the Roman mile was 5000 feet. It wasn't until much later that the English mile was redefined as 5280 feet.

One step is the distance one walks when measured from one foot to the other. A stride, on the other hand, is equivalent to two steps, or the distance between where one foot strikes the ground and where the same foot strikes the ground again. The Roman stride was nearly 6 feet, but the average stride today is usually considered 5 feet on level, unencumbered ground. Stride will vary depending on many variables such as leg length, terrain, weather, darkness, fitness, and many others.

Measuring your stride is sometimes referred to as finding your "tally." To find your tally, you will need to set up a course in your local terrain and practice. Use a long piece of string and measuring tape to set up a meandering route in the woods of some easily remembered distance such as 50 meters or 100 feet. It is important not to use a straight line course because your stride will need to naturally adjust for low branches, thick underbrush and other natural obstacles. Walk the string route several times over several days and keep track of the number of strides it takes to cover the course. Walk the route with your 24-hour pack in the morning while you are still energetic, and then also walk the route with your pack in the late afternoon after several hours of hiking or other physical exercise. Once you have completed the course several times, under several conditions, take the number of strides for each trial and obtain an average (add up the total strides and divide the sum by the number of trials. This will be your personal "tally" for determining distances in your terrain. If your course was 100 feet long and it took an average of 20 strides to cover the course, your tally is 20 strides for 100 feet, or five feet per stride.

Strides can vary substantially from one individual to another, so it is important for individuals to know their own personal stride length. Once one's stride has been determined, a method of counting strides over long distances becomes necessary. To do this, some have tied knots in string every 100 strides to keep all counting less than 100. Moving pebbles from one hand or pocket to another every 100 strides, and other similar techniques, have also been used. In SAR, especially when accurate count is important, a good method is to carry a small hand counter (also known as an inventory counter) and use it to count strides, or every 10 strides, or every 100, etc.

Applying counted strides from the field to a map is not always as simple as it seems. A person's stride changes in different terrain. Tall grass, uphill, downhill, sand, rocks, and other types of terrain affect one's stride. A topo map shows only a two-dimensional view of an area. In steep areas, horizontal distances on a map may not equal traveling distances in the field.

These and many other problems are significant considerations when estimating distance, but, unfortunately, no easy answer exists. Many rules of thumb have been proposed, but it is probably better if all SAR workers simply keep records of their traveling, estimate their personal differences, and make their own conversions for field work.

One appointed "tally" person per team can constantly keep track of distance traveled from a starting point. This can be valuable when estimating where in a search segment a clue is found, for example, or anytime a rough estimate of distance traveled is desired. Because of how much concentration it takes to constantly count strides during a search, it may not be prudent to ask only one person keep the tally, operate the radio, and navigate simultaneously.

Global Positioning System (GPS)

The Global Positioning System (GPS) is a space-based radio-navigation system consisting of a constellation of satellites and a network of ground stations used for monitoring and control. A minimum of 24 GPS satellites orbit the Earth providing users with accurate information on position, velocity, and time anywhere in the world and in all weather conditions. GPS is operated and maintained by the U.S. Department of Defense (DoD).

GPS has three parts: the space segment, the user segment, and the control segment. The space segment consists of the 24 satellites, each in its own orbit 11,000 nautical miles above the Earth. Each of the GPS satellites takes 12 hours to orbit the Earth. The user segment consists of receivers, which you can hold in your hand or mount in your vehicle. The control segment consists of ground stations (5 of them, located around the world) that make sure the satellites are working properly.

The principle behind GPS is the measurement of distance (or "range") between the receiver and the satellites. The satellites also specify exactly where they are in their orbits above the Earth. If the exact distance from a satellite in space is known, then we are somewhere on the surface of an imaginary sphere with radius equal to the distance to the satellite radius. If the exact distance from two satellites is known, then we are located somewhere on the line where the two spheres intersect. But when there is a third measurement from a satellite, there are only two possible points where we could be located. One of these is usually impossible, and the GPS receivers have mathematical methods of eliminating the impossible location.

The GPS satellites are positioned in orbit so that signals from six of them should be received nearly 100% of the time at any point on Earth. Signals from six satellites are required to get the very best position information. GPS satellites are equipped with very precise clocks that keep accurate time to within 3 nanoseconds, which is three billionths of a second. This precision timing is important because the receiver must determine exactly how long it takes for signals to travel from each GPS satellite to calculate its position. To measure precise latitude, longitude, and altitude, the receiver measures the time it took for the signals from a minimum of four separate satellites to get to the receiver.

For the system to accurately establish position, altitude, and velocity, the receiver must "acquire" four satellites. The acquisition of signals from three satellites can convey one's position on the earth's surface, but a fourth signal is required for altitude information. "Acquire" means that the unobstructed signals from four satellites

need to be received by the receiver. For this to happen there must be four satellites above the horizon above the receiver and the system is designed to achieve this everywhere on Earth. Because the GPS signal is in the 1 GHz (Gigahertz, or 1000 Megahertz) range, terrain (i.e., trees, hills, buildings, etc.), the metal from a vehicle (i.e., car roof, airplane fuselage, boat cabin, etc.), and even the human body can block the signal and make acquisition difficult or impossible. Clear, line-of-sight access between he receiver's antenna and the satellites is necessary for best results. Keep this in mind if you are trying to obtain GPS signals from a deep ravine or in a forest with heavy tree cover.

The GPS system can tell you your location anywhere on or above the Earth to within about 300 feet. Even greater accuracy, usually within less than three feet, can be obtained with corrections calculated by a GPS receiver at a known fixed location.

GPS receivers can be hand carried or installed on aircraft, ships, tanks, submarines, cars, and trucks. These receivers detect, decode, and process GPS satellite signals. More than 100 different receiver models are already in use. The typical handheld receiver is about the size of a cellular telephone, but the newer models are even smaller (Figure 10–38). The nearly 10,000 handheld units distributed to U.S. Armed Forces personnel during the Persian Gulf War weighed only 28 ounces.

Handheld GPS units are now available and being used by outdoor enthusiasts as well as SAR teams. However, it

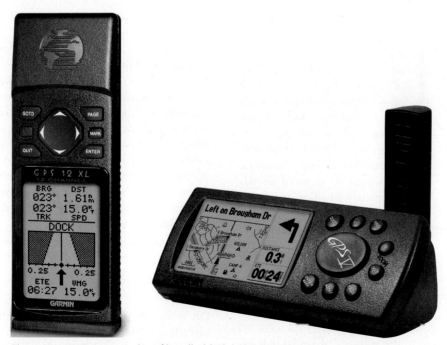

Figure 10–38 Two examples of handheld Global Positioning System (GPS) devices.

is critical to note the applications and limitations of such units before purchasing or using one in the field. The many challenges involved in the use of GPS by untrained personnel include the following:

- The device requires line-of-sight to the satellites and will not work in all terrains (i.e., deep canyons, heavy tree canopy, urban environment with tall buildings, etc.).
- GPS should not be used as the sole navigation device, but should complement other conventional approaches to navigation.
- The less than perfect accuracy is not always acceptable, especially for altitude.
- Human error (input error) is always a possibility.
- The position display can easily be misread, and the display can give the impression of far greater accuracy than the device is capable of.
- Especially considering today's GPS technology, which requires great current consumption, batteries can fail at any time. Typical battery life of most GPS units is between four and six hours.
- Many GPS units are not waterproof and require special protection during bad weather. The GPS units also need additional protection if crossing streams or near other water sources.

It is important to note that the GPS receiver is simply another tool in the land navigation skill "tool box" and it should never be considered a substitute for map and/or compass knowledge. In the hands of a skilled navigator, a GPS unit can provide significant benefits in the areas of expediency, precision, documentation, and reference. GPS is dependent on multiple variables, many of which are beyond the control of the user; these include power supply (batteries), satellite integrity, and signal strength. If one of these elements were to fail or be substantially weakened, the operator would be required to rely completely on alternate navigational skills. Regardless of the GPS equipment used and available, SAR personnel must be well versed in map and compass skills prior to utilization of a GPS unit.

The information contained herein is of a general nature and pertains to no specific model or type of GPS unit. The intention is to provide general information that will be pertinent to the majority of available mod-

els. It is highly recommended that SAR personnel attend a hands-on GPS training program and practice with GPS units in an outdoor setting before using the unit in a real-world SAR operation.

Common Components and Nomenclature

Although there are a variety of GPS units made by various companies, they all possess common components that are integral to their function.

Battery

Most GPS units take either two or four AA batteries that are housed in a plastic casing located in the base or back of the unit. GPS unit instruction manuals may state that the unit is "water resistant" or "waterproof." Read the specifications to determine the limits of each unit. While any appropriately sized batteries will work in the GPS unit, alkaline batteries generally produce the best results. Ni-cad and NiMH batteries are convenient because they are rechargeable; however, the rechargeable type of batteries usually do not have the full power of the alkaline batteries, plus the rechargeable batteries require the use of a charger. The more expensive lithium batteries may provide the best performance in cold-weather operations.

Always keep batteries stored at room temperature when not in use. It is also a good idea to carry at least one extra set of batteries as a backup. When outdoors, store the unit and spare batteries near the body within layers of clothing to avoid exposure to extreme cold or heat. In the event the batteries become very cold, re-warm them before use to avoid reduction in battery life. This can be done by holding the batteries in the palm of your hand for several minutes prior to use. Some GPS units may have an internal memory battery to retain information while the normal batteries are removed. These backup batteries will recharge automatically when the regular batteries are replaced. This process will take approximately 24 hours if the backup battery is completely drained. Memory batteries usually have a lifespan of about three months; after this time all user information and the almanac will be lost until the unit has reacquired a satellite signal and the information is renewed. Most of the newest generation GPS units do not require a backup battery because the data are stored in nonvolatile memory.

To limit the number and weight of the batteries, it would be wise to choose a GPS unit that uses the same battery as your light sources.

Keypad

On many of the older style GPS units the keypad is placed on the face while some of the newer models have placed many of the keys along the sides. Most of the keys will be adorned with a short label or some type of icon to signify its function, and many of the keys are also multifunctional. This means that a specific number of keystrokes can control a specific function or by depressing a key for a specified period of time will access another function. For example, pressing a key one time may display a certain menu, while pressing the same key two times in succession displays another. The interface keys are so diverse from one unit to the next that it is best to refer to the instruction manual to determine the functions associated with each key. If possible, try to find a unit that has a safety on the "on" button to help keep the GPS unit from being turned on by accident while in your pack.

LCD

The liquid crystal display (LCD) is the screen that shows the various menus or pages. Depending upon the make and model of the GPS, the LCD will vary in size, but it is the most sensitive component of the unit. Extreme heat will cause the screen to display nothing but a blackened image and in extreme cold little, if anything, can be seen. A sufficient impact upon the LCD can also cause it to "bleed" and malfunction.

Antenna

Almost all handheld GPS units house an internal antenna and provide the option of a plug-in external antenna. The antenna receives information called ephemeris from satellites in the form of a two-spread spectrum radio frequency signal (~1575 MHz). The antenna is often housed in the top of the GPS unit. Any obstruction between the antenna and the satellite will degrade the signal quality and hinder accuracy or proper functioning. This kind of signal degradation is often referred to as antenna masking. Reception is best at high elevations with 360 degrees of visibility; however, this does not mean that your GPS will not work while in densely forested areas. It is important to note that foliage does degrade signal quality and hence will lengthen acquisition time, possibly increase the estimated position error (EPE), and slow down ephemeris updates. Also note that if you are trying to use your GPS in a steep canyon, or an area of heavy foliage, it is more than likely that the antenna will not be able to receive appropriate signals from satellites for a correct display.

Satellite Characteristics

It is not necessary to know everything about the satellites in order to properly use a GPS unit, but some basic information may be useful, especially as it relates to terms that are frequently used to describe the GPS system.

NAVSTAR GPS Satellites

The satellites in the GPS are in carefully controlled orbits around the Earth at an altitude of approximately 11,000 nautical miles. The complete constellation consists of a minimum of 21 satellites and 3 working spares. Currently there are 27 total satellites in orbit and it is possible that there could be as many as 32. The goal of the system is to always provide at least four satellites somewhere in the visible sky. In practice there are usually many more than this, sometimes as many as 12.

Selective Availability (SA)

Before May 2000, all civilian GPS units received satellite information that contained built-in errors that limited accuracy. This error was designed for security reasons and was referred to as "selective availability" (SA). The use of SA has now been discontinued, so theoretically all GPS units can now achieve an accuracy of approximately 12 to 15 meters horizontal and vertical.

Differential GPS (DGPS)

DGPS is a method of improving the accuracy of a GPS receiver by adding a local reference station to augment the information available from the satellites. It also improves the integrity of the entire GPS system by identifying certain errors. The estimated accuracy while using DGPS is approximately 3 to 5 meters horizontal and vertical. In DGPS operation, a station, often called a beacon, transmits correction data in real time that is received by a separate box, called a beacon receiver, which in turn sends the correction information to the GPS receiver.

Wide Area Augmentation System (WAAS)

The Wide Area Augmentation System (WAAS) is the latest method of providing improved accuracy from the GPS system. It is similar in principle to the DGPS capability that is built into most of the recent GPS units except that a second receiver is not required. Instead of a beacon receiver, the correction data are sent via a geostationary satellite and are decoded by one of the regular channels already present in the GPS receiver. Thus, up to 2 of the 12 channels can be designated to decode regular GPS signals or can be used to decode the WAAS data. This works through the use of a set of ground stations all over the United States that collect correction data relative to the area of the country where they are located. All of the data are then packaged together, analyzed, converted to a digital correction format by a master station, and then uploaded to the geostationary satellite, which in turn transmits the data down to the GPS receiver. The GPS receiver then figures out which data are applicable to its current location and then applies the appropriate corrections to the receiver.

The WAAS system is still being set up and will be improved with more satellites in the future (possibly dozens worldwide). Because of the type of satellites used, a clear view of the southern sky is required to benefit from WAAS from the northern hemisphere. This means WAAS units are very useful on an airplane or perhaps a boat, but may be less useful to someone on the ground with a limited view of the horizon.

GPS Unit Screen Pages

Most GPS units display information in the form of screen "pages." Although various manufacturers display their pages slightly differently, they all have certain characteristics in common.

Satellite Page

The satellite page is usually the first functional screen or page to be displayed by the GPS unit (**Figure 10–39**). Although the satellite page will vary from unit to unit, most GPS satellite screens will be similar. Some of the newer GPS units will display more information and a select few will display less. The purpose of the satellite screen is to convey the current status of the connection between the GPS receiver and the GPS satellites.

Receiver Status The receiver status is the current type of satellite lock or mode. There are several messages that could be displayed to give the user a better idea of the current status of their GPS unit. These messages include:

- *Searching*—Unit is currently searching the sky for satellites.

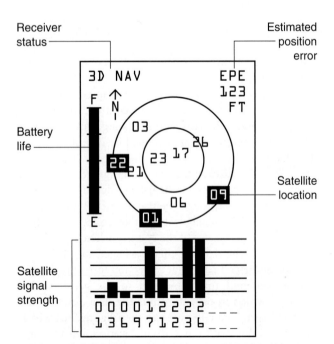

Figure 10–39 Satellite page on a Garmin GPS 12XL. (Courtesy of Garmin, Ltd.)

- *AutoLocate*—Unit is collecting new almanac data.
- *Acquiring*—Unit is collecting data prior to its first lock.
- *2D Nav*—Unit has a lock on horizontal position and is looking for a three-dimensional lock.
- *3D Nav*—Unit has a lock on both horizontal and vertical position and tracking normally.
- *2D Diff*—Unit has the two-dimensional lock using DGPS data.
- *3D Diff*—Unit has the three-dimensional lock using DGPS data.
- *Not Usable*—Unit was not able to compute a solution.
- *Poor Coverage*—Unit is attempting to compute a position but is having difficulty.
- *Enter Altitude*—Unit is requesting the user to input the approximate altitude to aid in acquiring a signal.
- *Simulator*—Unit is in simulator mode.

Battery Life There is a graphic representation of the battery life based upon alkaline batteries, with the exception of a select few GPS units that allow the user to define the battery type. Some units will not display the battery life if connected to an external power source, while others will display a full battery. Many newer units have placed this feature on a different page.

Satellite Signal Strength A bar graph represents the signal quality between particular satellites and the GPS receiver. The numbers on the bottom of the graph represent the individual satellites. The bars above each satellite number correspond to the signal strength of that satellite. If no bars are displayed, then no connection has been established. If a hollow bar is displayed, the receiver has found the satellite and is collecting data from it. When a solid bar is displayed, the receiver has collected data (ephemeris) from the satellite. Some GPS units have slight variations in their display. For example, a select few units use solid bars to identify when the receiver has acquired the satellite and a hollow bar to signify that it has collected the ephemeris. For almost all 12-channel GPS units, 12 openings will be displayed in the bar graph. The receiver will attempt to acquire all 12 satellites, but will choose the best four satellites from which to collect information. If the receiver is WAAS enabled, it will leave two openings strictly for WAAS satellites. Currently, WAAS satellites are distinguishable by a number designation above 32.

Satellite Position This diagram depicts the relative location of each satellite within range. Upon first turning on the GPS unit, these satellites will be arranged in accordance to the receiver's location and built-in almanac (stored data). The almanac will be fairly accurate if the receiver has acquired near the location before. This is often referred to as a "warm" start. If the user has traveled a distance of more than 300 to 500 miles with the unit off, then the almanac will have significant errors and the receiver will take longer to acquire. In many cases the GPS unit will prompt the user to redefine the general location to aid in acquisition (a "cold" start). The unit's satellite almanac will update once the GPS has collected ephemeris. Each satellite in the diagram is represented by its respective number and will correspond with the number shown in the satellite signal strength bar graph. The concentric circles represent the relative position of the satellites in the sky. The top of the screen typically represents north, so satellites represented at the bottom of the screen would be south of the receiver's current position. Some models allow control over where north is represented. The center of the diagram represents directly overhead, the first circle beyond the center denotes 45 degrees above the horizon, and the final circle corresponds to the horizon itself. So in the sample page, above satellite 09 would be on the southeast horizon.

Estimated Position Error (EPE) Sometimes labeled as "accuracy," the estimated position error is the manner in which the receivers attempt to give the user an idea of the approximate position discrepancy between what is given by the GPS unit and its true position. This number can be represented in either feet or meters depending upon the unit display properties found in the menu options. It is important to note that this number is a rough estimation and in many cases cannot be trusted. It is best to double the EPE number displayed to provide a safe margin of error.

Position Page

In many of the newer GPS units, the position information has been integrated with other pages and is sometimes called the trip computer page (Figure 10–40). The purpose of this screen is to provide the user with pertinent information concerning his or her position. This page displays several optional fields, meaning some may be modified to show different information. In this section the most widely used and pertinent of these fields will be discussed. Depending upon the unit used, these terms may be labeled differently (with or without acronyms), or not be available.

Optional Field Terminology

Position (POS) – The current position of the receiver displayed in the position format and datum designated by the user in the menu options.

Time – The current time displayed in the format designated by the user in the menu options.

Speed (SPD) – The current speed the unit is traveling displayed in the format designated by the user in the menu options (sometimes called, Speed Over Ground [SOG]).

Bearing (BRG) – The direction from current location to destination. In many new GPS models, this is displayed in cardinal direction, degrees, or mils. For use in land navigation it is best to set this for degrees. It is also important to note that the value will vary depending upon the north reference setting. If using a GPS unit with a compass, the north reference should be set at mag north.

Course Over Ground (COG) – Direction of the line connecting your previous position with your next position. This value is dependent on your definition of north. 'North' could be true north, magnetic north, grid north, etc., depending on the GPS setting (sometimes called: Course, Track [TRK], or Heading [HDG]).

Distance (DST) – The distance between the receiver's current position and the desired destination displayed in the format designated by the user in the menu options.

Altitude (ALT) – The current altitude of the receiver displayed in the format designated by the user in the menu options.

Estimated Time of Arrival (ETA) – The estimated time that the user will reach the desired destination, calculated by velocity made good.

Estimated Time Enroute (ETE) – The estimated time required to travel to desired destination, calculated by velocity made good (sometimes called: Time To Go [TTG], or Time To).

Turn (TRN) – The angle difference, in degrees, between the bearing to the destination and the current course

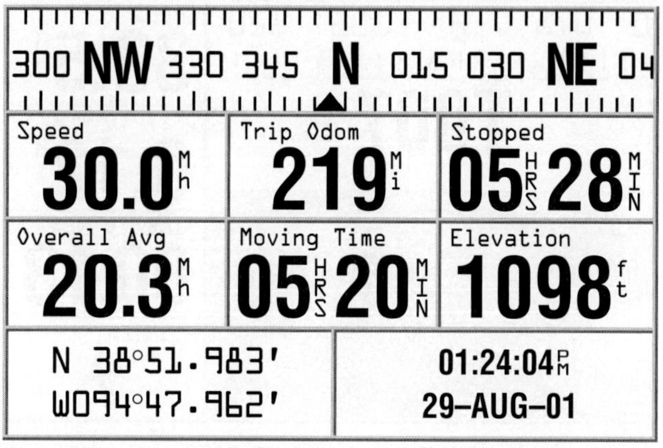

Figure 10–40 Position page on a Garmin V. (Courtesy of Garmin, Ltd.)

of the user. "L" represents turn left and "R" means turn right (sometimes called: Course To Steer [CTS]).

Velocity Made Good (VMG) – The speed the user is closing in on a destination along a desired course (sometimes called, Vector Velocity).

Cross Track Error (XTE) – The distance off desired course in either direction (sometimes called, Off Course or Course Error).

Odometer – A running tally of the distance traveled by the user.

Compass/Highway Page

The screen in **Figure 10–41** shows an example of the compass page (sometimes called the Pointer Page) on the top and the highway page on the bottom. Both of these pages are used as a reference page when navigating to a waypoint. Once again, it is important to note that this screen will vary somewhat depending upon the model of GPS.

Compass Page This page is labeled the compass page because of the compass-like diagram depicted. Although this diagram looks like a compass, it is not and should never be used as such. Some GPS models have an electronic compass built into them and although they can be utilized as a compass, they do not rival the accuracy or functionality of a traditional compass. The electronic compass will need to be selected within this page and calibrated before it can be used, otherwise the diagram of the compass will give the current track (TRK, see course over ground [COG]) like the models that do not have a built-in electronic compass. This feature will not work correctly if the receiver is not in motion. This happens because all the GPS is doing is displaying what direction the user has traveled from when it last updated its ephemeris. Most receivers have an update rate of once per second, but it is important to understand that TRK displayed is only as accurate as the position information. Within the compass diagram is the bearing indicator arrow. This arrow depicts the bearing and direction that the user must travel in order to reach the currently selected waypoint. Along with the compass diagram and direction indicator, several optional fields are displayed as well as the name of the destination or waypoint (see Position Page section for a description of these optional fields).

Highway Page This page looks similar to the compass page, with the exception that the highway diagram is in the place of the compass diagram. The highway diagram consists of a three-dimensional perspective road, with the receiver's position at the base of the road and the desired destination at the other end. If the user is heading directly towards the destination, the road will appear straight, and if the user drifts off course, the road will veer left or right to inform the user to compensate for the course deviation. As with the compass page, various optional fields are present as well as the name of the destination or waypoint (see Position Page section).

Map Page

This page contains a graphical representation of the unit's current position, nearby waypoints, possibly the user's track log, and a map of the area if loaded into the GPS unit. Each GPS manufacturer utilizes its own map software. This software is under constant development and is progressively expanding to meet the various needs and desires of the community. The layout of this page can vary significantly from model to model; however, nearly all models will have a pan feature (ability to go side to side), the ability to zoom in and out, and some type of scale. Some models will also have optional fields displayed such as the example in **Figure 10–42**. Review the owner's manual for specific instructions in using this page.

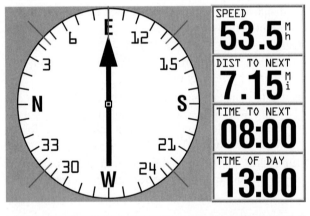
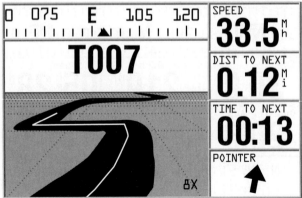

Figure 10–41 The compass/highway page of a Garmin V. (Courtesy of Garmin, Ltd.)

Menu Page

Most menu pages are accessed by simply scrolling through the different screens; however, some GPS units utilize an actual menu button to display this page. Within the menu the user will find a slew of various options for customizing the receiver and interfacing with other features. The submenus found within the main menu will vary from unit model to unit model. It is important to note which submenus are needed to customize the receiver to function properly when used during navigation.

Customizing GPS Settings

Using a GPS for land navigation requires several skills, including the ability to alter GPS unit settings and input waypoints and routes.

The purpose of altering the unit's settings is to not only personalize the user's preferences, but to also set the GPS up to work in conjunction with a map and compass. If the settings of the receiver do not correspond to the grid format or datum of the available maps, the position information will not be able to be translated from the GPS unit to the map. If the magnetic declination is not set to work with a compass, the discrepancy found when using both could confuse the user and lead to faulty navigation. The information given below will address where and when to alter the GPS unit's settings during land navigation. With all the different manufacturers and models of GPS units, it would not be practical to give the exact button configurations for every type. It is best left for the user to consult the receiver's user manual to learn the exact location and button configuration for the specific unit. Most of these settings will be found in the main menu.

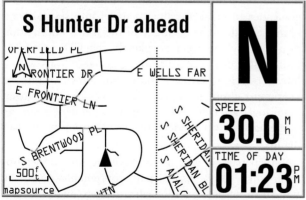

Figure 10–42 Map page of a Garmin V. (Courtesy of Garmin, Ltd.)

Units

This setting determines what types of units will be displayed by the GPS. The typical unit settings include: statute (i.e., miles, feet, inches), metric (i.e., kilometers, meters, millimeters), and nautical miles (marine-based units). Most models default to the statute system. For some models there is one field to alter the unit settings, and the settings are established throughout the entire receiver. Many of the newer GPS units allow the user to customize variable information fields to display different unit settings. For example, the distance may be given in meters (metric system), while the altitude displayed in feet (statute system).

Datum

A datum is a mathematical model of the Earth's shape and dimensions that is used in conjunction with a grid projection to create a coordinate system used for plotting position on the Earth's surface. Different maps often have a different datum that affects the projection format. If the corresponding map datum is not selected within the GPS unit, the coordinates given by the receiver could be inaccurate up to 900 meters depending upon the datum selected. The map datum is normally given in the marginal information of a USGS topographical map listed under horizontal datum. Most GPS units default to WGS84.

Position Format

The position format is the grid projection used to designate a coordinate system for plotting a position on the Earth's surface. When using a GPS in conjunction with a map, the user needs to select the position format that corresponds to the one to be utilized with the map. Maps typically have several grid systems on them. The most common within the United States include Latitude/Longitude (hddd.ddddd°, hddd°.mm.mmm′, and hddd°.mm′ss.s″), and Universal Transverse Mercator (UTM) grids. Most GPS units default to Latitude/Longitude.

Time/Universal Time Coordinate (UTC)

The GPS receiver will automatically determine your local time from UTC once it has collected these data from the satellites. A select few receivers require the correct time deviation of the area's local time from the UTC to be inputted. If an incorrect time deviation is input, the position information will be inaccurate. Some GPSs have the ability to adjust the UTC offset, and it is always a good idea to check and ensure the correct data are entered. It is also important to remember to compensate for daylight savings time during this operation. Many units will automatically do this, and some have the option of being set to automatic update or user specified.

Magnetic Declination

Magnetic declination (also known as variation) is the angular difference between true north and magnetic north. This variation comes into play when using a compass with a map during navigation. When using a GPS device in conjunction with a compass, it is important to ensure that the correct declination is loaded into the receiver; otherwise the GPS may give a faulty bearing. Typically this setting is referred to as the "North Reference." Most GPS units have an auto feature in that the proper declination is set as soon as the unit has acquired. The most common options in the receiver for the north reference are that of: True North, Mag North, Grid North, and User. True north uses the north value without compensating for magnetic variation. This is fine to use as long as the user is not using the GPS information in conjunction with a compass (unless the user compensates for the magnetic variation in some manner). Mag north will automatically calculate the proper declination once the GPS has acquired, and then the unit bearing information is ready to be used with a compass. The Grid north option will reference north, based upon the grid projection of the area. In most cases this option should not be used. The User option allows the user to select a north point. If User is selected, it is important that the declination be adjusted when operating the receiver in a different area or with a different map.

Waypoints

Waypoints are position coordinates that the GPS unit will store in its memory. Different models have a different limit on the number of waypoints that can be stored. Most units can store a minimum of 250 waypoints, while the newer units usually have a capacity for up to 1000. Different models also have different means for marking a waypoint; the user manual should be referenced to see how this is done. When marking a waypoint with the GPS, you will have the option of designating a name or symbol for ease of reference in the future. Most models will default the name with a number identification from 001 to 999 depending on available openings. For example, if the user inputs a waypoint at 001, then the next default waypoint name will automatically go to 002. Once the name and symbol is designated, the waypoint will be stored in the unit's database for future use. Most units store only the horizontal data, but a select few also can store the elevation. To aid in accuracy, some receivers also have an averaging feature that allows the unit to assign the waypoint to a more accurate position. Once the unit has done this, it will assign a figure of merit (FOM) to indicate the probable accuracy of the position information.

The user can also input coordinates of a position without having to travel there. For most units this is done by accessing the main menu and selecting the waypoints or landmarks submenu. It is best to refer to the receiver's user manual to see how this is done. Before this is done, the user needs to ensure that the position format and datum are set to the map from which the coordinates are derived. The user will then be given several data fields to input including: waypoint name, possibly symbol if supported, position coordinates, and user comments if supported. Once the user has input the proper information and saved it, the waypoint will be stored in the receiver's memory for future reference.

Yet another means to plot a waypoint is to use an existing waypoint as a reference point, and then input the distance and bearing from this reference point. This information is normally gleaned from a map and compass. This method of plotting a waypoint is often referred to as projecting a waypoint, and is less reliable than the methods described earlier.

Routes

A route is a collection of waypoints strung together to reach a final destination. Many users find this option unnecessary because the final destination can simply be input into the receiver as a waypoint. Routes can come in handy if a direct approach to the final point is not possible or if the distance to the final point is significant. To circumnavigate around an obstacle, simply input waypoints that head towards the final point but will take a course around the obstacle. Once the user has reached the first waypoint, the GPS unit will direct the user to the next waypoint and so on until the final point is reached. The number of waypoints is dependent upon the type and size of the obstacle to be avoided. Waypoints should be determined by using a map to plot the best possible route. Once this is done, the user should input a waypoint for each section of travel that requires a direction change. If traveling a large distance, it is a good idea to break the line of travel into several waypoints to aid in the accuracy of the travel information displayed by the receiver, namely the ETE and ETA. Routes also can be used to designate rest stops with a line of travel. To create a route with the GPS unit, the user must input all applicable waypoints and group them together. How this is done is dependent upon the particular receiver model and can be found in the user manual.

SAR personnel who are expected to use GPS equipment—like any specialized equipment—must be trained in its use, practice with it often, and possess a full appreciation of its limitations.

SAR Terms

Bearing The direction of an object measured in degrees from north.

Declination The angle between the direction the magnetic needle points (magnetic north) and true north.

Ephemeris A table giving the coordinates of GPS satellites at a number of specific times during a given period.

Geographic Coordinate System Navigating using a system of reference lines called parallels of latitude and meridians of longitude.

Global Positioning System (GPS) A space-based radio-navigation system consisting of a constellation of satellites and a network of ground stations used for monitoring and control.

Topographical (topo) maps Type of map that portrays the shape and elevation of the terrain with lines, while showing a graphic representation of selected man-made and natural features on a part of the Earth's surface plotted to a definite scale.

Universal Transverse Mercator System (UTM) Navigating using a special grid used worldwide.

References

Bowditch, N. (2002). *The American Practical Navigator: 'Bowditch' 2002 Bicentennial Edition*. Arcata, CA: Paradise Cay Publications.

Burns, B., Burns, M., & Hughs, P. (1999). *Wilderness Navigation: Finding Your Way Using Map, Compass, Altimeter, & GPS*. New York, NY: Mountaineers Books.

Cox, M., & Fulsass, K. (eds.) (2003). *Mountaineering: Freedom of the Hills*, 7th ed. New York, NY: Mountaineers Books.

El-Rabbany, A. (2002). *Introduction to GPS: The Global Positioning System*. Norwood, MA: Artech House.

Ferguson, M., Kalisek, R., & Tucker, L. (1997). GPS land navigation. In: *A Complete Guidebook for Backcountry Users of the NAVSTAR Satellite System*. New York, NY: Glassford Publishing.

Gatty, H. (1999). *Finding Your Way Without Map and Compass*. Mineola, NY: Dover Publications.

Hodgson, M. (2000). *Compass & Map Navigator*, revised ed. Guilford, CT: Globe Pequot Printers.

Jacobson, C. (1999). *Basic Essentials Map & Compass*, 2nd ed., revised. Guilford, CT: Globe Pequot Printers.

Johnson, M. (2003). *The Ultimate Desert Handbook: A Manual for Desert Hikers, Campers, and Travelers*. New York, NY: Ragged Mountain Press/McGraw Hill.

Kals, W.S. (1983). *Sierra Club Land Navigation Handbook: Sierra Club Guide to Map and Compass*. San Francisco, CA: Sierra Club Books.

Kjellström, B. (1994). *Be Expert With Map and Compass*. Somerset, NJ: John Wiley & Sons.

Letham, L. (2001). *GPS Made Easy: Using Global Positioning Systems in the Outdoors*, 3rd ed., revised. New York, NY: Mountaineers Books.

Manning, H. (1986). *Backpacking: One Step at a Time*, 4th ed. New York, NY: Vintage Books.

McManners, H. (1998). *The Complete Wilderness Training Book*. New York, NY: DK Publishing.

Peters, J.W. (2002). GPS Navigation Guide. In: *http://www.GPS Navigator Magazine.com*, Eugene, OR. Accessed October 2004.

Petzoldt, P. (1974). *The Wilderness Handbook*. New York, NY: W.W. Norton & Company, Inc.

Randall, G. (1998). *The Outward Bound Map & Compass Handbook*, revised ed. Guilford, CT: The Lyons Press.

Rawlins, C., & Fletcher, C. (2002). *The Complete Walker IV*, revised ed. New York, NY: Alfred A. Knopf, Inc.

Chapter 11

SAR Resources and Technology

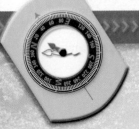

Upon completion of this chapter and any course activities, the student will be able to meet the following objectives:

List at least three advantages and three disadvantages for five types of operational resources that may be used for SAR. (p. 177-192)

List three ways to categorize SAR resources. (p. 176)

List three human and animal resources. (p. 177-184)

Describe differences between tracking/trailing and air-scenting canines. (p. 183)

List at least two uses for aircraft in SAR operations. (p. 185)

Resources

A "resource," when used in regards to search and rescue, refers to a person, group, or piece of equipment that has the ability to contribute to an operation or organization. A resource is simply an asset that lies ready for use or can be drawn upon for aid. A single person is termed an "individual resource," whereas a collection of individuals and their equipment are called a "group resource." A dog team is a resource and so may be a fisherman with a fish-finder. Anyone or anything that could serve as an asset in a SAR event may be considered a resource.

At its most fundamental level, search and rescue requires participants to be versed in a wide variety of skills and information. However, operational effectiveness in SAR occasionally requires the utilization of individuals and/or groups that have special knowledge. Here, some common and some not so common areas of specialization are discussed. Although this text does not go into great detail describing each particular search and rescue resource, the following information is intended to offer a general description of the various specialties and equipment that may be called upon to help resolve a SAR problem.

There are many ways to categorize SAR resources, but common methods most often depend on the type of specialization of the particular resource. In the end, categorizing resources boils down to three basic subdivisions:

- Human and animal
- Informational
- Equipment and technology

It is a combination of these three subdivisions that provides SAR personnel with the potential resource base to solve operational problems. Rarely does a single resource offer only one option or application to a task. Rather, it is a thorough understanding of resource capability and complementary applications that gets the job

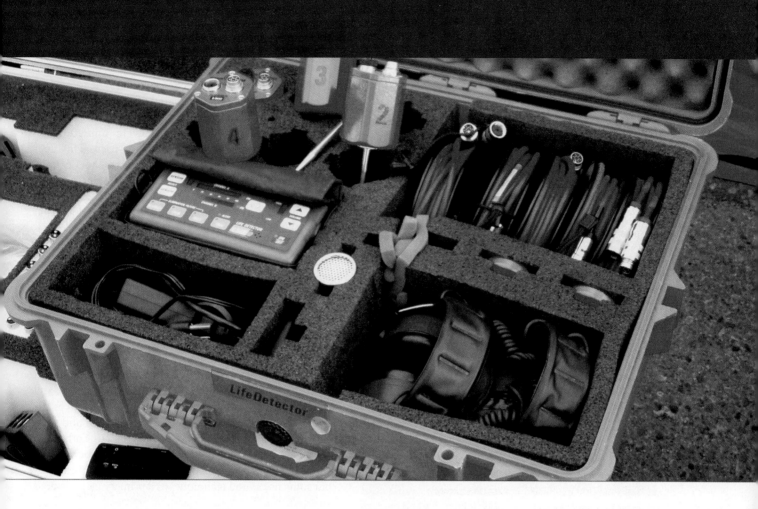

done. The intent here is to familiarize SAR personnel with what is available and the potential application of these resources.

It is impossible to identify all the potential information sources that are available to individual SAR teams. This chapter is intended only as a primer to provide an overview of the vast array of options available regarding what might be useful in SAR incidents and to expose SAR personnel to some of the resources with which they might become involved. In this age of information technology, nearly all data imaginable exist somewhere. It is up to the individuals and teams who need these data to determine exactly how to get it.

Human and Animal Resources

The emphasis under this category is on the capability of the resource. Equipment or an unusual environment may be involved, but it is usually only incidental to the application of some specialized, required skill or capability.

Searchers

Three types of human search resources are discussed: hasty teams, grid search crews, and human trackers. Each has its own uses, benefits, and limitations.

Hasty Teams

Hasty teams are small (usually 3 members), well-trained, highly mobile, self-sufficient, clue-conscious teams that provide the backbone for state-of-the-art search efforts. They utilize fast, non-thorough search tactics in areas most likely to produce clues or, better yet, the subject(s), quickly. The efficiency and usefulness of hasty teams are based upon how quickly they can respond and the accuracy of the initial information.

Ideally, these teams should include two or three individuals who are: track and sign aware; clue and subject oriented; familiar with the local terrain and dangers; completely self-sufficient; able to skillfully interview witnesses; possess pinpoint navigational skills; capable of traveling quickly into the field; and be at least advanced first aid trained. Hasty teams usually operate under standard operating procedures so that they do not have to wait for specific instructions, and they carry all the equipment they might need to help themselves and the subject for at least 24 hours.

Sources of hasty teams usually include organized SAR teams and some emergency response agencies.

Grid Search Crews

Using a more systematic approach to searching, grid search crews primarily use vision to search in a well-defined, usually small, segment of land or water

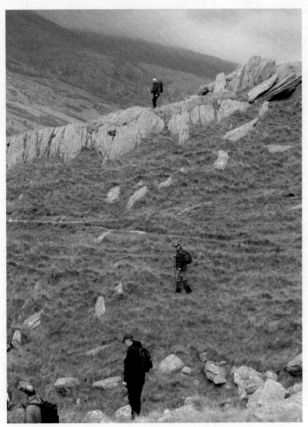

Figure 11–1 Grid searching is resource-intensive and tends to be very damaging to evidence. Therefore, it is generally less preferred to other methods which utilize fewer personnel in a more efficient manner.

(Figure 11–1). The classic approach to grid searching involves several individuals (almost always too many) standing in a line, and then walking together through an area in search of either evidence or subjects. However, such resource-intensive approaches to searching are generally less preferred to those which utilize fewer personnel in a more efficient manner (e.g., hasty teams, tracking, dogs, aircraft, etc). In addition, tight grid searching (see Chapter 15, Search Operations) tends to be very damaging to evidence and generally difficult to coordinate.

Tight grid search teams perform either tight grid searches (thus, the name) or evidence searches. The objective of tight grid teams is to search a segment to a high probability of detection (POD). The objective of the same group in an evidence search is to search very thoroughly in a very small area for inanimate objects, not live subjects. Although grid teams can be invaluable in the right situation, they are usually so damaging to the environment and evidence that they are only called as a last resort. This type of resource also requires many

searchers, often making such teams difficult to coordinate and manage. Unlike many other resources, grid teams may consist of a mixture of trained and untrained searchers and, thus, may have severe limitations in terms of when and where they can be used. This does not mean, however, that all unskilled searchers can accomplish the same results. As a minimum, at least half of any grid team should be trained in navigation, search techniques, team organization, communication, and other skills that can allow the supplementary use of untrained personnel. It is also important to note that when grid teams are used in a segment, any clues not discovered in the area are very likely destroyed forever.

Loose grid search teams are very similar to tight grid teams except they may not maintain visual contact with adjacent searchers while searching. Thus, these teams must have more skilled members who can travel and act somewhat independently. This relative independence requires that members of this type of team be skilled at navigation, communication, self-sufficiency, survival, and general search techniques. The often large distances between searchers allows fewer people per team and so is easier to administrate and coordinate with other resources. These types of teams often mix sound (i.e., yelling and whistle-blowing) into their visual searches, but some use sound techniques as a primary tactic (sound sweeps).

Since loose grid search teams need to be self-reliant and skilled, sources of this type of resource usually include organized SAR teams and other emergency services agencies that can supply skilled personnel. Tight grid search teams, on the other hand, can be supplemented with personnel from any physically capable source, even if the individuals are untrained in SAR.

Human Trackers

Trackers use primarily their visual senses to search for evidence left by a person's passing (Figure 11–2). They "cut" or look for <u>sign</u> (discoverable evidence) by examining the area where the subject would likely have passed. This process of looking for the first piece of evidence from which to track is called <u>sign cutting</u>. Following the subsequent chain or chronology of sign is called "tracking." In SAR, most trackers use a stride-based approach called the "Step-by-Step" Method. This method is simple, methodical, and emphasizes finding every piece of possible evidence left by a subject.

Tracking is a very visual skill and requires a great deal of practice and experience to achieve even a limited level of effectiveness. However, all searchers should be trained to a minimum level, referred to by many as "track aware." This entry level allows all searchers to at least be aware that tracks and related evidence exist. First, searchers must know to look for this type of evi-

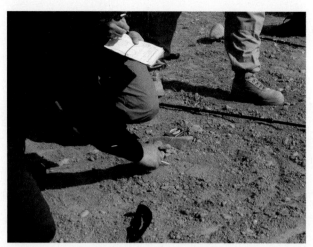

Figure 11-2 Human trackers use primarily their visual senses to search for evidence left by a person's passing.

dence. Second, they must learn how to find it. In the end, the most important role for tracking is undoubtedly its ability to quickly determine the direction of travel of the subject and, thus, limit the search area.

Organized SAR groups are a good source of trackers, as are the United States Border Patrol and some other law enforcement and military agencies. However, care should be taken to assess the individual's unsubstantiated tracking ability. In most SAR situations, depending on someone who claims to be able to track but cannot actually do it is far worse than not having a "tracker" at all. For more information on tracking, see Chapter 13, Tracking.

Technical Rope Rescuers

The word "technical" precedes components of search and rescue where very specialized techniques are applied to the study of a science, art, or craft. Technical rope rescue applies to those specific rescue techniques that involve rope and its related equipment.

Rope rescue is required in many different environments and is often what novices envision when thinking about rescue in general. In reality, rope rescue is a complex tool used in the rescue function to achieve a goal that cannot otherwise be achieved. Rope rescue is a very specialized discipline that involves equipment such as ascenders, pulleys, friction devices, and carabiners; it includes skills such as tying knots, rigging a mechanical advantage system, and rappelling.

When rope rescue is required, there is almost always an elevation differential necessitating the use of rope rescue equipment to either raise or lower one or both of the rescuers and subjects. Because it does not take much of a fall to seriously injure a person, rope rescue is considered both hazardous and exciting.

Organized SAR teams are a good source of rope rescue resources, both in terms of equipment and personnel. However, fire service, law enforcement, park services, and often emergency medical agencies have substantial rope rescue capabilities that should not be overlooked.

I N F O
"Sign cutting" is the process of looking for the first piece of evidence from which to track.

SAR Tips

More information on rope rescue and evacuation can be found in Chapter 16 (Rescue).

Management

Management resources are often among the most important to the success of an incident, especially when extended operations and planning are required. Several specific types of management resources are often keys to effective command and control.

Search Planning and Management

The specific functions required to effectively plan and manage a search, especially an extended or large one, often require highly trained individuals. In particular, the following functions (using ICS nomenclature) should be staffed by specialists:

- Incident Commander
- Investigation Unit Leader
- Communications Unit Leader
- Information Officer
- Operations Chief
- Logistics Chief
- Plans Chief

Excellent training is available for each of these areas of specialization and individuals with these skills can be invaluable during a SAR event (Figure 11-3). However, do not overlook individuals who may not be formally trained in SAR, but still possess the necessary skills and/or contacts to get the job done.

Organized SAR teams are good sources of these specialists and should be planned ahead of time, much in the same way that tactical resources are done, because they are not always available within the immediate area or jurisdiction.

Logistical Support

Food, shelter, and other logistical concerns are often difficult obstacles during a SAR event. Using specially skilled personnel in this support function can often make a substantial difference in the comfort and safety of all human resources.

Sources of these specialists are often numerous and can be provided by civic organizations, the Red Cross,

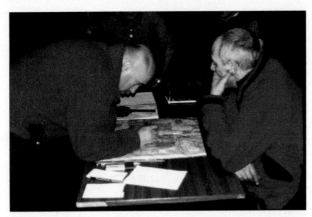

Figure 11–3 Management resources are among the most important to the success of any incident and should not be taken for granted. Photo courtesy of M. Gibbings.

the Salvation Army, church groups, auxiliaries of emergency services agencies (i.e., fire department auxiliary), military bases, and private vendors.

Investigators/Interviewers

Investigation is a management skill that is required in every SAR event. Getting the information required to institute an effective and efficient search takes a great deal of practice and skill. In the end, a properly conducted investigation will often make the difference between success and failure. One crucial skill involved in investigation is extracting information from people through asking questions or interviewing. A novice will ask extraneous questions, sometimes not ever getting to the right ones, and will usually take far too long to extract the pertinent information. The most skilled interviewers know exactly what questions to ask, how to ask them, and whom to ask. A properly conducted interview often abbreviates the entire investigation process and produces both planning (i.e., what should we do?) and searching (i.e., where should we look?) information.

Law enforcement agencies are classically the source for the best interviewers because interviewing is an integral part of their job. However, search and rescue organizations and individual specialists can also have much to offer.

Communications Support

In addition to the internal communications systems of responsible organizations and support agencies, specialized communication support, such as portable radios, cell phones, and radio operators, is often available from:

- REACT units
- CB clubs
- HAM operators

In many areas, one phone call to the right person can get all the necessary communication resources supplied at an incident.

Facilities

An important component of the incident command system, especially when the command structure grows large in size, is predesignated incident facilities. When many people must be fed, housed, and rested, the physical requirements can be both numerous and extraordinary. Some thought should be given to accommodating the following resources during the planning stages of larger incidents.

- Extra telephones and lines
- Computer and fax equipment
- Photocopy equipment
- Transportation (trucks, buses, aircraft, etc.)
- Sanitation facilities (dumpsters and portable toilets)
- Temporary shelter (tents, canopies, mobile homes)
- Portable heaters or air conditioners

As the size of an incident grows, so do the requirements of the physical facilities. Resources that improve the comfort and usability of these facilities can be invaluable as the incident increases in size and complexity.

Critical Incident Stress Management (CISM) Teams

There are hundreds of CISM teams in the United States, and many more in other parts of the world. CISM teams are made up of mental health professionals, trained emergency services personnel (peers), and clergy who provide an organized means by which individuals who have experienced a "critical incident" can be helped. A critical incident is an event faced by emergency workers that creates unusual or acute emotional reactions which interfere with their ability to function.

Environment-Specific Personnel

The harsher the environment, the more difficult it is to meet operational SAR objectives. Harsher and more hazardous environments also require personnel to be able to overcome both environmental and operational challenges simultaneously. Thus, specialized groups have evolved to address those special situations.

More information on the specific hazards of the various environments as well as how to travel through them may be found in Chapters 8 (Safety in SAR Environments) and 12 (Travel Skills: Foot Travel for SAR Personnel).

Mountaineers

Mountainous or alpine environments often involve both technical terrain (i.e., steep slopes, scree slopes, rock cliffs, etc.) and inclement weather in addition to their relative remoteness. The combination of dangerous terrain, diverse, severe weather, and extreme isolation makes this environment one of the most dangerous on the planet for SAR.

SAR personnel working in this environment are required to be prepared for just about anything. It may be warm, it may snow, or it may rain. It may be calm, or wind may make it difficult to stand. Simple hiking may be suitable for most travel, but rock and ice climbing, snowshoeing, and belaying may also be required. The catch phrase is, "be prepared for anything," including unusual medical conditions (Figure 11–4). For example, acute mountain sickness, also known as altitude illness, is a condition related to working at high altitudes that can be fatal if not recognized and treated properly.

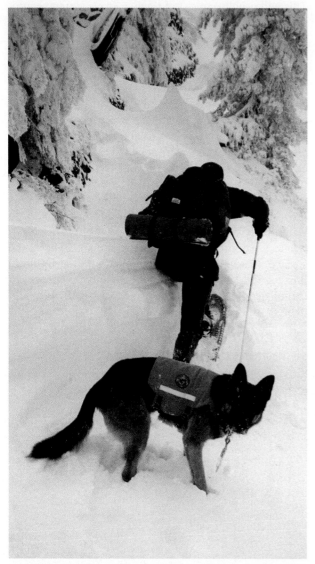

Figure 11–4 SAR personnel working in the mountain/alpine environment are required to be prepared for just about anything.

SAR units that specialize in the skills and equipment required to effectively and safely operate in remote alpine environments can be found throughout the United States, but are mostly located in the Rocky and Coastal Mountain areas of the west. Many of these units are affiliated with the Mountain Rescue Association (MRA), a nonprofit organization dedicated to the research, development, and distribution of search, rescue, communications, and medical information, primarily as it relates to the alpine environment.

Ice, Snow, and Cold

Just about every SAR unit has to deal with a cold environment at one time or another, but some have the additional challenge of dealing with extreme cold, ice, and snow frequently. Alpine and arctic units must often travel through cold environments, over ice and snow, to meet their objectives. For these units, and others working in similar environments, technique and equipment measures beyond those taken by most units may be required. Avalanche shovels, cords, transceivers, and probes are the tools of the SAR trade in snow-covered alpine terrain. Crampons, snowshoes, Nordic skis, and arctic clothing are also frequently required by members of units operating in cold, snow, and ice-covered environments. Hypothermia and frostbite are a common concern, and cold weather emergency service units must be adept at recognizing and treating them.

The National Ski Patrol is an educational organization dedicated to serving the public and the ski industry by promoting ski safety and providing educational services so the membership can deliver emergency care. Ski Patrollers often become involved in SAR in the cold and snow environment and, much like the MRA, serve as a good place to turn for information regarding training.

Subterranean (Cavers)

The underground environment is special in that nowhere else can a person experience such absolute darkness, the distinctive odor of wet rock and mud, constant cool temperatures, and perfect silence. Perhaps this is what has drawn people into caves for thousands of years, thus requiring someone to go in after individuals who have become lost or injured.

Caves and mines are common in today's society. Construction projects, mining, and spelunking (caving) are daily occurrences requiring individuals to exist and travel safely underground. SAR in these areas is particularly specialized because the environment necessitates equipment and skills that are considered only conveniences in other places. The absolute darkness requires multiple sources of reliable light, the dampness and cool temperatures require addressing the extreme potential for hypothermia, and the confined nature of the environment requires safety equipment to prevent injury. Many of the skills and equipment from other SAR disciplines are used in the subterranean environment (i.e., ropes, rescue hardware, etc.), but modification of techniques and equipment are also required to maintain safety and effectiveness.

Today, confined space and cave rescue units are well equipped to deal with lost or injured people in the underground environment. Teams that specialize in confined space rescue usually limit themselves to the urban setting and specific environments such as tanks, basements, and the like. However, cave rescuers specialize in the natural underground environment and will likely be the resource of choice in a caving incident. Not only will local cavers be familiar with the general environment, but they will also likely know the layout of the particular cavern involved.

In 1941, the National Speleological Society (NSS) was formed. From their association with others with similar interests, local cavers formed chapters (grottos) and, from there, potential rescuers found a place to exchange ideas. The first people called to rescue a lost or injured caver were other cavers, so local grottos often formed their own formal or informal cave rescue groups. Over the years, regional networks and eventually a national network evolved.

In 1977, the National Cave Rescue Commission (NCRC) was organized as a commission of the NSS. The NCRC is not a response organization, but rather a communications network, operated by volunteers, developed to coordinate cave rescue resources throughout the United States. In addition, the NCRC also serves as an equipment cache for specialized cave rescue equipment, a clearing house for cave rescue information (i.e., training, equipment, personnel, etc.), and a sponsor of training seminars.

The Mine Safety and Health Administration is a federal agency charged with establishing and enforcing standards for the health and safety of mine workers in the United States. They are a good source of information regarding equipment and safety in the subterranean environment. Additional resources that might be helpful in supplying equipment are mining equipment stores and outdoor recreational equipment retailers.

Aquatic (Water SAR)

Aquatic environments include everything from surf to rivers and lakes. Each specific type of aquatic environment has its unique characteristics and hazards, including those shared with other environments (i.e., hazardous materials, confined space, caves, etc.).

All responders to the aquatic environment must be trained and equipped for the specific types of situations in their area. For instance, coastal teams must be able to negotiate heavy surf and possibly strong currents; teams in the mountains or near fast flowing rivers/irrigation canals must train in swift water river rescue techniques with the possible use of rope systems. U.S. Air Force Pararescue personnel are equipped to drop mid-ocean to assist distressed boats or downed aircraft; the Navy trains surface swimmers to rescue pilots who have either ditched or ejected over water.

The most common surface operations for aquatic rescuers will likely be of the swift water variety (Figure 11–5). This will usually consist of rigging a rope system; equipping the rescuer with wet suit, helmet, knife, gloves, harness, boogie board, and fins; preparing a standby rescuer (or diver), similarly equipped; rigging safety ropes downstream; and then trying to reach and retrieve the victim.

Water rescue, particularly swift water, is one of the most dangerous areas of technical rescue. Although advances in technology have made water rescue safer, rescuers still need to receive special training before undertaking rescue in this environment. There are numerous cases where rescuers have drowned trying to save a victim because improper equipment and techniques were used or because of inadequate training. Rescuers must learn how to recognize hidden hazards associated with water, such as current, water level, lowhead dams, backwashes, hydraulics, and any hazard not apparent on the surface. In addition, moving water has the capability of pinning individuals against rocks, submerging them in turbulence, or impaling them on rocks, branches, and debris. All water rescuers should be trained in self-

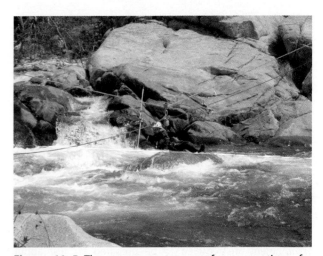

Figure 11–5 The most common surface operations for aquatic rescuers will likely be of the swift water variety.

rescue techniques, and should be familiar with local water conditions.

Where the victim submerges below the surface of the water, similar rigging, techniques, and equipment will need to be applied by divers. Diving is tenfold more dangerous to rescuers than surface operations, and should, therefore, be approached much more cautiously and only by those completely familiar with its hazards.

Aquatic rescue expertise can usually be procured from local water rescue units or individuals, public safety dive-rescue units, or organized dive organizations (e.g., Diver's Alert Network, National Association of Underwater Instructors, SCUBA Clubs, etc.). For information on Public Safety Diving and water rescue, contact the International Association of Dive Rescue Specialists.

Hazardous Materials

Hazardous materials, often called "haz mat," refers to any substance or chemical that may be harmful or dangerous to humans. The realm of hazardous materials touches so many aspects of emergency response that the federal government has enacted legislation (Superfund Amendment and Reauthorization Act [SARA], Title III) and regulations (Code of Federal Regulations [CFR] 1910.120), which require all responders who have the possibility of encountering hazardous materials to have at least basic and recurrent recognition training. For personnel who will mitigate and manage a hazardous material incident, additional training is required.

Although all rescuers (in an ideal world) should have hazardous materials recognition training, haz mat technicians with considerable training and skill are needed to handle anything more than the most minor spill or leak. In the United States, this type of resource is usually available through the fire service.

Confined Space

According to the National Fire Protection Association (NFPA), a confined space is a space that has all of the following characteristics:

1. Is large enough and so configured that a person can enter and perform assigned work.
2. Has limited or restricted means for entry or exit.
3. Is not designed for continuous human occupancy.

Examples of confined spaces include tanks, vessels, silos, storage bins, hoppers, vaults, wells, trenches, cisterns, and pits.

To perform a rescue in a confined space requires very specialized equipment and skill. In addition, federal legislation and regulations apply to operations in most types of confined spaces. Why does the federal government care so much about this particular environment? Because this environment has claimed disproportion-

ately more workers' and rescuers' lives than other environments, and has earned the respect and attention of both rescue personnel and regulatory agencies.

If rescue operations in a confined space are necessary, or anticipated, qualified confined space rescue personnel must be procured, and the local fire department is a good place to start. Industrial complexes and utility companies may also have resources available.

Animals

Although many animals may have some use in a SAR operation, two stand out as being used regularly around the world in search and rescue: dogs and horses.

Dogs

A dog team is comprised of one or more dogs (usually only one) and a human "handler." There are two types of dogs that are commonly used in SAR: tracking/trailing dogs and air scenting (searching) dogs. Each type differs in its approach to searching and its value depends upon varying factors. Considerations, such as when in the search the animals will be used (early or late), weather, and skill of the handler, all enter into determining the type and effectiveness of the team.

Humans give off a constant stream of scent, like an invisible smoke, which is mostly made up of skin cells that are constantly being shed (40,000 per minute). These cells, their associated bacteria, and body secretions are detectable by a dog as they either float through the air or come to rest in the environment. Air scenting dogs detect the scent as it floats through the air, while tracking/trailing dogs detect the scent (along with crushed vegetation) as it comes to rest on the ground (or snow, or rubble, or water, etc.). Tracking/trailing dogs frequently work on lead, require a scent article to establish the scent, and follow very closely on the trail of where a person traveled, regardless of the wind. Air scenting dogs, on the other hand, work off lead to follow a subject's scent to its source and do not require a scent article. Specifically bred and trained air scenting dogs can even discriminate between individual humans.

The most skilled dog handlers train for years with the same animal in order to assure that it will be an eager worker with an agreeable temperament, have good manners, and learn to communicate with its handler. The communication flow is two-way, however. The dog learns what is desired and expected of it, and the handler learns to read what the dog is sensing. The ability of a handler to know when the dog is on the trail or has "alerted" to scent is acquired through many hours, and often years, of practice (Figure 11–6). It is this ability, and the degree to which it is honed, that differentiates a trained SAR dog handler from a dog owner.

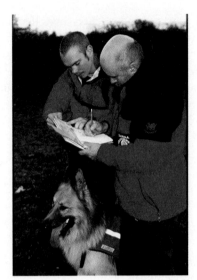

Figure 11–6 The most skilled dog handlers train for years with the same animal in order to assure that it will be an eager worker with an agreeable temperament, have good manners, and learn to communicate with its handler. Photo courtesy of M. Gibbings.

As with most specialized resources, dog teams are only as good as their training and experience. It is not unreasonable for a SAR manager to ask about a dog team's experience and training, and they should have no problems describing it. However, there are no universally set standards or qualifications for dogs and their handlers. Although some qualifications have been set by various organizations (i.e., NASAR), strict adherence is rarely required. It is also important to note that the best dog teams have handlers who are skilled at far more than just dog handling. Just like with other resources, cross training in navigation, communication, and other SAR skills is important.

Dog teams are a highly efficient resource and are often quite effective as first responders or as part of a hasty team. Dogs work well at night when visual searching is difficult, and usually require very little support beyond transportation. They work well in most environments and have been used successfully to locate subjects and clues buried in snow, rubble, and even under water (the scent floats to the surface). Generally, dog units are available through organized SAR units, law enforcement agencies, and specialized SAR dog organizations such as CARDA (California Rescue Dog Association), NASAR (National Association for Search and Rescue), and Dogs East.

Equine

Horses and mules act primarily as a means of transportation for equipment and at least one rider who may be a searcher. Unlike many other vehicle-resource combinations, horses and skilled riders can travel far with very little support in difficult terrain. So, horses can be valuable for transporting supplies and equipment as well as for searching remote or rough terrain. The problem is that these equestrian units can be quite damaging to the terrain and certain evidence, and it is difficult to search for small or subtle bits of evidence from horseback. As long as their limitations are known, horses can be a valuable asset, especially in the right circumstances. In addition, while horses generally do not actively search (like a dog), they have been known to alert in some way when in close proximity to a lost subject.

Law enforcement agencies, local "dude ranches," and horseback guide services are all good sources of horses and experienced riders. Some areas of the country also have organized equestrian units that specialize in the use of horses for SAR.

Informational Resources

Informational resources are those data bases and technical information sources that can be accessed when research is necessary for both planning and operational decision making. Information sources such as technical manuals, the Internet, poison control centers, U.S. Weather Service (NOAA), state and local SAR data bases, lost subject behavior studies, and accident statistics from the National Safety Council all provide a rich source of data for complex problem solving in SAR.

As an example, weather information can be difficult to acquire without specialized training like that offered to pilots. Federal Aviation Administration (FAA) resources such as Flight Service Stations (FSS) and Air Route Traffic Control Centers (ARTCC) are usually available around the clock with current weather and predictions. However, radio and TV news organizations, specialized cable weather channels, the U.S. Department of Commerce's National Oceanic and Atmospheric Administration (NOAA), and military bases can all provide accurate current and forecast weather information.

There is probably no better source for weather information in the United States than an experienced, current pilot who can access the federal aviation system's (FAA, FSS, ARTCC) weather information. Usually, all he or she might need is a telephone (800-WX-BRIEF in the United States).

Equipment and Technology

In SAR, equipment and technology can combine to deliver operational and support capabilities that as little as 10 years ago were not even possible. Specialized transportation such as aircraft and specialty vehicles, electronic devices, and extraordinarily capable communications equipment are just a few examples of this constantly expanding realm of resources being applied to meet SAR objectives.

Aircraft

Aircraft can serve the same purpose as grid searchers only from a greater distance, at a greater speed, over a larger area, and usually with a lower level of thoroughness.

Within a search effort, aircraft can serve both as a tactical tool to look for clues and as transportation for personnel and equipment. Both fixed-wing and rotor-wing aircraft have their place in SAR and, as other resources, have their advantages and limitations. Among the most obvious limitations are the expense and complex use requirements of aircraft. Aircraft not only take very specialized personnel and cost a great deal to operate, they also have very strict weather and environmental restrictions. For instance, it would be difficult to search from an aircraft in a snowstorm, and terrain may prevent searching certain areas from the air. However, most of these difficulties can be adequately addressed and minimized in a well-developed preplan.

Helicopters are useful for the movement of supplies and equipment, search area evaluation (planning), and for actual searching (Figure 11–7). The military is a common source for this type of resource, usually through a local base or the Rescue Coordination Center (RCC), but many private and/or volunteer providers also offer services.

The MAST (Military Assistance to Safety and Traffic) program was created by Public Law 93-155 in November 1973. Under this law, the U.S. Army and Air Force have identified certain units to assist local governments in maintaining an effective emergency service. The MAST program is a temporary measure to fill local needs in areas where civilian assets are insufficient or nonexistent, and units are authorized to provide direct support in coordination with local governments, medical facilities, and law enforcement agencies. After approval for mobilization, MAST units are directed to conduct specific missions.

When MAST units are used on SAR missions, as opposed to local medical evacuations, they are recruited and controlled by the Air Force Rescue Coordination Center (AFRCC). The MAST program is also recognized for other humanitarian efforts. For instance, the northwestern

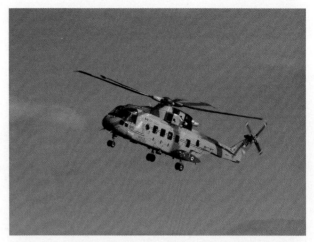

Figure 11–7 Helicopters are useful for the movement of supplies and equipment, search area evaluation (planning), and for actual searching.

United States utilizes MAST organizations for such tasks as helicopter transportation of premature infants to neonatal care facilities, the transfer of critically burned patients to burn centers, and the air evacuation of traffic accident victims. MAST organizations in other parts of the country may provide similar services; however, there is no central controlling office or address. Indeed, not all Army and Air Force operations have a MAST program. In those areas where there is adequate private helicopter assistance, the MAST units may not be active. For example, citizens in the state of West Virginia usually utilize private aeromedical providers (i.e., HealthNet) for medical transports.

Fixed-wing aircraft are useful for search area evaluation and for actual searching under certain terrain and vegetation conditions.

Sources include:

1. Military: primarily through Rescue Coordination Center or local military base
2. Civil Air Patrol: through RCC or local CAP unit
3. Government contract
4. Private and volunteer clubs and groups

Specialized Vehicles

This type of resource includes local units or individuals with vehicles capable of responding in special terrain/ environmental conditions, such as:

- Over-snow vehicles
- Four-wheel drive vehicles
- All-terrain vehicles
- Mountain bikes

Sensor Technologies

Locating equipment has many different applications. Their uses range from determining where a subject lies within a collapsed building to locating a rescuer who needs assistance. Locating technology is useful for coordinating searches over vast areas because it can help determine which areas have been searched and provide a geographic reference to base operations.

The newest and most sophisticated locating equipment employs advanced computers, listening devices, cameras, and satellites to assist with locating a subject or tracking a rescuer. The capabilities and applications of recently developed advanced locating and tracking equipment have made rescue operations much more efficient. However, there are still many rescue needs that have not been satisfied with the existing technology. Many of the systems presented here have been developed for military or scientific purposes and then adapted to SAR applications. This section describes some advances, capabilities, and limitations of locating technology.

Thermal Imaging (Infrared)

These advanced technology devices were developed for the military and are now used by police to track criminal activity in the dark. Thermal imaging devices use infrared technology to sense heat. Typically, infrared equipment will display a monochrome or color image highlighting as little as 0.1°F difference between an object and its background. This allows a human body to be seen in complete darkness or in a smoke obscured environment. The more intense the heat source, the brighter the image appears in the display. The display will produce a silhouette type image of a person, but will not show detailed features.

Fire fighters have adapted thermal imaging cameras to look for victims through smoke at a fire. This application incorporates infrared viewing technology into a either fire fighter's helmet or a handheld device. These devices are primarily designed for structural fire fighting but may be adapted for technical rescue. Thermal imaging devices are now available that weigh less than one pound.

The operating principle of this type of device is the same as the forward looking infrared (FLIR) units described below. All objects radiate a certain amount of heat, which travels outward as detectable energy. Because of differences in the amount of heat being radiated, the viewer detects each difference as more intense or less intense image. Thermal-imagery devices can be used in daylight or darkness, and can be extremely useful because of their ability to see through smoke, dust, heavy rain, falling snow, fog, camouflage, and light vegetation.

Thermal imaging equipment has multiple applications, but it is expensive and may have significant limitations (Figure 11–8). Infrared radiation cannot be detected through concrete, rock, brick, wood, or even thick sheet rock (drywall) walls. Thus, infrared locating technology has very limited value at structural collapse sites.

The handheld devices are ruggedly designed for limited exposure to areas near a fire or water. They can usually be used for one to two hours before the batteries die. Some units must be turned off hourly to cool down, since their airtight design does not allow for easy cooling of internal components.

Forward Looking Infrared (FLIR)

Thermal, infrared imaging and forward looking infrared (FLIR) units are used to scan wide areas, most often from aircraft, and have numerous applications for SAR. In water rescue operations, they can be used during the day or night to scan the surface for a subject. They are useful on wide rivers, lakes, or other large bodies of water where it may be difficult to pinpoint the location of a subject. Handheld thermal image cameras, similar to TV cameras, can also be used by rescuers in helicopters or on the ground. The more powerful FLIR units, utilized mostly by aircraft, are very expensive.

FLIR was first used in law enforcement in 1984 and utilizes thermal airborne imaging in a wide application of search environments. The technology involves registering temperature differences of houses, trees, cars, and people (so slight as to be almost nonexistent) and projecting these minimum resolvable temperature differences onto a TV monitor. The system has now become a widely accepted law enforcement resource.

The units themselves (a tough polymer/plastics "Cyclops"-looking ball) can be easily adapted to the

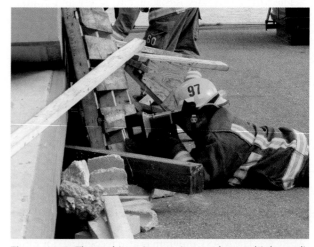

Figure 11–8 Thermal imaging equipment has multiple applications, but it is expensive and may have significant limitations.

mount on a normal helicopter's search- or spot-light bracket. Installation takes minimal time and it can be affixed to nearly any helicopter. The detector moves up and down as well as from left to right, and is controlled by a handheld (computer linked) joystick that has various buttons and toggles to control field of view switching (wide or narrow), optimal signal presentation, and travel sweep. For many units, the best operating altitude is between 600 and 800 feet (180 and 250 meters) where a 300- to 450-foot (100 to 150 meter) wide ground swath can be observed.

On the imaging screen (if white is selected as warm) the eerie, almost photonegative-type image will show tree branches on a cold winter's night as warmer (almost white) with tree trunks (which lose less heat) being darker. Houses show up distinctively radiating white through glass windows, while cars show a distinctive glow wherever their engines are situated.

Tests and actual searches tend to be more successful at night when ambient temperatures are most uniform and no artifacts of localized heating by sunlight distort findings. Forested areas can be penetrated well, although dense leaf growth or evergreen cover requires greater operator skill to detect visual differences. The units have been tested and used under actual conditions of fog, rain, snow, and extreme cold with excellent results. Images of people, dogs, and various forms of wildlife are clearly visible, as are tracks in the snow (less than ~15 minutes old). In field tests, ground team members have been asked to quickly identify themselves by showing a portion of their skin. Individuals wrapped in sleeping bags that were difficult to detect were immediately visible when they showed their faces or put a hand or arm out.

Trees, roads, fields, shacks, or buildings all have marginally different temperatures that the monitor translates into a very clear picture. These can be recorded on videotape and replayed later. Even the smallest heat sources, like the place where a vehicle has stopped and started again, and even where individuals have stopped and then continued can be detected.

Subjects who cannot verbally communicate their location, such as unconscious individuals, may be spotted using infrared devices. Some thermal imaging units can see several feet below the surface of the water. This capability could assist with locating a submerged victim, a victim in very shallow water, or even a body, since it may still emit enough heat to activate these units for hours after death.

Helicopter-mounted FLIR units can sense heat variations as far as 10 miles or more, but may cost over $100,000. The handheld models, which use a less powerful lens, cost in the range of $16,000. More expensive models can see up to 500 yards.

Light Amplification (Night Vision)

Another technology for nighttime searching is light amplification devices. Unlike the infrared technology that can "see" humans in complete darkness, night vision units require some ambient light, whether it be residual light at dusk, light from street lamps, or, in some cases, infrared light. For example, light amplification devices can be used to search a river at night if there is some light projected onto the search area from the shore. The newest units, however, can work on overcast nights because they are very sensitive to infrared light that penetrates clouds.

These devices do not project detectable energy. They amplify the existing or ambient light at night to project an image on the scope or viewer. Ambient light may come from moonlight, starlight, or the glow from cities and towns. Light from flares, searchlights, and laser illumination improves the viewing capability, but should not be viewed directly by the device. Image-intensification devices are adversely affected by fog, smoke, heavy rain, and falling snow.

Night vision technology was originally designed to help helicopter pilots see the ground during the night. For SAR applications, it allows rescuers to distinguish objects at distances as far as 200 yards. The units provide viewers with an electronically enhanced video image that enables them to see people, buildings, vehicles, and the landscape. Some night vision units magnify images one to two times while amplifying the light up to 100,000 times. These units, however, cannot see through foliage or dense smoke or fog, as the infrared units can. Night vision units come in binocular, monocular, scope, and goggle styles. Low-end models cost approximately $500.

The standard military models (AN/PVS-7A and B) of NVGs are equipped with an infrared light source and a positive control switch that permits close-in viewing from 10 inches to infinity. This allows a person wearing the device under low light conditions to do everything from read a map to drive a vehicle. The units weigh about 1.5 pounds and are capable of continuous operation over a 15-hour period before battery replacement is required. Some also have a high light cutoff feature that shuts power down to the goggles when they are exposed to bright light. Therefore, it is important to note that during night helicopter operations where NVGs are in use by the aircraft crew, it is absolutely essential that ground personnel *do not* shine or flash lights directly at the aircraft. Rather, the appropriate method of signaling such an aircraft is to shine a light, or lights, toward the ground.

Cost of the units can vary from $1,000 to $4,000. But, despite this substantial price tag, the technology has found a place with numerous police and government agencies, and has proven quite useful in SAR.

Videography, Photography, and Photo Interpretation

Of course, videographic and/or photographic evidence indicating the whereabouts of a search subject would be outstanding, but acquiring it takes a great deal of planning, equipment, and skill. For instance, trail- or road-blocks could be replaced with remote video cameras, but the setup and monitoring of such equipment could be more trouble than its worth. Aerial photographs could show evidence like human-made signals, tracks, discarded evidence, or wreckage, but acquiring such photographs would take a great deal of resources (i.e., aircraft, pilot, photographer, photographic equipment, etc.) and an enormously skilled interpreter (one to analyze the photographs). So, the argument becomes, "Is it worth the trouble" rather than "Can we do it?"

Additional problems arise for SAR managers with these types of resources. For instance, how is the location of evidence on an aerial photograph transferred to a map that can be utilized by field search crews? What is the scale on a particular aerial photo? Questions like these are not insurmountable, but require a great deal of forethought and planning to address.

Real-time video has had widespread acceptance in certain settings such as building collapse and confined space rescue. Small, maneuverable cameras can be slipped into small spaces to visually examine a void where victims may be trapped or where rescuers may soon enter. Also, rescuers now can have a video camera built into their helmets to broadcast a constant visual image to supervisors who view the hazardous environment from relative safety. Such use of video technology not only enhances the safety of rescuers, it also allows viewing of areas that otherwise may never have been viewed. The application for field SAR units has yet to be exploited.

Sonar

Sonar (sound amplification) technology can be useful in some underwater searches. Very few SAR teams use this technology at present, partly because of the expense of the equipment and partly because of the challenge of deploying it quickly by trained operators. Sonar is typically used by boaters to determine the depth of water or locate fish ("fish-finder") but similar technology specific for use in SAR is available (**Figure 11–9**). It plots objects detected underwater on a display monitor located in the rescue boat. With proper training, rescuers can learn how to differentiate the profile of a human body from fish, debris, and other objects in the water. A body on the bottom—a likely location—can be very difficult to

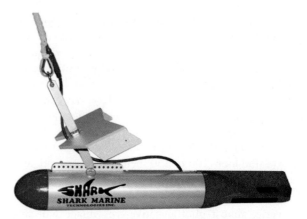

Figure 11–9 Side-scan Sonar has been used very effectively in SAR work in the underwater environment.

locate using sonar because of the very slight differential created by the width of the body as compared with other objects on the bottom. Improvements in technology, however, have improved this capability significantly.

Sound and Vibration Detection

Devices for listening, for example, those able to hear sound over great distances (such as powerful unidirectional, low-level microphones), from remote locations (wired or wireless microphones), through various media (concrete, collapsed structures, etc.), and in low sound situations, occasionally become available for use in SAR situations. Like any unusual resource, their limitations and use should be thoroughly investigated so that, should the need arise, SAR personnel are prepared to benefit fully from the technology. Everyone should always be on the lookout for not only applications for new technology, but also new applications for old technology. Sound detection devices are a good example of the latter.

The requirements of the urban SAR (USAR) environment give rise to a great opportunity to reevaluate current technology in order to meet new needs. For instance, vibration and sound detection devices are being used in collapse structures to listen for the cries, and even the breathing and heartbeats, of trapped victims. This type of application of technology, of course, is expensive, but when such resources are required, nothing else will suffice.

Avalanche Beacons/Transceivers

In the early 1970s, avalanche rescue beacons, or transceivers, were introduced into the United States. Since then, these devices have become the most-used personal rescue devices in the world. The reason is that, when used properly, there is no faster, more efficient, or more effective way of locating buried avalanche victims; numerous documented cases of lives being saved have been attributed to their use.

Costing anywhere from $50 to $200 (U.S.), these devices are available from most outdoor and winter equipment shops. Their use is simple. Avalanche beacons emit a signal on one or two frequencies when they are set on "transmit" (2275 Hz and/or 457 kHz, but 2275 Hz seems to be more of the standard in the United States). If the wearer of one of these devices were to become buried in an avalanche, rescuers could turn their beacons on "receive" to pick up, and home in on, the signal from the buried unit. Various search patterns combined with evaluation of the strength of the signal are then used to narrow down the location of the buried beacon. The signal carries about 100 feet, but frequent practice, well-maintained, and properly used beacons are necessary to make the system work. Although skilled practitioners can usually find a subject in less than five minutes after picking up the signal, the use of these devices is not straightforward. Effective use takes frequent practice and thorough knowledge of the devices and their limitations.

Communications Equipment

An abundance of highly advanced communications equipment is available to rescuers today. Communications equipment provides a vital link between rescuers, especially if they are separated visually. It allows them to communicate needs, findings, distress calls, and even images of the incident to other rescue personnel or to a remote location. A functional communications system is essential to maintaining organization and safety at any rescue scene.

Communications equipment is particularly important to rescuers entering dangerous environments. The lack of proper communications has been an issue in cases involving injuries and death to rescuers. Often, rescuers who enter a confined space, for example, are out of visual and audible contact with non-entry personnel. During such incidents, if the entry rescuers were to experience a life-threatening situation and need assistance, communications technology might be the only means of requesting help.

Communications technology can transmit a signal over a radio frequency or hard wire cable. Radio signals can be blocked by walls and metal, and are limited by distance or other barriers. Communications systems that use radio frequency transmission are considered at most 95% reliable. Hard wire communications are the only media considered nearly 100% reliable, but they

are limited by practical considerations, such as the length of the communications cable.

The type of communications system used should be dictated by the needs of rescuers and the types of situations they anticipate. For instance, rescuers who are entering a confined space or cave containing walls and other barriers that may inhibit radio frequency transmission should utilize hard wired systems if they are available. This section discusses communications equipment designed and used for a variety of different rescue systems.

Radio Frequency (RF) Systems

The standard handheld and mobile communications units used by most emergency services and rescuers transmit over radio frequency (RF). The frequency of different systems varies from 25 MHz to the 800 MHz band. RF systems have strengths and weaknesses that make them more applicable in certain rescue situations than in others.

RF-based communications systems generally can transmit over a large area. Given a constant transmission power, the lower frequency signals travel farther than the higher frequency signals, but they do not penetrate barriers as well as a higher frequency signal. For example, a 40-MHz signal from a standard mobile radio can travel 50 or more miles without a signal repeater, but it is very unlikely that an 800-MHz signal with the same power could match this without ideal atmospheric conditions. Conversely, it is much harder for a 40-MHz unit to transmit through an area surrounded by concrete than it is for an 800-MHz unit. Well designed RF systems with repeaters can transmit hundreds of miles. Also, RF systems generally allow the user to choose between a number of channels or talk groups.

There are many limitations associated with RF systems. Higher frequency RF units depend on signals bouncing around to reach the person on the other end. Obstructions such as concrete, metal, tunnels, and atmospheric conditions (e.g., an electric storm) can prevent a transmission from reaching other users. Static interference can make transmissions unintelligible. Outside interference may also leak in from others using similar frequencies.

RF is the best method of communication in incidents where rescuers are geographically scattered over an area or for surface-level communications at a small-scale incident. It is one of the best methods of communications for rescuers involved in: wilderness search; urban search; trench rescue; water rescue (surface communications only); or any other surface-level operations environment. It is generally not as reliable for operations involving: subsurface communications (i.e., confined space such as a sewer system, or subway); underwater communications; or communications deep within a building heavily partitioned with walls and floors. In these situations, the RF signal may have trouble getting outside to a repeater or other rescuers. However, some technology discussed below can help to conduct or carry a RF signal out of a confined area.

Trunked Radio Systems

New, advanced technology trunked systems offer rescuers many advantages over older technology systems. The older, conventional radio systems are still widely used today, but are limited in the number of channels available to emergency personnel. Conventional radio systems match one channel per frequency. For example, a jurisdiction that is allocated four emergency frequencies by the Federal Communications Commission (FCC) would have four emergency channels.

Newer trunked systems, however, can allocate twenty or more "talk groups" to the four frequencies. Trunked systems do not require one frequency for every single talk group. Instead, the system picks an open frequency when a user transmits over a channel. Trunked systems work on the concept that even though there are a multitude of talk groups available to users, it is extremely unlikely that more than a few of them are in use simultaneously at any given time.

Trunked systems can offer hundreds of talk groups, even though the system may only use a small number of discrete frequencies. The heart of a trunked system is a computer that assigns a user an open frequency. However, the computer selection process is invisible to the user. The multiple talk group capability of trunked radio systems offers many advantages at small- and large-scale search and rescue incidents.

Typically, there are many high-priority operations occurring simultaneously at a disaster site. Coordination of the operations is very difficult, especially if only one or two channels are available to rescuers. Trunked technology could offer multiple talk groups. For instance, the operations section could utilize one talk group, while the command staff could utilize another.

A trunked system can be designed to allow communications among multiple agencies. This allows fire, police, public works, and other agencies to communicate with one another, and facilitate communications during a disaster. The technology also allows other jurisdictions responding for mutual aid to be attached to the radio system so that no patching of frequencies is necessary. One limitation with the trunked system is that if the signal does not reach the central trunked system receiver, the transmission will not reach other radios that are connected to the system. Also, if the computer goes down, most of the system becomes inoperative.

Hard Wired Systems

Hard wired systems are considered to be the most reliable available because users are directly connected (**Figure 11–10**). Some systems use a console to interconnect several users. This allows for duplex communications, where two or more of the rescuers can talk simultaneously and everyone hears them (similar to a conference telephone call). The systems generally use headsets, sometimes with throat microphones, which are attached to the wire that runs to a central console. The headsets and microphones are very compact, and the transmit button can be placed in a rescuer's palm or the system can be voice activated. These features facilitate movement within a confined space or inside a protective suit.

Hard wired systems can be used effectively at incidents where RF signals cannot penetrate, such as confined spaces. The wire carries the signal and virtually ensures that a rescuer can be heard at any time. Many rescuers find the greatest advantage of these systems is the psychological reassurance of knowing that they will always be able to communicate, especially when they are out of visual contact with non-entry personnel.

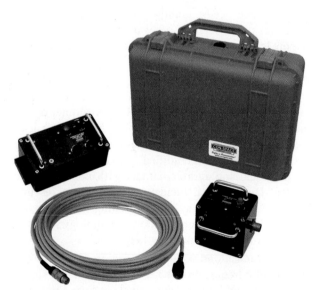

Figure 11–10 Hard wired systems are considered to be the most reliable communications systems available because users are directly connected. Photo courtesy of CON-SPACE Communications, Inc.

INFO
Trunked radio systems can allocate many "talk groups" to just a few frequencies, offering many advantages over conventional radio systems that match one channel per frequency.

SARTips

Several hard wired units have emergency buttons that can be activated if a rescuer needs assistance but is unable to talk. Some are intrinsically safe, making them useful at incidents where the atmosphere is flammable or explosive, such as silos, sewers, vats, storage tanks, or ship hulls. The main power supply for intrinsically safe units remains outside of the explosive environment. The fully shielded wire carries only a few millivolts. Newer hard wired systems are also insulated from outside electrical signals that can create interference or static.

Hard wired communications systems can also be used by divers. Underwater communications is particularly important in dark or dirty water where visibility is severely restricted. This technology allows divers to communicate and coordinate their efforts. It also allows divers to communicate with rescue personnel on the surface. These systems give psychological reassurance to divers.

The major limitation with any hard wired system is the length of the wire. Depending on the system, the wire is generally limited to 500 to 1500 feet. For longer distances, a repeater may be necessary to boost the signal. Most hard wired systems are also limited to four or five users, unlike RF systems that can accommodate thousands of users. However, sometimes two hard wired systems can be connected at the control console to increase the number of users.

Users of hard wired systems must also deal with dragging wire, which may become snagged or tangled. One approach to this problem involves feeding the line or lines (including additional lines such as air hose, and power lines) into 2-inch tubular webbing. This webbing system can be made into various length sections that can be combined as needed for extension. The slick texture of the nylon webbing makes it less vulnerable to becoming stuck or jammed on obstacles or bends within a confined space.

Communications Wire/Rope

Many rescue incidents require a safety line to be attached to rescuers at all times. Rescuers involved with confined space entry, diving (especially under ice and in caves), rappelling, or swift water entry often must utilize safety lines. Sometimes the rescuers also need to take a hard wired communications line with them. Additionally, they may have to take an air hose for air supply (surface supplied air). The three separate lines may present a hazard to the rescuer if they become tangled, twisted, or caught.

Communications wire/rope is a technology that combines two of these lines into one, to reduce the risk of tangling. It is usually made as a kernmantle, with a wire running through the inside of the kern (the rope's core). Rope strength is not significantly compromised by the encased wire, allowing it to serve as a safety line. Each end of the wire/rope has a locking coaxial-type connection so that it can be attached to a radio, headset, or other communications console.

Most communications wire/rope has a breaking strength around 5000 pounds depending on the diameter of the rope. However, military-grade wire/rope is rated as high as 9000 pounds. The rope is made from synthetic fibers and is waterproof. Since the wire runs through the center of the rope, it is intrinsically safe for rescue operations in flammable environments. But, under high stress, the wire portion of the rope could be damaged by the greater elasticity of the rope. Communications wire/rope is available in various diameters and lengths and generally costs approximately $3 per foot if it is encased in kernmantle rope.

Cellular and Satellite Telephones

Following major disasters, telephone systems may be totally disabled or severely limited. Communications cables may be down, incoming and outgoing calls may jam circuits, and switching stations may be destroyed. Many rescue teams have begun to use alternative telephone systems such as cellular and satellite phones to work around the potential telephone problems.

When hard wired systems are out of service, cellular phones are one alternative. This assumes that the cellular receiving sites are not destroyed or overtaxed. However, with the increasing number of cellular phones in use by the public, cells may also become jammed and prevent rescuers' calls from getting through. Cellular transmissions may not get through if the user is in an area where signals cannot reach a receiving cell.

Another option to bypass the entire local telephone system is a satellite telephone. Satellite telephones can bypass the jammed circuitry of a disaster scene. These expensive units are particularly useful for rescuers in remote areas where neither hard wired nor cellular receiving sites are available.

Additional Resources

Of course, there are many other specialized equipment resources with which SAR personnel might come in contact. For instance, many specialized pieces of equipment used by the military might come in handy in SAR situations. Mine detectors, for example, have been used in avalanche rescue. The same might be said for thermistors, which are sensitive to changes in temperatures in the medium over which they are passed. Mechanical sniffers are sensitive to odors and have been used to detect bodies in disaster settings, and magnetometers, which work on deviations in the earth's magnetic field, have been used to find rocks, metal, and even bodies covered in snow.

If the potential exists for resources to be required, especially of the expensive and/or highly technical type, it is up to SAR personnel to seek out reliable sources and confirm availability. First notice of an incident is not the time to investigate resource availability. Plan ahead, know where to go, know who to ask, and know whether what you need is available—all before anything is needed.

SAR Terms

Grid search Search practice involving search crews relying on vision to line search a well-defined, usually small segment.

Hasty teams Small (usually 3 members), well-trained, highly mobile, self-sufficient, clue-conscious search teams.

Sign Discoverable evidence located in an area where a subject would likely have passed.

Sign cutting The process of looking for the first piece of evidence from which to track.

References

American Rescue Dog Association. (2002). *Search and Rescue Dogs: Training the K-9 Hero,* 2nd ed. Indianapolis, IN: Howell Book House.

Brown, M.G. (2000). *Engineering Practical Rope Rescue Systems.* Clifton Park, NY: Delmar Learning.

Carss, R. (2000). *The SAS Guide to Tracking.* Guilford, CT: The Lyons Press.

Cox, M., & Fulsass, K., eds. (2003). *Mountaineering: Freedom of the Hills,* 7th ed. New York, NY: Mountaineers Books.

Frank, J.A., ed. (1998). *CMC Rope Rescue Manual*, 3rd ed. Santa Barbara, CA: CMC Rescue.

Getchell, A. (1995). *The Essential Outdoor Gear Manual: Equipment Care and Repair for Outdoorspeople*. New York, NY: International Marine/Ragged Mountain Press.

Hawley, C. (2000). *Hazardous Materials Response and Operations*. New York, NY: Delmar Learning.

Hill, K. (1997). *Managing Lost Person Incidents*. Chantilly, VA: National Association for Search and Rescue.

Mitchell, J.T., Everly, G.S., & Everly, G.S., Jr. (2001). *Critical Incident Stress Debriefing: An Operations Manual for CISD, Diffusing and Other Group Intervention Services*, 3rd ed. Ellicott City, MD: Chevron Publishing Corporation.

Ray, S., & Bechtel, L. (1997). *River Rescue: A Manual for Whitewater Safety*, 3rd ed. Boston, MA: Appalachian Mountain Club Books.

Roop, M., & Vines, T. (1998). *Confined Space and Structural Rope Rescue*. St. Louis, MO: Mosby, Inc.

Taylor, A., & Cooper, D.C. (1990). *Fundamentals of Mantracking: The Step-by-Step Method*, 2nd ed. Olympia, WA: ERI, International.

Vines, T., & Hudson, S. (1999). *High Angle Rescue Techniques*, 2nd ed. St. Louis, MO: Mosby, Inc.

Walbridge, C., & Sundmacher, W. (1995). *Whitewater Rescue Manual: New Techniques for Canoeists, Kayakers and Rafters*. New York, NY: International Marine/Ragged Mountain Press.

Washburn, A.R. (2002). *Search and Detection*, 4th ed. Linthicum, MD: Institute for Operations Research and the Management Sciences.

Chapter 12

Travel Skills: Foot Travel for SAR Personnel

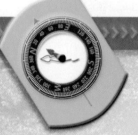

>>>>> **Objectives**

Upon completion of this chapter and any course activities, the student will be able to meet the following objectives:

Describe traveling skills used in varying environments during SAR operations. (p. 199-207)

Describe the preparation and conditioning needed to perform while wearing a SAR ready pack. (p. 195-196)

Describe the general use of an ice axe. (p. 198-199)

Describe a method for safely crossing a stream or river on foot. (p. 201-202)

Describe the rest step in mountaineering. (p. 197)

Travel Considerations

Just because you have good motor skills and balance does not insure your capability to travel in the wilderness or work in the rigorous environments posed by a search and rescue mission. There are many "tricks-of-the-trade" that not only insure comfort and optional speed, but, most importantly, provide the degree of safety required for SAR work.

To get from one place to another in SAR, there are a number of guidelines to consider that will make the mission safer and easier for everyone in the field.

Technical and Non-Technical Travel

Foot travel may be required in one of two forms during a SAR incident: non-technical and technical. SAR personnel have very little control over where or when this type of travel takes place. Assignments are made and SAR personnel simply carry them out. Specific skill and knowledge of proper travel technique can increase comfort and reduce injury.

Walking and non-technical travel (searching, getting to the search area, etc.) may be necessary in one or more general environments (desert, mountain, arctic, river, tropical, forest, etc.).

Climbing or more technical travel (accessing a search area, examining a high-risk area, technical rescue, etc.) may also involve one of many environments (ice, rock, talus, etc.). Again, proper technique improves safety and ease of travel.

Recreation

Traveling on foot for recreational purposes can also involve technical and non-technical actions, but with far different motivations and goals. Here, the traveler has total control over where and when travel takes place.

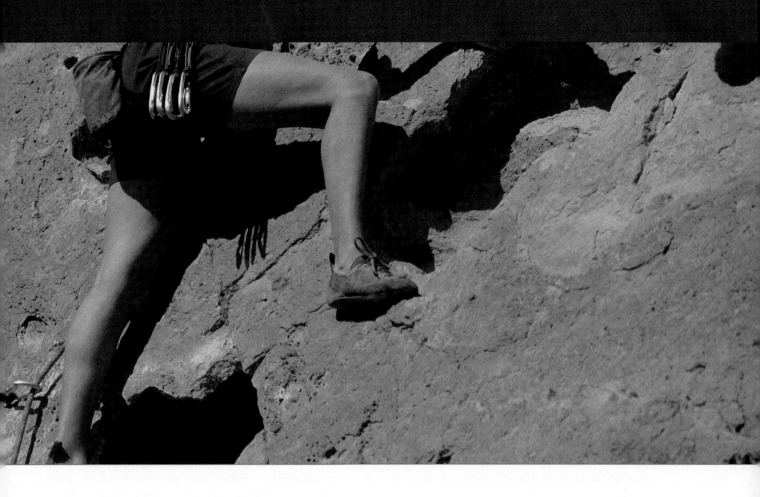

This is a distinct advantage in terms of safety. Technique still plays a large part, but planning is far more important because it is not nearly as rushed as during a SAR incident. Dangerous routes can be avoided by planning around them.

Walking, hiking, hill walking, or non-technical travel is most often used to easily and safely move through an area chosen for esthetic characteristics (pretty sights, nice views, good camping or picnic areas, etc.) or because it offers a desired physical or mental challenge or benefit.

Urgent or Emergency Situation

Walking may be the only way out of a dangerous situation for SAR personnel, especially if the individual is lost. For example, a hiker with an injury may be in danger of exposure or infection without definitive medical care. Since care is rarely available in the hiking environment, travel is required to transport the individual to the care. If the hiker is lost, travel is complicated substantially, even if he or she physically can walk. Motivation in this situation comes from survival senses, and is rarely related to travel skill and knowledge. Con-

siderations regarding travel in an emergency (to travel or not to travel) are covered in Chapter 6, Survival and Improvisation.

Walking

As mentioned in Chapter 5, Physiology and Fitness, conditioning is an important component of SAR involvement. Since walking is the primary mode of transportation in a SAR incident, being conditioned to walk or hike for long distances may mean the difference between effectiveness and futility. Conditioning should include nutrition and hydration for a comprehensive approach to being prepared for travel in SAR work.

Five things are needed to prepare for traveling in SAR work: fitness (cardiovascular and muscular endurance, muscular strength, and flexibility), energy, water, rest, and technique. The first four of these topics are discussed in detail in Chapter 5, Physiology and Fitness. However, because technique can influence so many other aspects of outdoor travel, some basic guidelines will be provided here.

Physical Fitness

Physical preparation for travel is straightforward. Under ideal conditions, SAR personnel are in excellent physical shape, fueled with nutritious food, enjoy normal hydration, and have slept eight hours before an arduous mission. While that isn't quite realistic, good rest and nutrition substantially improve performance over those in poor condition, who eat and drink poorly, and get little or no rest before call-out. In fact, maximum performance in SAR is only one of the many benefits of proper nutrition, rest, and exercise.

Gear

SAR personnel also need to be prepared for traveling by knowing how to dress, pack, and plan. Clothing for specific environments is covered in Chapter 7, Clothing. It is important to note that proper dress is mandatory for effective and safe travel. SAR personnel should wear their clothing in layers and make adjustments to provide for climate, temperature, and precipitation. How to pack is covered in Chapter 9, SAR Ready Pack and Personal Equipment.

Planning

Planning a trip and route finding are also important, but this, of course, is not something that can be done before a SAR incident. After receiving an assignment in a SAR mission, there may be a brief opportunity for planning. Whether traveling to an assigned area or traveling within an area requiring SAR, the route should be carefully planned. Once you determine that travel on foot will be required, it is your responsibility to identify the best type of travel (snowshoe, ski, hike, climb, etc.) and plan the best route. Maps and experienced individuals can be valuable tools for travel planning, but keep in mind that no matter what you use, you must plan your travels, know the route, and follow your plans.

Being Prepared

The following points summarize how SAR personnel prepare for the rigors of traveling in a SAR environment:

1. A SAR incident could occur at any time, so you should be prepared at all times.
2. Maintain a level of physical conditioning commensurate with your specific SAR responsibilities. In other words, field personnel should maintain a high level of conditioning.
3. Eat proper foods in appropriate amounts and get plenty of rest.
4. Maintain hydration by drinking plenty of water before and during a mission.
5. Be properly clothed for the type of travel anticipated.
6. Pack and carry the appropriate equipment for the type of travel anticipated.
7. Before traveling in a SAR mission, plan your travels and know your route.

Walking Technique

Land travel techniques are based largely on experience. However, experience can be partially replaced by practices learned through instruction and observation.

Skill and technique are as important for SAR travel as fitness. Without the proper techniques, the best conditioned person in the world could easily reach his or her limits while traveling. After your physical limits are reached, you tend to lose effectiveness as a searcher. So, there is a direct correlation between conditioning, skills, and effectiveness in the field.

On short journeys, it is not essential to walk properly or efficiently. However, walking for several miles during a SAR mission with a heavy load where lives depend on your ability to travel is another matter.

Route When the exact route or approach to an objective is not important to the desired outcome, SAR personnel can improvise and travel the easiest and simplest route. When deciding exactly which path to take (route finding), several options are usually available. A compass heading is often used to get from one place to another, but can be difficult in rugged terrain. Novices could stick to this type of route because it is easy and requires little thought, but the terrain could be difficult. SAR personnel who have some experience will first determine their objective, and then figure an easy route to that goal by finding the path of least resistance.

Often, a curved route of greater distance can be easier and faster to travel than a straight path. Following a route of constant elevation (contour line) is easier to traverse because it requires less energy than moving uphill and downhill. Traveling by altimeter uses this approach and can be a valuable skill in your navigational arsenal. Game trails, roads, and man-made trails may take the traveler a greater distance, but also may allow quicker walking and, therefore, less overall travel time.

Factor terrain, weather, and vegetation into the decision to take a longer, but quicker and easier route to an objective. Whatever the situation, consider everything and you can almost always find a better path.

Pace Pace and rest are crucial to travel efficiency. Maintain a realistic pace to save energy. It increases durability and keeps body temperature stable because it reduces the practice of quick starts and lengthy rests. More importantly, a moderate, realistic pace is essential in high altitudes to avoid hypoxia (lack of oxygen), which can lead to lapse of judgment and hallucinations. In addition, practice rhythmic breathing to prevent headache, nausea, lack of appetite, and irritability. Rhythmic breathing is simply a consistent breathing cycle to a set pace. Maintaining regular breathing and pace ratio allows for more relaxed walking and often takes the mind off of the drudgery of monotonous travel.

Fatigue in the SAR environment is dangerous. It increases the chances of accident and injury, and weakens judgment. Everyone needs to rest, no matter how physically fit. Do not force rest, enjoy it. If you are barely making it to the next rest stop before collapsing, you need to rest more often. Inexperienced travelers tend to rest too often and underestimate their abilities. Rest stops should be short since it requires added energy to begin again after cooling off. A rest of about 10 minutes per hour while traveling over easy terrain is usually acceptable.

Occasionally, the terrain may be so difficult and the energy required to travel so great that rest is required between each step. This is when you can use the "rest step" (**Figure 12-1**). Adopted from mountaineering, the "rest step" or "lock step" is a technique of taking small steps, locking each knee and synchronizing the breathing, to allow for a brief respite before taking the next small step. This technique is slow, but may be the only way to travel over difficult terrain, especially at high altitude. Think of it as steady, consistent, and slow travel, instead of erratic stop-and-go movement. A novice SAR hiker can virtually eliminate all long rest stops with this technique and actually make very good travel time.

Many novice SAR personnel make the mistake of walking too fast, usually thinking of the distance to be covered, the urgency of the situation, or the perceived shame of traveling slower than others. Speed is dictated by the area to be covered and the time available (or assigned). Walking too fast decreases the probability of detection (see Chapters 14 and 15) as well as reducing energy stores. In *Mountaineering: Freedom of the Hills*, the authors suggest that if a pace cannot be sustained hour after hour, it is too fast. In addition, they state that you are going too fast when it takes great effort to take the next step or when the lungs are gasping for air. Whatever the problem and whatever the cause, walking fast may be common in recreational hiking, but it is inexcusable and unsafe in SAR work.

In a group, pace is determined by the slowest traveler. Excess energy is far better than dealing with severe fatigue. Spacing between individuals in a group is also important while walking. When distance has not been dictated by the search assignment or desired coverage, the rate of travel and the terrain determines the distance between travelers. On most trails, at average walking speeds, this distance is about 6 to 10 feet apart. SAR team members should always see other team members they are traveling with and should certainly stay within earshot of each other.

Even though downhill walking is less fatiguing than uphill, traveling downhill is not without its problems. Toes are jammed into the front of the shoes, knees are jarred, and the entire body begins to ache from dropping the weight of the body onto a locked knee and leg at each step. Blisters seem to multiply as the best fitting footgear is tested, and energy is expended preventing a steady speed increase. What do you do? Start by tightening your laces to decrease the movement of the foot inside your footgear. This reduces blisters but also reduces circulation to the feet.

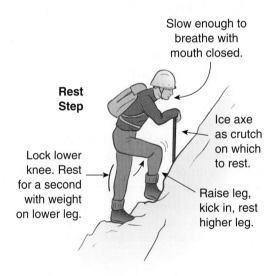

Rest Step

Slow enough to breathe with mouth closed.

Ice axe as crutch on which to rest.

Lock lower knee. Rest for a second with weight on lower leg.

Raise leg, kick in, rest higher leg.

Figure 12-1 The rest step is a mountaineering technique developed to maintain pace with heavy loads, at high altitudes or in rough, steep terrain. It involves taking small steps, locking each knee and synchronizing breathing, all to allow a brief respite between each step. The technique is slow, but in rough, steep terrain, especially at altitude, it provides for good footing and minimal waste of energy.

Taking this approach in cold weather requires constant monitoring of the feet. Second, fill the toe area of the footgear with socks or other padding to cushion the impact of the feet and place the foot lightly on the ground during walking. Placing the feet lightly takes much muscle energy and requires resting just as much as traveling uphill.

Generally, tighten shoe- or bootlaces for any travel over terrain where the foot inside the shoe can put pressure in any direction except down. Pressing the foot in any direction but down subjects the feet to stress for which they may not be prepared (no calluses) (see Chapter 7, Clothing).

A walking stick and ice axe can be valuable adjuncts to the SAR traveler. The walking stick, in addition to being useful for support during travel, can be substituted for everything from a tent pole to a weapon. One of the more common uses of a walking stick in SAR work is as a tracking stick (see Chapter 13, Tracking).

The use of the ice axe in SAR is derived from its roots in mountaineering (Figure 12–2). The axe is carried primarily for use in mountainous conditions, usually at higher elevations, when ice and snow conditions are coupled with severe terrain. Classically, carry the ice axe to aid in balance while walking (downhill, uphill, glissading, etc.), as a braking device during a fall or glissades, or as an anchor in snow. When using the device properly, it can save your life and aid in rescuing others.

On any slope where a slip may lead to a quick descent or a slide down a mountainside, carry the ice axe in a position ready to make an arrest. The ready position is as follows:

1. Place one hand, preferably the stronger one, on the head of the axe with the thumb under the adze and fingers over the pick.

2. Place your other hand on the shaft next to the spike.

If walking with the axe in one hand, use your stronger hand. If you slip, your immediate action is to grasp the shaft with the free hand and go into the arrest position (Figure 12–3). When the fall occurs, the faster you brake, the better your chances of stopping. Move quickly! The faster you slide, the harder it is to stop. Immediately press the pick into the slope just above the shoulder so the adze is near the angle formed by the neck and shoulders.

The shaft should cross the chest diagonally with the spike held firmly close to the opposite hip. Hold a short axe (i.e., for ice climbing) in the same position, although the spike will not reach the opposite hip. Your chest and shoulders should press strongly on the shaft and your spine arched slightly to distribute weight primarily at the

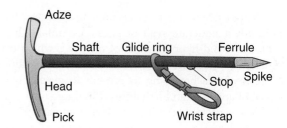

Figure 12–2 Parts of an ice axe.

shoulders and toes. Legs should be stiff and spread apart, toes digging in (if wearing crampons, keep your toes off the surface until almost stopped), and hang on the axe. Basically, the ideal arrest position is sliding on the stomach, feet downhill, with the weight on the pick (shoulders) and the toes. The hand on the shaft must be toward the spike end so that the axe does not pivot on the pick and cause injury.

Guidelines for Using an Ice Axe to Arrest a Fall

1. Do not try to lift your body off the ice while pressing the pick into the ground. Keep the axe close to the chest and keep your face down. The ice and snow at that level is uncomfortable, but lifting the body can decrease control.

2. Do not press the spike end into the ice to attempt an arrest because this could rip the axe out of your hand or pivot the shaft over your head and make it useless for arresting.

3. Keep the axe below the shoulders at all cost. The pressure that one can apply for braking is substantially decreased when holding the axe over the shoulders.

4. If you fall onto your back with feet downhill, grasp the axe properly and turn toward the hand that holds the pick end of the axe. Assume the prone, feet downhill, arrest position.

5. If you fall onto your back with your feet uphill, press the pick into the ice beside your hip with the shaft held across your body. Use the pick as a pivot and turn your body to the head uphill position by rolling onto your stomach. Pull the pick into the proper shoulder position and continue to press into the ice until stopped.

6. Hold on to the axe. Losing your axe in mountainous terrain where ice and snow impede safe travel is paramount to throwing away your clothes. In both, you are in a dangerous environment without the very tools necessary for safe travel.

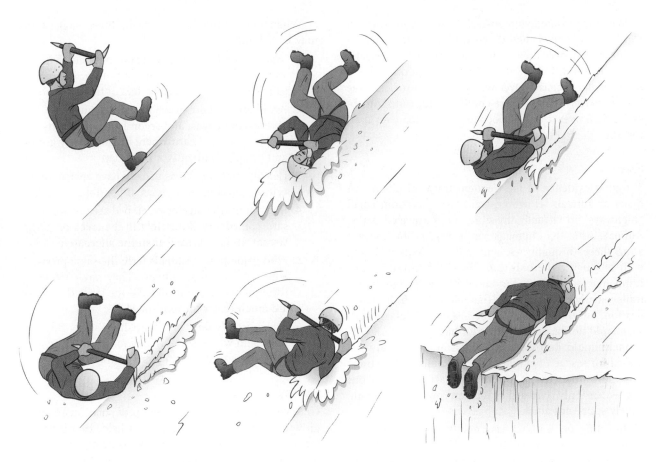

Figure 12–3 Use of an ice axe to arrest a fall.

General Wilderness Travel

Wilderness travel requires constant awareness. A novice views a landscape from the top of a hill with care and interest, and says, "Let's go." The experienced person carefully surveys the surrounding countryside. A distant blur may be mist or smoke; a faint, winding line on a far-off hill may be man-made or an animal trail; a blur in the lowlands may be a herd of deer or cattle. One—or perhaps all—of the information gathered visually could serve to make traveling easier and safer.

Two fundamental rules regarding wilderness travel need to be mastered in order to expend a minimum of energy and time. First, keep the weight of the body directly over the feet. Second, keep the sole of the foot flat on the ground to improve traction. These fundamentals are most easily accomplished by taking small steps at a slow, steady pace. Avoid an angle of descent that is too steep and use to your advantage any indentations or ground protrusions, however small.

Consider hard ground to be firmly packed dirt that will not give way under the weight of a person's step.

When ascending, apply the above fundamentals with the addition of locking the knees on every step in order to rest the leg muscles. When encountering steep slopes, traversing them is easier than climbing straight up. Turn at the end of each traverse by stepping off in the new direction with the uphill foot. This prevents crossing the feet and possible loss of balance. In traversing, the full sole principle is done by rolling the ankle away from the hill on each step. For narrow stretches, the herringbone step may be used; that is, ascending straight up a slope with toes pointed out and using the principles stated above. Descending is usually easiest by coming straight down a slope without traversing. Keep your back straight and the knees bent in such a manner that they take up the slack of each step. Again, remember the weight must be directly over the feet, and place the full sole on the ground with every step.

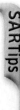

OPERATIONS
Two Basic Rules of Wilderness Travel
- Keep the body weight directly over the feet.
- Keep the sole of the foot flat to improve traction.

When confronted with obstacles within your route of travel, such as rocks and downed trees, make every attempt to walk over them rather than on them, especially in uphill travel. Even walking around such obstacles is occasionally preferred over walking onto a rock or tree and then over. It takes more energy to step onto the obstacle then over it than it does to simply step over it altogether.

Trails

A trail is evidence of the frequent travel of either humans or animals. However, trails can vary from small "highways" to virtually invisible, rarely traveled paths. Animals other than humans can be responsible for creating these throughways, and can be credited, often, with producing the only passable paths through environments too difficult for many people. "Man-made" trails usually have markings that allow easy trail identification, but these marks can be lost or unreadable and, so, should not be depended on for navigation. SAR personnel should keep in mind that trails are rarely designed for rescue operations. They should look at trails as opportunities to use avenues of least resistance, but not as the only avenues available. Trails also provide "likely spots" for clues.

Traveling on trails is easy and deserves little time dedicated to technique, but some guidelines can be helpful. First, recall the importance of spacing when traveling in a group. Give fellow team members room to move and room to stop without being trampled. Loosen laces to facilitate foot circulation while traveling on good, flat trails, and tighten them when on more severe terrain. Take rest breaks off of the trail so that others can easily pass. Keep your eyes open for evidence left by other people, which may include clues left by the lost subject.

Brush

Technique for traveling through brush is not nearly as important as learning to avoid it altogether. Proper travel technique through brush is directed at getting through it quickly or traveling around it, unless, of course, it needs to be searched. This type of vegetation is usually found in gullies and drainages where water and rich soil are prevalent. Brush can be small trees, shrubs, or vines that cause difficulty in travel because they prevent thorough examination of the ground and impede walking. In downhill walking situations, brush can be dangerous because a foot may catch the vegetation and cause a fall. Thorns may also be present in this type of vegetation, which can cause injuries ranging from minor abrasions to major incisions that can lead to a dangerous infection in the field.

When you cannot avoid brush, these suggestions may be helpful:

1. Walk around the brushy area, if possible. Even walking miles on a trail or road can be easier and safer than several hundred feet of heavy brush.
2. Avoid areas where brush flourishes, such as ravines, drainages, and second-growth, short-timbered areas. Learn where brush usually grows and be able to identify it on a map.
3. Heavily timbered areas usually have sparse under brush. Travel in these areas, if possible.
4. If travel in drainage or creek bed area is necessary, consider walking right in the creek or stream. It may be safer than the alternative.
5. Find game trails. Animals have the same problems with brush as humans. They rarely travel through brush and if they do, the trails they leave are much easier for foot travel.
6. Brush usually does not flourish on scree, ridgelines, and where snow is always around. Consider these routes if they can be traveled safely.

Grassy Slopes

Grassy slopes are usually made up of small tussocks of growth rather than one continuous field. In ascending, techniques should include taking advantage of any indentations or protrusions for traction. It is better, however, to step on the upper side of these protrusions or tussocks where the ground is more level than on the lower side. Descending on grassy slopes is best accomplished by traversing with care taken to visualize every step so as not to twist or turn an ankle. Be especially careful because wet, grassy slopes are treacherous with nearly any type of boot sole.

Grassy areas tend to easily show signs of travel. Seek evidence of travel on grassy areas to determine the whereabouts of the lost subject.

Scree and Talus Slopes

Scree slopes consist of small rocks and gravel that have collected below rock ridges and cliffs. The size of the scree varies from small particles to the size of a fist. Occasionally, it is a mixture of all sizes of rocks, but most scree slopes are comprised of rocks the same size. Ascending scree slopes is difficult, tiring, and should be avoided when possible. All principles of ascending hard ground apply, but each step must be picked carefully, so the foot will not slide down when weight is placed on it. This is best done by kicking in with the toe of the upper foot forming a step in the scree. After determining the step is stable, carefully transfer weight from the lower foot to upper and repeat the process. The best method for descending scree is to come straight down the slope with feet in a slight pigeon-toed position using a short shuffling step with the knees bent and back straight. When several travelers descend a scree slope together, they should be as close together as possible, one behind the other, to prevent injury from dislodged rocks. Since there is a tendency to run down scree slopes, care must be taken to ensure that this is avoided and control is not lost. When traversing a scree slope with no gain or loss of altitude, use the hop-skip method, which is simply a hopping motion in which the lower foot takes all the weight and using the upper foot for balance.

<u>Talus slopes</u> are similar in makeup to the scree slopes, except the rock pieces are larger. The technique of walking on talus is to step on top of, and on the uphill side of, the rocks. This prevents them from tilting and rolling downhill. All other previously mentioned fundamentals apply. Usually talus is easier to ascend and traverse, while scree is a more desirable avenue of descent.

Streams/Rivers

SAR personnel may find it necessary to cross a stream or river when traveling through some terrain. These rivers and streams can range from small, ankle-deep brooks to large rivers that may be so swift that a person can hear boulders on the bottom being crashed together by the current (**Figure 12–4**).

Safely crossing any waterway at a recognized ford is always the preferred approach, but this may be impossible. Take time to examine the possibilities before deciding to jump into any stream.

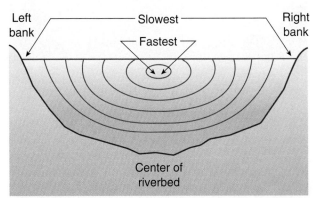

Cross Section of River

Figure 12–4 Cross section of a river showing relative current speed.

Careful study is required to find a place to safely cross a stream. If there is a high vantage point beside the river, a team member should climb the rise and look over the river. Do not be afraid to move parallel to the river to find a safe crossing point. Finding a safe crossing may be easy if the river breaks into a number of small channels. Survey the area on the opposite bank to make sure travel will be easier after crossing. If the waterways are of glacial origin, postpone crossing until early morning when the flow will probably decrease.

When selecting a crossing site on a fast moving river, the traveler should:

1. When possible, select a travel course that leads across the current at about a 45-degree angle downstream.

2. Never attempt to ford a stream directly above, or close to, a deep or rapid waterfall or a deep channel. Cross the stream where the opposite side comprises shallow banks or sandbars.

3. Avoid rocky places, since a fall may cause serious injury. However, an occasional rock that breaks the current may be of some assistance. The depth of the water is not necessarily a deterrent. Deep water may run more slowly and be safer than shallow.

4. Have a plan of action for making the crossing before entering the water. Use all possible precautions, and if the stream appears treacherous, cross using a technique that stabilizes the traveler in the water. Some of these techniques include: rope assisted, pole assisted, and team crossing.

5. Avoid pointing the feet downstream. A foot or ankle can easily be trapped under a rock or in a root, causing a fall. Falling in moving water with a foot entrapped can quickly lead to death.

Before attempting any crossing of any water at all, unfasten the waist strap to any pack and remove one arm from the shoulder straps to facilitate an expedient ditching of the pack should swimming be required after a fall.

Examine the exact route carefully before crossing. If making a rock-to-rock jumping attempt, be sure of the route and be careful of slippery footing. Perhaps sand could be thrown on the slippery spots. An ice axe or walking stick can make the difference between a safe crossing and a tragedy. Poke the axe or stick into the water ahead of you, searching for dangerous holes in the bottom or lean upstream onto the shaft as an added point of support during crossing.

The speed and force of water is quite easy to underestimate. The sound of flowing water coupled with calm surroundings tends to make rivers and streams seem almost serene. However, the power of moving water is one of the strongest forces in nature, and should not be taken lightly. Never work against that power; work with it. In a battle against powerful natural forces, you can never win.

Never tie ropes to the river crosser in belayed crossings. Hold the line in your hand so you can drop it should the rope impede travel or cause entrapment.

If you do find yourself in fast moving water swimming downstream after a fall, make sure to put your feet downstream, swim on your back, and ditch your pack. Paddle with your hands toward shore and do not make an attempt to stand until reaching shallow water very near shore. Attempting to walk in fast moving water can entrap a foot and force you underwater with very little chance of survival.

When walking in water, consider taking off your footgear and even your socks. It may be cold, but the brief discomfort during the crossing is usually better than cold, wet feet for the rest of the day from soaking wet boots and socks. If removal of the footgear is impractical, try inserting a vapor barrier (plastic bag, etc.) inside your boots or shoes and over your socks. This will aid in keeping your feet warm during the crossing. Never try to put bags over your boots or shoes for a water crossing. It is a waste of time because the first step will break a hole in the material, rendering it far less than waterproof. In addition, the material may get caught underwater and cause an unexpected fall.

Whatever method is used to cross a stream or river, tailor the approach to the weakest member of your group. Look long and hard before attempting a wet crossing, and be sure to exhaust all chances of a dry ford.

Desert

Before traveling in the desert, weigh the decision to travel against the environmental factors of terrain and climate, condition of SAR personnel, hazards, and the amount of water (and food) required (Figure 12–5).

The time of day for traveling is greatly dependent on two significant factors. First and most obvious is temperature, and second is type of terrain. For example, in rocky or mountainous deserts, the eroded drainages and canyons may not be seen at night and could result in a serious fall. Additionally, man-made features such as mining shafts or pits and irrigation channels could cause similar problems. If the temperature is not conducive to day travel, and the option is available, SAR team members should travel during the cooler parts of the day (in early morning or late evening). During the winter in the mid-latitude deserts, the cold temperatures make day travel most sensible.

There are three types of deserts: mountain, rocky plateau, and sandy or dune deserts, all of which can present difficult travel problems.

Mountain deserts are characterized by scattered ranges or areas of barren hills or mountains, separated by dry, flat basins. High ground may rise gradually or abruptly from flat areas to a height of several thousand feet above sea level. Most desert rainfall occurs at high elevations and the rapid runoff causes flash floods that erode deep gullies or ravines and deposit sand and gravel around the edges of the basins. Basins without shallow lakes will have alkaline flats, which can cause problems with chemical burns and can destroy clothing and equipment.

For desert travel, a compass is a valuable piece of equipment. Without a compass, you must use landmarks for local navigation and this can lead to difficulties. Mirages cause considerable trouble. Ground haze throughout the day may obscure vision. Distances are deceptive in the deserts; travelers have reported difficulty in estimating distances and the size of objects. Objects have a way of vanishing in some cases when the eye is moved for an instant, and in other cases, many peaks or hills look alike, causing difficulties in determining the original object.

The persistent winds of desert areas seem to provide no cooling effect, and many desert workers have reported that the wind "got on their nerves." More significant is the fact that the constant wind usually carries an amount of sand or dirt particles that can get in eyes, ears, nostrils, and mouth, and can cause irritations that are often severe.

There is no question that those who are familiar with working in hot areas are more likely to be capable of

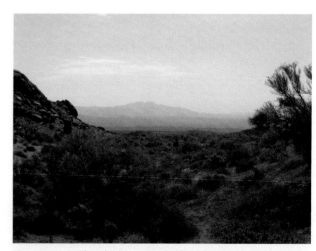

Figure 12–5 The decision to conduct SAR operations in the desert must be carefully weighed against the numerous risks and hazards that exist.

putting up with the heat of the desert. However, it is the nature of SAR work that teams are mobilized with little or no notice, and are exposed to extreme conditions of weather without adequate acclimatization. This poses quite a problem for SAR managers. They should draw their personnel from acclimatized teams, but this is rarely possible. Everyone operationally involved in these types of missions must understand the hazards and how to handle them. Everyone needs to be mindful of the extreme threat that heat can pose. Any group preparing itself for SAR work in hot climates should undergo specialized training prior to engaging in such work. This training should graduate in difficulty until members learn the necessary skills for operations within their area.

Specific skills and knowledge necessary for desert SAR work should include, but not be limited to, the following:

1. Knowledge of heat stress and its impact on the body and mind. The effects of heat stress are cumulative. Working day after day, even with intermixed rest, catches up to you.

2. Energy conservation and discipline for desert work. SAR assignments must be conservative, especially prior to acclimatization. If unacclimatized SAR personnel must work hard in the heat for one hour, then they must rest for the next two hours.

3. Pacing. Rest before you need to, start up slowly and wind down slowly, rest during the hot part of the day, work at night, and get sufficient sleep.

4. Water and electrolyte management. It is important to take water and trace mineral supplements (Gatorade®, etc.) at the same time; one without the other may only worsen the situation.

5. Avoiding dehydration and heat problems. Adequate hydration helps you to avoid: heat stroke, heat exhaustion, heat cramps, heat weakness, sun blindness, electrolyte imbalance, etc.

Jungle Environments

The inexperienced person's view of jungle travel may range from difficult to nearly impossible. However, with patience and good planning, the best and least difficult route can be selected. In some cases, the easiest routes are rivers, trails, and ridgelines. However, there may be hazards associated with these routes.

Rivers and streams may be overgrown, difficult to reach, impossible to raft or ford, and may also be infested with leeches. Trails may lead to a dead end, or into thick brush or swamps. Ridges may end abruptly at a cliff. Vegetation along a ridge may also conceal crevices or extend out past cliffs, making the cliff unnoticed until it's too late.

The machete is a good aid in the jungle, but SAR personnel rarely carry such a device. Brush is better parted than cut, but if the machete is required, it should be used in a down-and-out angle, instead of flat and level, as this method requires less effort.

In a jungle-like environment, team members should take their time and not hurry. This should allow them to observe their surroundings and get a better insight as to the best route of travel. Individuals should pay attention to the ground for the best footing locations as well as evidence from the passage of others, that is, the missing subject. Avoid grabbing bushes or plants when walking because some vegetation is poisonous and these actions may disturb animals. Step carefully; falling can be a painful experience because of the many plants that have razor sharp edges, thorns, and hooks. In jungle-like areas, wear gloves and fully buttoned clothes for protection from the same hazards.

Quicksand may be a problem. In appearance, quicksand looks just like the surrounding area with an absence of vegetation. It is usually located near the mouths of large rivers and on flat shores. The simplest description of quicksand is that it is a natural water tank filled with sand and supplied with water. The bottom consists of clay or other substances capable of holding water. The sand grains are rounded, as opposed to normal sharper edged sand, which is caused by the same water movement that prevents it from settling and stabilizing. The density of this sand-water solution will support a person's body weight, but there is a danger of drowning if a person panics. In quicksand, use the spread-eagle position to help disperse the body weight to keep from sinking and use a swimming motion to gain solid ground. Avoid panicky quick movements. Don't struggle! Just spread out and swim or pull yourself along the surface.

Snow

Travel in snow and ice is often required by SAR personnel. The greatest hazard in snow and ice areas is the intense cold and high winds. Both can lead to physical problems such as hypothermia and frostbite as well as a loss of dexterity and coordination. Judging distance can be difficult because of the lack of landmarks and the clear, cold air. Image distortion is a common phenomenon.

Where strong winds prevail, "white-out" conditions may exist and personnel should avoid travel during these times. A white-out condition occurs when there is complete snow cover and wind-driven snow or humidity causes uniform light to be reflected from both the ground and sky. The result is little or no depth perception, so everything appears white. If traveling during bad weather in the snow, take great care to avoid becoming disoriented or falling into crevasses, over cliffs, or high snow ridges.

In arctic areas, strong winds often sweep unchecked across tundra areas (due to lack of vegetation) causing white-out conditions. Because of blowing snow, fog, and lack of landmarks, a compass is a must for travel. Yet, it still may be difficult to navigate a true course because the magnetic variation (declination) in the high latitudes (polar areas) is often extreme. During the summer months in these same arctic regions, the terrain is usually a mass of bogs, swamps, and standing water, and crossing them is difficult at best. Rain and fog are common, and insects such as mosquitoes, midges, and black flies can cause travel problems. If the skin is not completely covered or if travelers do not use a head net or insect repellent, insect bites may be a major threat to health and mental well-being.

Summer travel in timbered sub-arctic environments should not present any major problems. However, travel on ridges is preferred, because the terrain is drier and there are usually fewer insects. During the cold months, snow may be deep and travel is difficult without some type of snowshoes or skis. Travel is generally easier on frozen rivers, streams, and lakes, which may have less snow, making them easier to walk on.

In mountainous country, it is often best to travel along ridgelines because they provide a firmer walking surface and there is usually less vegetation with which to contend. High winds make travel impractical if not impossible at times. Glaciers have many hidden dangers. Glacial streams may run just under the surface of the snow or ice, creating weak spots, or they may run on the surface and cause slick ice. Crevasses running across glaciers can be a few feet to several hundred feet deep. A thin layer of snow often covers crevasses, making them practically invisible. Unwary team members can fall into crevasses and sustain severe injuries or death. If glacial travel is required, it is best to use a probe pole or ice axe to test the footing ahead.

In ice and snow conditions, river and stream travel can be hazardous. Comparatively straight rivers are that way because of the volume of water flow and extremely fast currents. These rivers tend to have very thin ice in the winter, especially where snow banks extend out over the water. If an object protrudes through the ice, the immediate area will be weak and should be avoided. Where two rivers and streams come together, the current is swift and the ice will be weaker than on the rest of the river. Very often after freeze up, the source of the river or stream dries up so rapidly that air pockets form under the ice and can be dangerous. During the runoff months (spring and summer), rivers and streams usually have a large volume of very cold water that can cause cold injuries. Stream banks are often choked with alder, devil's club, and other thick vegetation, making traveling very slow and difficult.

In snow environments, optimum travel conditions may vary from hour to hour. Test indicators may show the best method of travel, such as depth that a person sinks into the snow. The best snow condition is one that supports a person on or near the surface when wearing boots and the second best is calf-deep snow conditions. If possible, avoid traveling in thigh or waist deep snow and wear snowshoes when conditions dictate.

South and west slopes offer hard surfaces late in the day after exposure to the sun has melted the snow slightly and the surface is refrozen. East and north slopes tend to remain soft and unstable. Walking on one side of a ridge, gully, clump of trees, or large boulders is often more solid than the other side. Dirty snow absorbs more heat than clean snow; slopes darkened by rocks, dust, or uprooted vegetation usually provide more solid footing. Travel can be best in the morning to take advantage of stable snow conditions. Since sunlight affects the stability of snow, travel may be best when done in shaded areas where footing should remain stable.

In areas covered by early seasonal snowfall, travel cautiously between deep snow and clear ground. Snow on slopes tends to slip away from rocks on the downhill side, forming openings. These openings, called "moats," are filled by subsequent snowfalls. During the snow season, moats below large rocks or cliffs may become extremely wide and deep, presenting a hazard to any SAR personnel.

Snowshoes

Use a striding technique for movement with snowshoes. In taking a stride, lift the toe of the snowshoe upward to clear the snow and thrust forward. Conserve energy by lifting the snowshoe no higher than is necessary to clear the snow. If the front of the snowshoe catches, pull the foot back to free it and then lift it before proceeding with the stride. The best and least exerting method of travel is a loose-kneed rocking gait in a normal rhythmic stride. Take care not to step on or catch the other snowshoe.

On gentle slopes, ascend by climbing straight upward; traction is generally very poor on hard-packed or crusty snow. Ascend steeper terrain by traversing and packing a trail similar to a shelf. When climbing, place the snowshoe horizontally in the snow. On hard snow, place the snowshoe flat on the surface with the toe of the upper one diagonally uphill to get more traction. If the snow supports the weight of a person, it may be better to remove the snowshoes and temporarily proceed on foot. In turning, the best method is to swing the leg up and turn the snowshoe in the new direction of travel.

Step over obstacles such as logs, tree stumps, ditches, and small streams. Take care not to place too much strain on the snowshoe in shallow snow. There is danger of catching and tearing the webbing on tree stumps or snags. Wet snow will frequently ball up under the feet, making walking uncomfortable. Knock this snow off with a stick or pole.

Generally, ski poles are not used in snowshoeing; however, one or two poles are desirable when carrying heavy loads, especially in mountainous terrain. Do not fasten the bindings too tightly, or circulation will be impaired and cause frostbite. During stops, check the bindings for fit and possible readjustment.

Uphill Travel

Maximum altitude may be obtained with less effort by traversing a slope. A zigzag or <u>switchback</u> route used to traverse steep slopes places body weight over the entire foot as opposed to the balls of the feet as in a straight line uphill climb. An additional advantage to zigzagging or switchbacking is alternating the stress and strain placed on the feet, ankles, legs, and arms when making a change in direction.

When making a change in direction, the body is temporarily out of balance. The proper method for turning on the steep slope is to pivot on the outside foot (the one away from the slope). With the upper slope on the right side, kick the left foot (pivot foot) directly into the slope. This transfers the body weight onto the left foot while pivoting toward the slope. The slope is then positioned on the left side and the right foot is on the outside.

In soft snow on steep slopes, stamp in pit steps for solid footing. On hard snow, the surface is solid but slippery, and level pit steps must be made. In both cases, make the steps by swinging the entire leg in toward the slope, not by merely pushing the boot into the snow. In hard snow, when one or two blows do not suffice, use crampons. Space steps evenly and close together to facilitate ease of travel and balance. Additionally, the lead climber must consider the other team members, especially those who have a shorter stride.

A team should travel in single file when ascending, permitting the leader to establish the route. The physical exertion of the climbing leader is greater than that of any other team member. The climbing leader must remain alert to safeguard other team members while choosing the best route of travel. Change the lead function frequently to prevent exhaustion of any one individual. Team members following the leader should use the same leg swing technique to establish foot positions, improving each step as they climb. Each foot must be firmly kicked into place, securely positioning the boot in the step. In compact snow, the kick should be somewhat low, shaving off snow during each step, thus enlarging the hole by deepening. In very soft snow, it is usually easier to bring the boot down from above, dragging a layer of snow into the step to strengthen and decrease the depth of it.

When necessary to traverse a slope without an increase in elevation, the heels rather than the toes form the step. During the stride, the climber twists the leading leg so that the boot heel strikes the slope first, carrying most of the weight into the step. The toe is pointed up and out. Similar to the plunge step (Figure 12–6), the heel makes the platform secure by compacting the snow more effectively than the toe.

Descending

The route down a slope may be different from the route up a slope. Route variations may be required for descending different sides of a mountain or moving just a few feet from icy shadows onto sun-softened slopes. A good surface snow condition is ideal for descending rapidly since it yields comfortably underfoot. The primary techniques for descending snow-covered slopes are plunge stepping and descending step by step.

The plunge step (see Figure 12–6) makes extensive use of the heels of the feet and is applicable on scree as well as snow. Ideally, the plunging route should be at an angle, one that is within the capabilities of the team and affords a safe descent. The angle at which the heel enters the surface varies with the surface hardness. On soft snow slopes, almost any angle suffices; however, if the person leans too far forward, there is a risk of lodging the foot in a rut and inflicting injuries.

On hard snow, the heel will not penetrate the surface unless it has sufficient force behind it. Failure to firmly drive the heel into the snow can cause a slip and subsequent slide. The quickest way to check a slip is to shift the

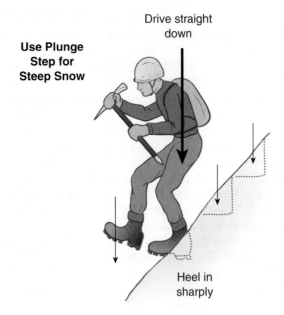

Use Plunge Step for Steep Snow

Drive straight down

Heel in sharply

Figure 12–6 Plunge step used to descend scree or snow.

weight onto the other heel, making several short, stiff-legged stomps. This technique is not intended to replace "the ice arrest" technique, which is usually more effective. When roped, plunging requires coordination and awareness of all team members' progress. Limit the speed of the team to the slowest member. Plunging may not work when wearing crampons due to the snow compacting and sticking to them.

Use the step-by-step descending technique when the terrain is extremely steep, snow significantly deep, or circumstances dictate a slower pace. On near-vertical walls, it is necessary to face the slope and cautiously lower oneself step by step, thrusting the toe of the boot into the snow while maintaining an anchor or handhold with the axe. Once the new foothold withstands the body's full weight, repeat the technique. On moderately angled terrain, the team can face away from the slope and descend by step-kicking with the heels.

A belay, or anchor, can be set up in several different ways using the ice axe and your body. One of these is termed the "Boot Axe Belay." The boot axe belay can be set up rapidly and used when a team is moving together and belaying is only required at a few spots. Practice the boot axe belay until a sweep and jab of the ice axe can set up the stance within a couple of seconds. The axe provides an anchor to the slope and the slope and the boot braces the axe. Both give a friction surface over which the run of rope is controlled.

To prepare a boot axe belay, stamp out in the snow a firm platform, large enough for the axe and uphill boot. Jam the ice axe shaft as deeply as possible, at a slight up-

hill angle (against the anticipated fall) into the snow at the rear of the platform. The pick is parallel to the fall line, pointing uphill, thus applying the strongest dimension of the shaft against the force of a fall. The length of the pick prevents the rope from escaping over the top of the shaft.

The belayer stands below the axe, facing at a right angle to the fall line. Stamp the uphill boot into the slope against the downhill side of the shaft at a right angle to the fall line, bracing the shaft against downhill pull. The downhill boot is in a firmly compacted step below the uphill boot so that the leg is straight, stiffly bracing the belayer. The uphill hand is on the axe head in arrest grasp, bracing the shaft against downhill and lateral stress. From below, the rope crosses the toe of the boot, preventing the rope from trenching into the snow. The rope bends around the uphill side of the shaft, then down across the instep of the bracing boot, and is controlled by the downhill hand. To apply braking through greater friction, the downhill or braking hand brings the rope uphill around the heel, forming an "S" bend.

Crampon Technique

Crampons are a lightweight frame of steel spikes that can be attached to one's boots. To put the crampons on, the harness is attached by positioning the buckles to cinch on the outward sides of the boots. Special care must be taken to strap the crampons tightly to the boots, running the strap through each attachment prong or ring. If crampons do not have heel loops, ankle straps should be long enough to be crossed behind the boot before being secured to prevent boots from sliding backward out of the crampons. Many crampons have been lost because this precaution was not taken. When trimming new straps, make allowance for gaiters, which sometimes cover the instep of the boot. When putting the crampons on, lay each crampon on the snow or ice with all rings and straps outward. Then place the boot on the crampon and tighten the straps. Even modern neoprene-coated nylon straps should be checked from time to time to make sure they are tight, have not been cut, and are not trailing loop strap ends that could cause the wearer to trip.

If crampons may be needed, they should be carried. Weather conditions change rapidly; an east-facing slope may be mushy enough for step-kicking during the morning, but can become a smooth sheet of ice in the afternoon shade. Furthermore, using crampons may contribute directly to the team's safety by enabling it to negotiate stretches of ice faster and with less fatigue than having to chop steps. Your situation determines whether or not to wear crampons. Wearing crampons should not be considered mandatory because of venturing onto a glacier; neither should a team attempt to save time by never wearing crampons on steep, exposed icy patches just because they are fairly short. Another important guideline is to don crampons before they are needed to avoid teetering in ice steps. On mixed rock and ice climbs, constant attaching and removing of crampons takes so much time that the objective may be lost.

Wear crampons throughout the entire climb if the terrain is 50% or more suitable for crampons (crampons may skid or be broken on rock surfaces). Crampons may not be required if the snow or ice patches are fairly short, good belays are available, and rock predominates. These alternatives are merely suggestions and the decision must be based on the conditions at hand.

Take crampons off when the snow begins to ball up badly in them and no improvement in snow conditions is anticipated. On the ascent, it may be possible to clear away the soft surface snow and climb on the ice below, but this is usually impractical and futile on the descent. Occasionally the climber should kick the crampons free of accumulated snow. The time-worn practice of striking the ice axe shaft against the crampons to knock out the snow is effective, but hard on the axe and perhaps the ankle. In situations where the crampons must be worn even though the snow balls up in them, shuffling the feet through the snow instead of stepping over the surface tends to force the accumulated snow through the back points. The normal kicking motion of the foot generally keeps the crampons snow-free on the ascent and while traversing.

On the descent, drive the toe of the boot under the surface of the snow ahead of the heel, walking on the ball of the foot. Keep the weight well forward and use short skating steps allowing the foot to slide forward and penetrate the harder sub-layers.

Flat-footing involves a logical and natural progression of coordinated body and ice axe positions to allow the climber to move steadily and in balance while keeping all vertical points of the crampons biting into the ice. The weight is directly over the feet, the crampon points stamped firmly into the ice with each step, with the ankles and knees flexed to allow boot soles to remain parallel to the slope.

On gentle slopes, the climber walks straight up the hill. Normally, the feet are naturally flat to the slope and the axe is used as a cane. If pointing the toes uphill becomes awkward, they may be turned outward in duck-fashion. As the slope steepens, the body is turned to face across the slope rather than up it. The feet may also point across the slope, but additional flexibility and greater security are gained by pointing the lower foot downhill. Use the axe to maintain balance and carried in the cane position or the arrest grasp with either the pick or point touching the slope. Movement is diagonal rather than straight upward, and the climber takes ad-

vantage of terrain irregularities and graded slopes. Change your direction as in step-kicking on snow by planting the downhill foot, turning the body toward the slope to face the opposite direction, and stepping off with the new downhill foot.

On gentler slopes, use the flat-footed approach throughout. On steeper slopes, it is more secure and easier to initiate the turn by kicking the front points and briefly front-pointing through the turn. At some point in the turn, the grip on the axe must be reversed. The exact moment for this depends on the climber and the specific situation. However, the climber's stance must be secure when temporarily relinquishing the axe as the third point of support.

On steep slopes, which approach the limit of practical use of this style of ascent, the climber relies on the axe for hold security as well as for balance. Hold the axe in the arrest grasp with one hand on the head and the other on the shaft, above the point. Plant the well-sharpened pick firmly in the ice at about shoulder height to provide one point of suspension while a foot moves forward and the crampons are stamped.

Descent follows the same general progression of foot and axe positions; descend the fall line, gradually turning the toes out as the slope gets steeper. As the slope steepens, widen the stance, flex the knees, and lean forward to keep weight over the feet, and finally, face sideways and descend with the support of the axe in the arrest position. On very steep or hard ice, it may be necessary to face the slope and front-point downwards. When walking flat-foot downhill, all crampon points should be stamped firmly into the ice. It may be necessary to strive to take small steps allowing the climber to maintain balance during moves; long steps require major weight shifts to adjust balance.

Climbing

Balance climbing is the type of movement used to climb rock faces. It is a combination of the balance movement of a tightrope walker and the unbalanced climbing of a person ascending a tree or ladder. During the process of route selection, climbers often mentally climb the route to learn what might be expected. Climbers should not wear gloves when balance climbing.

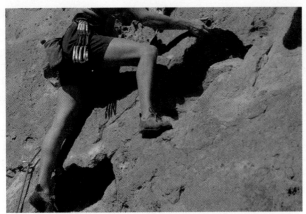

Figure 12–7 When climbing, the feet, not the hands, should carry the weight (with rare exception). The hands are for balance.

Body Position

The climber must keep good balance when climbing (the weight placed over the feet during movement). The feet, not the hands, should carry the weight (with rare exception). The hands are for balance (Figure 12–7). The feet do not provide proper traction when the climber leans in toward the rock. With the body in balance, the climber moves with a slow, rhythmic motion. Whenever possible, use three points of support, such as two feet and one hand. The preferred handholds are waist to shoulder high. Resting is necessary when climbing because tense muscles tire quickly. When resting, keep the arms low where circulation is not impaired. Use of small intermediate holds is preferable to stretching and clinging to widely separated big holds. Avoid a spread-eagle position, where a climber stretches too far (and cannot let go).

Types of Holds

Push holds are desirable because they help the climber keep the arms low. However, they are more difficult to hold onto in case of a slip. A push hold is often used to advantage in combination with a pull hold.

Pull holds are those that are pulled down upon and are the easiest holds to use. They are also the most likely to break out.

Jam holds involve jamming any part of the body or extremity into a crack. This is done by putting the hand into the crack and clenching it into a fist or by placing the arm into the crack and twisting the elbow against one side and the hand against the other side. When using the foot in a jam hold, take care to ensure placing the boot so it can be removed easily when climbing is continued.

The holds mentioned above are considered basic and from these any number of combinations and variations can be used. The number of these variations depends only on the limit of the individual's imagination. Following are a few of the more common variations:

- The counter-force is attained by pinching a protruding part between the thumb and fingers and pulling outward or pressing inward with the arms.
- The lay-back is done by leaning to one side of an offset crack with the hands pulling and the feet pushing against the offset side. Lay-backing is a classic form of force or counter-force where the hands and feet pull and push in opposite directions, enabling the climber to move up in a series of shifting moves. It is very strenuous.
- Underclings permit cross pressure between hands and feet.

- Mantleshelving, or mantling, takes advantage of down pressure exerted by one or both hands on a slab or shelf. Straightening and locking the arm raises the body, allowing a leg to be placed on a higher hold.
- Chimney climbing is a body-jam hold used in very wide cracks. Use the arms and legs to apply pressure against the opposite faces of the rock in a counter-force move. The outstretched hands hold the body while the legs are drawn as high as possible. Flexing the legs forces the body up. Continue this procedure as necessary. Another method is to place the back against one wall and the legs and arms against the other and "worm" upward.

Friction Climbing

A slab is a relatively smooth portion of rock lying at an angle. When traversing, point the lower foot slightly downhill to increase balance and friction of the foot. Use all irregularities in the slope for additional friction. On steep slabs, it may be necessary to squat with the body weight well over the feet with hands alongside for added friction. Use this position for ascending, traversing, or descending. A slip may result if the climber leans back or lets the buttocks down. Wet, icy, mossy, or scree covered slabs are the most dangerous.

Friction holds depend solely on the friction of hands or feet against a relatively smooth surface with a shallow hold. They are difficult to use because they give a feeling of insecurity, which the inexperienced climber tries to correct by leaning close to the rock, thereby increasing the imbalance. They often serve well as intermediate holds, giving needed support while the climber moves over them. However, they would not hold if the climber decided to stop.

SAR Terms

Crampons A lightweight frame of steel spikes that can be attached to one's boots.

Scree slopes Areas consisting of small rocks and gravel that have collected below rock ridges and cliffs.

Switchback A zigzag pattern used to traverse steep slopes.

Talus slopes Similar in makeup to the scree slopes, except the rock pieces are larger.

References

Cox, M., & Fulsass, K., eds. (2003). *Mountaineering: Freedom of the Hills,* 7th ed. New York, NY: Mountaineers Books.

Johnson, M. (2003). *The Ultimate Desert Handbook: A Manual for Desert Hikers, Campers, and Travelers.* New York, NY: Ragged Mountain Press/McGraw Hill.

Manning, H. (1986). *Backpacking: One Step at a Time,* 4th ed. New York, NY: Vintage Books.

McManners, H. (1998). *The Complete Wilderness Training Book.* New York, NY: DK Publishing.

Petzoldt, P. (1974). *The Wilderness Handbook.* New York, NY: W.W. Norton & Company, Inc.

Rawlins, C., & Fletcher, C. (2002). *The Complete Walker IV*, revised ed. New York, NY: Alfred A. Knopf, Inc.

Chapter 13
Tracking

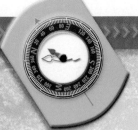

Objectives

Upon completion of this chapter and any course activities, the student will be able to meet the following objectives:

Define the following:
    Track or print. (p. 210–211)
    Sign. (p. 211)
    Sign-cutting. (p. 212)
    Step-by-step tracking. (p. 212, 214–215)

Describe the use of a tracking stick/walking stick in tracking. (p. 214–215)

Describe the method of labeling a track. (p. 215)

Describe the responsibilities of each of the members of a tracking crew (point, flankers). (p. 215–216)

Tracking in Perspective

Tracking, by simple definition, is following signs or tracks left by someone or something. It is used to detect the path (direction, movement) of someone or something. However, tracking, when applied to SAR, becomes a more complex skill. It not only concerns itself with detection, but with interpretation of clues.

Unfortunately, tracking is underutilized in SAR situations. More often than not, SAR personnel ignore sign and track because they are unaware of its potential. SAR personnel are too often guilty of literally walking on the very evidence for which they search because of looking for the subject or staring at a map. A story has been printed on the ground and we, as "track aware" searchers, must discover its existence, and then learn to interpret it (Figure 13–1). This is not to say that once tracking is applied to SAR situations, every lost subject will be found. Rather, tracking will give the subject a much better chance to survive and it can help to prove (or disprove) that a lost person is within a designated search area.

Reading this material will not make anyone an expert tracker. Tracking is an acquired skill and it takes determination, patience, and a willingness to learn. Becoming a highly skilled tracker takes thousands of hours of practice. It may be a high price to pay, but when the consequences involve human life, no investment of time is too much.

Definitions and Terminology

A <u>track</u> or <u>print</u> is an impression left from the passage of a person that can be positively identified as being human. Further, a track may be *complete*, meaning that the entire impression is visible; *partial*, meaning that it is

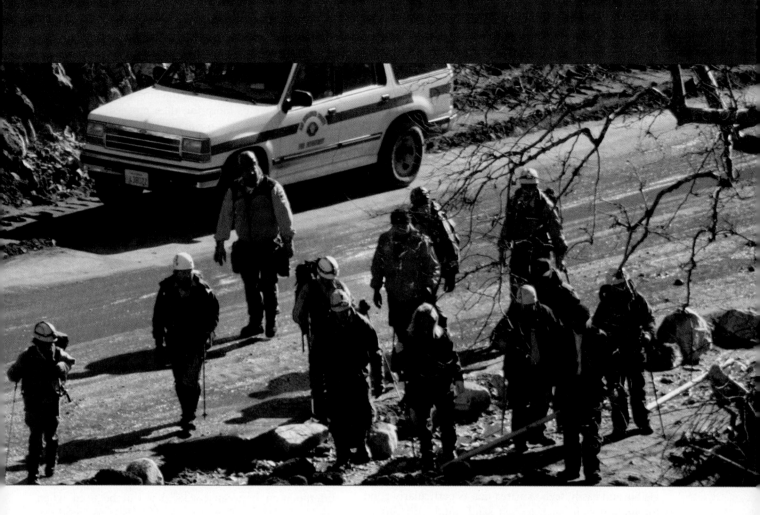

not visible in its entirety; and/or *identifiable*, meaning that, complete or partial, it has at least one characteristic that differentiates it from others similar to it. <u>Tracking</u> is simply defined as following someone, or something, by stringing together a continuous chain of their sign. <u>Sign</u> is any evidence of change from the natural state that is inflicted on an environment by a person's

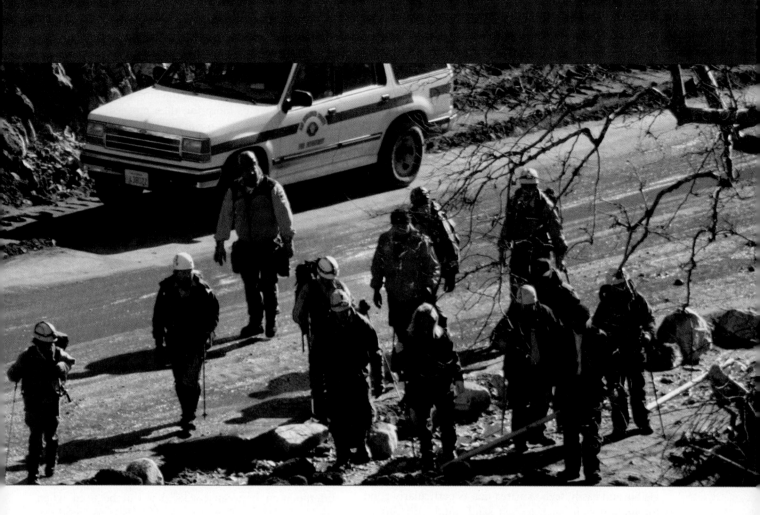

Figure 13–1   A story has been printed on the ground and we, as "track aware" SAR personnel, must discover its existence and learn to interpret it.

passage. A track, whether complete or partial, is many individual pieces of sign combined in such a way as to form a print. The technique is first to find some sign, then interpret it, and ultimately act on it. Simply put, tracking is the ability to put sign together, after investigation, in chronological order over a large area.

To be of any use, sign must be discovered. Seeing it is usually fairly easy because there is so much of it. A walking person leaves sign approximately every 18 to 20 inches, or over 3000 times per mile, so catching even a small percentage of it shouldn't be much trouble. The problem lies not in finding sign, but in determining which is relevant and which is not. The novice tracker, for example, often sees plenty of relevant sign, yet disregards it because he or she believes it to be insignificant. The experienced tracker sees the same information but has learned to glean its meaning.

If sign is considered evidence, then common law enforcement terms can be applied to distinguish different types. Sign can be separated into two categories: conclusively human, and corroborant. *Conclusively human* sign is a disturbance which, on its own, can positively be said to have been caused by a person and not an animal. *Corroborant* sign is disturbance that is not decisively human and could have been caused by an animal. This type of sign may corroborate other evidence but, when considered on its own, is not conclusive. It cannot be positively determined to have been caused by a person, but may confirm or substantiate other evidence with which it may be found.

Sign cutting is looking for sign in order to establish a starting point from which to track. Tracking involves following a chronology of sign, or consecutive tracks, step-by-step. Sign cutting is searching for the *first* sign or track. Another principal difference between the two is that tracking is done by traveling the same direction as the person who laid the track, and sign cutting is done traveling perpendicular to the direction of travel of the person being followed. Sign cutting is done by looking for sign in a path that would intersect that of the person who laid the track. It is most effective when performed in an area where the sign being sought is most visible and easily seen. An area that is particularly good for finding sign, such as wet sand, mud, soft dirt or snow, is sometimes called a *track trap* or *"cuttable" area*. Track traps are often man-made by scraping an area clean so as to show sign easily (**Figure 13–2**).

Sign cutting can substantially reduce the search area by detecting sign that indicates direction of travel. This can be a very efficient application of resources, particularly at the onset of an incident when urgency is high and resources are sparse.

Jump tracking is a form of tracking that involves finding a big, obvious footprint, then proceeding along the presumed direction of travel until another obvious track is found. Jump tracking involves guesswork, luck, essentially no skill, and can be dangerous when a life depends on skillful tracking. One of the biggest problems in tracking has always been the destruction of sign by unknowing, yet energetic, searchers. Jump tracking offers great potential for this type of clue erasure. Since virtually all humans can jump track without training, this is not the type of tracking that will be discussed here.

Step-by-Step tracking is a disciplined teaching system where a tracker sees each step in sequence and proceeds no further than the last visible track, using the stride to determine where next to look for sign. This system, above all, makes all searchers clue conscious and track aware (aware that track and sign exist). It is the standard for which an experienced tracker will strive at all times. In theory, a tracker attempts to find every piece of evidence left by his or her quarry. In a real situation, this is not always possible and even the best trackers must accept small gaps in the continuous chain of evidence. The words "small gaps" best distinguish the Step-by-Step method from jump tracking.

Bracketing is an occasionally acceptable method of interpolation between tracks that can be used when standard Step-by-Step approaches fail to produce. Bracketing is meant as a stopgap measure that uses a predetermined stride to skip one step in sequence in order to find the next, and then use it to find the one skipped. In terms of the Step-by-Step approach, bracketing is cheating because it involves moving past the last visible sign in order to continue the track. Bracketing, however, is not a license to jump track and should be used only infrequently to maintain continuity on an important track. Students may come to this on their own but will never receive permission to do it.

Programs that teach the Step-by-Step method do not teach tracking, per se, but an approach that offers the tools to teach one's self the skills of tracking. Anyone can learn to track. All it takes beyond learning the basics of the Step-by-Step approach, if you are motivated, is practice—hours and hours of practice. You may never become an expert tracker but, at the very least, the Step-by-Step approach will make you track and sign aware and, therefore, be a better searcher.

Anyone can learn to track. It simply takes a willingness to learn, patience, determination, hard work, and practice. It is like any other important endeavor. Keep in mind that everyone does not have to become a "tracking guru." Just having the interest and open-mindedness to attend a Step-by-Step program will likely improve one's value as a searcher.

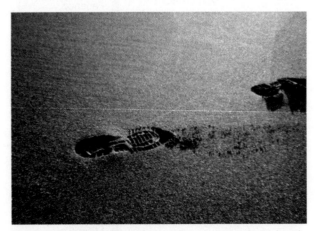

Figure 13–2 Well-defined track on firm, moist sand on a beach. Trackers very rarely get to deal with prints this perfect.

Equipment for Tracking

Tracking essentially requires very little equipment. A pair of eyes that, aided or not, provide nearly 20/20 vision is the only prerequisite. However, experience has indicated that some accessory equipment can be quite helpful.

1. Clothing should be appropriate for the terrain and weather, and durable enough to withstand ventures into dense brush and rugged terrain. A broad-brimmed hat may be handy for protecting the eyes from the sun, or shading tracks when the sun is high in the sky. Above all, the tracker must be able to work comfortably in whatever environment he or she is thrust.

2. A walking or sign cutting stick is a must, especially for novice trackers. A light, durable stick, approximately 40 inches long is best but longer may be preferred. This stick, which is used to focus the attention of a tracker, should have at least two "O" rings or rubber bands on it for measuring distance and stride (some use many more than two rings).

3. A measuring device such as a tape measure can be valuable when measuring print size or stride. Some attach a measuring tape to their stick, but most simply carry a metal, carpenter's-type, tape measure in their pocket.

4. A small notepad and pencil are needed to record measurements and fill out track reports. A good drawing of a print will be indispensable.

5. Trail tape can be carried to cordon off evidence or sign, or to prevent the trampling of a good track. Plastic surveyor's tape works well, but care must be taken to see that it is retrieved after it has served its purpose. Royal blue is the best color for this purpose.

6. A flashlight can be important when light is not at an optimum. Since light plays such an important part in the ability to see, it is easy to appreciate how an artificial light source is helpful.

7. A mirror can be used to redirect natural light low across sign when the sun is high in the sky.

Tracking is not an equipment-intensive pursuit. Sight, patience, perseverance, and determination are requirements. The listed specific equipment is helpful, but the brain and the body are the primary tools of the trade.

Credo of the Novice Tracker

The fundamental principle on which tracking is based is sound training. The rules upon which all future tracking experience is based lie within the following credo. These very basic rules also serve as the "ABCs" of the Step-by-Step method of tracking.

Any track or sign is considered evidence until proven otherwise. Treat all track and sign as if they were positively identified as being that of the person being sought. *Once a track or sign has been destroyed, it cannot be reconstituted.* It is lost forever. The destruction of a track, clue, or any sign not only chips away at the finite body of available information, it reduces the chances of meeting your objective. If that objective is finding a lost person, destroying tracks, clues, or any sign can literally mean the difference between life and death.

Beyond simply finding and interpreting sign, a tracker is obliged to protect it. Remember, any clue is important, no matter how small or seemingly insignificant. Do not move from one place to another without being track aware. An untrained person stepping on good sign or track is unfortunate. A tracker or searcher doing the same is inexcusable.

Light

Since tracking is an intensely visual skill, it is easy to understand how light can play an important role. Tracking is far simpler when the light is of the proper intensity and from the right direction. However, Mother Nature does not always supply the optimum lighting conditions required for tracking during a SAR incident. When learning to track, using the sun properly is one of the most important things to learn. Tracks are easiest to see when the sun is at a low angle, for example, early in the morning and late in the afternoon (Figure 13–3). The low angle causes longer shadows that bring out the details of any depression on the ground, making sign easier to see. Clouds, diffuse light (through pollution or clouds), and the sun high overhead all diminish the shadow effect. Put simply, sign and track are usually easier to see while

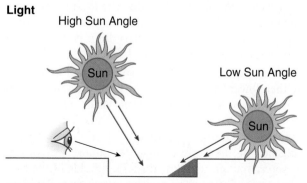

Light

High Sun Angle

Low Sun Angle

Sun

Sun

Figure 13–3 Tracks are easiest to see when the sun is at a low angle, such as early in the morning and late in the afternoon.

facing the light source, and with that source at a low angle to the ground.

Since facing the light source can make tracks easier to detect, moving around into a position to optimize the angle to the sun is to be encouraged. Be careful, however, that you do not trample evidence in your search for the proper angle from which to view. The angle will not matter if you have nothing to look at but your own footprints.

Tracking at Night

Because light plays such an important role in tracking, it is easy to see how tracking can be performed at night when the light source is completely under the control of the tracker. An artificial light source can be rotated completely around the track from a low angle to allow for the best view, thus emphasizing otherwise unnoticed sign. An additional benefit of tracking at night can be realized if the lost individual stops moving (to sleep, for instance), thereby allowing night trackers to catch up.

In addition, since darkness at night hides most of the distractions seen during the day, your light source can serve to focus your attention and concentration where it should be.

A diffuse hand lantern works best when tracking at night. Some success has been achieved with Coleman® lanterns with deflectors that keep the light out of the tracker's eyes. Also, the battery-powered fluorescent lanterns have been used effectively. The key, however, is not brightness. The flashlights commonly carried by law enforcement personnel that serve as "attitude adjusters" and fire starters (with light beam only) are generally worthless as tracking lights. These bright lights diminish night vision and are too intense to bring out subtle sign on an otherwise dark night. The ideal night tracking light should not be so bright as to ruin night vision, yet last a long time (good battery life), be lightweight and durable, and offer a diffuse beam.

Some experienced trackers have attached headlamps to their lower legs, just below the knee, or to their tracking sticks to obtain the best angle while walking. The U.S. Border Patrol often uses lights attached low on a vehicle for cutting sign on a road. The proper light attached at the correct angle can allow a driver, or observer/spotter, to follow track on the side of the road for a great distance at a faster speed than could be achieved on foot.

Sign Cutting and the Step-by-Step Method

Most trades have their specialized tools. In tracking it is the sign cutting stick. It is difficult to believe that such a simple tool can be so effective, but it is true. When properly used, a sign cutting stick can seem to make sign pop out of thin air. In reality, all it does is force you to look where you want to be looking, instead of everywhere else.

The Step-by-Step method of tracking is stride-based. That is, a tracker gets from one track to the next by determining stride (distance from heel of rear print to heel of front print) then searching one stride from the last track found. This requires some type of device for measuring stride and, for this, the sign cutting stick works well.

When the stride length is indicated on the sign cutting stick by placing the "O" ring or rubber band one stride length from the end, the marker can be placed at the heel of the last track and the end of the stick pointed in the direction of travel. The end of the stick, then, becomes a pointer towards where the next sign or track is expected to be found. The stick causes the tracker's attention to be focused on a small piece of ground rather than a large area. Finding sign is easier when the "search area" is limited. A sign cutting stick does just that.

To use the sign cutting stick, do the following (**Figure 13–4**):

1. Find or make a stick that is approximately 40 inches long or longer. On it, place at least two rubber bands (or rubber "O" rings) that can be moved on the stick, but will stay in place if desired. For one-time uses, a large twig can be procured from the environment and marked with a knife, pencil, or other marker.

2. At the earliest opportunity while tracking someone, determine his or her stride by measuring the distance from the heel of the rear print to the heel on the front print. Position a marker on your sign cutting stick (either a rubber band, "O" ring, or other mark), so that the distance from the tip of the stick to the marker is the same distance as the stride.

3. On the last print found, hold the stick so that the stride mark is held close to, but above, the rear of the heel. Move the tip of the stick through an arc that covers the area where the next track should fall.

4. While sweeping the stick very slowly, study the area directly in front of the tip for sign. Take about twenty seconds to sweep from the 10 o'clock to 2 o'clock positions. Somewhere during the sweep, the tip of the stick should be pointing to the heel

Use of Tracking Stick

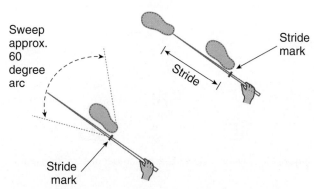

Figure 13–4 Typical sign cutting stick in use.

Labeling Tracks

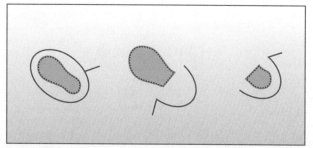

Figure 13–5 Tracks should be marked in two ways: Indicate whether they are right or left, and circle them if they are fully identifiable.

of the next print. It may be obvious or it may be difficult, but it is there. If you don't find anything during the first sweep, make the next sweep even slower. Constantly be alert to the possibility that the subject being tracked may abruptly change direction or alter his or her stride.

A person's eyes are accustomed to wandering as he or she chooses, without the owner/operator being consciously aware of the mechanics involved. Basically, the eyes will do as they please unless directed to do otherwise, which is why we need the assistance of our most valued tool (and friend), the sign cutting stick. This potent tracking aid assists in training the eye to concentrate on the small piece of real estate, about one square foot, where the next track will fall. As simple as this procedure seems, it is extremely difficult to learn because the eyes are in intimate contact with the brain, which (for most people) is capable of performing several functions at once. The eyes, however, are capable of looking only at one spot at a time. While most of us will use and move the stick as we're taught, too often we allow our eyes to nervously dart several steps ahead or to the side, hoping to get lucky and find that big, easy sign. The point is this: Most of us are cursed with a cheating mind and a wandering eye, and as long as we let them control our actions, we will never learn to track. Force your eyes to return to finding that difficult sign in front of the stick and concentrate there ONLY. This is where you will learn the trade.

Labeling Tracks

It is important when using the sign cutting stick to know if the track being sought is a right footprint or a left one. By marking the last track found, a tracker can immediately tell which (left or right) should be next.

Tracks should be marked in two ways: Indicate whether they are right or left, and circle them if they are fully identifiable (**Figure 13–5**). To mark a track, or partial track, left or right, start by using the sign cutting stick to etch a semicircle to the rear of the track. To a tracker, this arc indicates that there is a track immediately ahead, and STAY OFF. A short hash mark is placed at the right end of the arc to indicate right, and at the left end of the arc to indicate left.

Trackers are rarely lucky enough to get a series of full prints to follow. They must depend on chaining together a collection of sign. When a print is found that is positively identifiable, that is, there is enough print visible to indicate shoe type and sole pattern, it should be completely encircled. This should indicate to others that they are to stay away so that a drawing can be made and the evidence preserved.

The Tracking Team

A common approach to following a track by the Step-by-Step method is with three-person teams or crews (**Figure 13–6**). The three-person team, comprised of a Point Person and two Flankers, has several advantages:

1. It allows for consultation in difficult situations because three heads are better than one. If you can convince another hard head that what you are seeing is sign, then you are twice as likely to be right.

2. When training, it builds confidence, reduces errors, and benefits students by allowing a verbal exchange of the details of what is seen rather than just mutual observation of a clue.

3. It allows rotation of the Point Person who is physically on the ground searching for sign.

Tracking Team

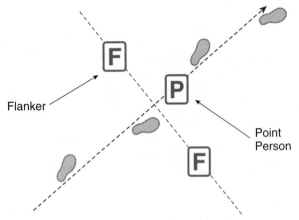

Flanker

Point
Person

Figure 13–6 The Step-by-Step method of tracking uses a three-person team comprised of a Point Person and two Flankers.

Tracking Team *Field of view*

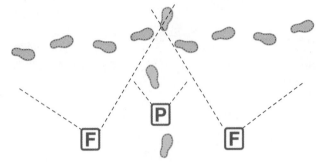

Figure 13–7 Field of view of each member of a tracking team.

Point is a tiring position, especially when sign is limited.

4. It allows the team to split up if several trails diverge. Any team member can call the team back together when one finds that he or she is on the correct track. Actually, this is sign cutting and can lead to bad habits during the learning phase, so be careful.

The general responsibilities of the team members are as follows:

Point

- Stays just behind the last track found, uses a sign cutting stick to search for the next one, and marks the tracks as the team progresses.
- Keeps Flankers from obliterating sign by getting ahead.
- Coordinates efforts of team.

Flankers

- From more of an upright position, the Flankers watch the side for incoming tracks that might confuse the situation (Figure 13–7).
- They watch for a sudden turn of the trail being followed.
- They help the Point Person find the next track from their vantage positions.

Tracking, like other types of searching, is not something that can be done all day long without rest. For a tracker to be effective, he or she must rest at regular intervals and rotate through the Point position with other trackers. Searching for anything while exhausted and fatigued is actually detrimental to the search effort. Sign and track—like all evidence in a search—must be discovered to be useful. Pressing on while fatigued is ad-

mirable, but a tired tracker may miss things that could affect the entire effort. When lives may weigh in the balance, this is unacceptable.

One often misunderstood component of the tracking team is the continuous exchange of ideas and information that should take place between team members. An interplay of opinion between the Point and Flankers allows ideas that may have to be filtered through the thoughts of the others. This interaction could be as simple as the Point continuously talking about what is seen, and can include each of the Flankers challenging the Point so that all opinions on any discovery can be considered. After everyone has spoken their piece, a consensus can be achieved. This ends up being an efficient way of preventing an overbearing individual from pushing the team in an undesirable direction. When everyone is involved in what is going on, there is a better chance that the team is heading the right way. Do not construe this to mean that silence is never desirable, however. Occasionally, when great concentration is required, silence may indeed be golden.

If you take the time to describe, in detail, what you see and why you think it relates to your subject's track, you'll be much less likely to con yourself into moving to the next step without just cause.

Detecting Sign

Whenever a person walks through an area, whether it is at home or in the wilderness, evidence is left of that passage. A person must contact his or her environment in order to travel by foot. In fact, walking, the most common type of unaided travel, requires a person to come into contact with his or her environment approximately once every 18 to 20 inches. Some disturbance (sign) is made through that contact and the first phase of tracking incorporates detecting this sign. The next phase of tracking includes following a track after finding the initial sign.

Sign: The Specifics

The subtle details of sign are beyond the scope of this text, but much can be learned from any one footprint. Some of the information available from a single print includes:

1. Length and width can help identify the print and distinguish it from others that may be similar. Size of a print can also give a rough idea of the person's size.

2. The general type of sole (if discernible) can help distinguish it from others as well as offer an aid in describing the print to searchers.

3. Measurements of specific parts of a sole pattern can help positively identify a print. That is, lug sizes, areas of wear, or pattern dimensions can help distinguish one print from others.

4. Several prints in a row can help determine direction of travel and stride, which can aid in finding subsequent prints.

Even though it is rare to find a complete clear print, fragments of prints and sign are common in most terrain. Because of this, as much information as possible must be learned from each piece of sign. Tracking is not a race to see who finishes first; it is an exercise in accuracy and efficiency. There is no excuse for losing the trail. Getting there quickly is worthless if you end up at the wrong place.

Drawing a print, particularly a complete and identifiable one, can help others to know which footprint to seek (**Figure 13–8**). The drawing can be copied and handed out to searchers so that one specific print can be sought, thus lessening the possibilities. When time allows, drawing a print, or a part thereof, is always a good idea. A standard track report form that offers an area to draw and describe a print is good for this purpose. An example Track ID Form is provided in Appendix 3.

It would be impossible to mention all the different types of sign that exist because sign varies so much with terrain, weather, time of day, vegetation, and other factors. Here only the most common types of sign and their general categories are addressed.

Sign depends greatly on the environment in which it is produced. A marsh may produce completely different sign than would a desert, for instance, but some similarities do exist. These similarities must be understood by all trackers, but it is still important that a tracker be familiar with the sign most common to his or her region.

In addition, as mentioned earlier, sign can be conclusively human or corroborant. Conclusively human sign is a disturbance that, when considered on its own with no other evidence, can be said to have been definitely caused by a person and not an animal. Corroborant sign, on the other hand, is disturbance that is not decisively human and could have been caused by an animal. This type of sign may corroborate other evidence, but, when considered on its own, is not conclusive. It cannot be determined to have been definitely caused by a person, but it may confirm or substantiate other evidence with which it may be found. While conclusively human sign is often discovered by very unskilled trackers (jump tracking), corroborant sign is not. Frequently, corroborant sign is obvious to a skilled tracker yet invisible to the novice, and when a novice does discover such disturbance, it is usually misinterpreted. Also, corroborant sign, which by itself proves nothing, would most certainly have been caused by the person being tracked if it were to fall exactly between two other pieces of sign at approximately a stride's distance. Because of this, corroborant sign can be as important in the long run as conclusively human sign and should never be overlooked or ignored.

Communicating Prints: Track ID

It is essential for a tracker to be able to do three things with a print once it has been positively identified:

1. Communicate the track to others.

2. Differentiate the track from other similar tracks.

3. Document the description for later use.

The last two items can be easily accomplished by simply studying the print, measuring it, and then drawing it (**Figure 13–9**). Photographing the track can be important, but more can be learned by drawing it. This can bring details to the attention of the tracker that other-

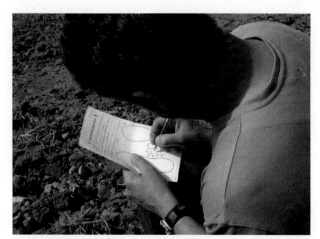

Figure 13–8 Drawing a footprint, particularly a complete and identifiable one, can help others to know what print to seek.

wise might have been missed, and can emphasize subtle marks that might be difficult or impossible to see in a photograph. Photographing a track is a good idea, but should not replace a sketch.

Study and measure every aspect of a print and indicate the measurements on the drawing. Measure at least: the length of the track; the widest part of the sole and the heel; the length of the heel; the stride (heel to heel), if possible; widths of any lines or marks; distances between lines or marks; number and size of any geometric shapes; and the number of lugs or other sole characteristics. Be careful to note any nail holes or stitches that are evident in the print as well as the number and sizes of any marks or lines. Search for and note any cuts, worn spots, or other details unique to the print. Everything visible should be noted and documented on the sketch. Any one of these characteristics might be what differentiates this track from others and is, therefore, important.

Beware of suggesting a size for the print (i.e., size 3 or 4) from measurements made in the field. Manufacturers vary widely in their approach to sizing footgear and no standards really exist. Rather than convey an estimated size, relate the measurements.

The drawing can be copied and distributed to other searchers, but occasionally the print may need to be described via radio. Tracking is almost entirely visual, whereas radio communication is entirely verbal. The skills required to perform both well are related but not the same. Practice at each is important.

When verbally communicating a track, certain ideas should be kept in mind to minimize confusion and maximize efficiency.

- Make sure to identify yourself and give your location as well as the direction of travel (with compass) of the track, if necessary.

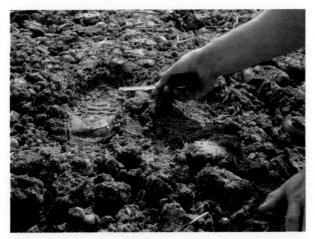

Figure 13–9 Study and measure every aspect of a print and indicate the measurements on the drawing.

- Keep it simple. Paint a mental picture by using words that are familiar to everyone and to which everyone can relate. Use words that are easy to understand and whose meaning is limited.

- Begin with a general description. Is it a flat (no heel) or a heel (a distinct heel)? Continue with a term that describes the general class of footgear, if possible. (i.e., athletic shoe, sandal, work boot, hiking boot, dress shoe, cowboy boot, etc.) Beware of speculation as to the type, and know the differences before using the terms.

- As a secondary consideration, briefly describe the type of terrain and ground conditions as well as the age of the track, if possible. This might give an indication of the detail to expect.

- Give the specific details describing the sole pattern starting at one end of the print (tell which). Such details should include, but not necessarily be limited to, the following:

  – Although all measurements should be documented, in the interest of clarity and brevity, only the length and width of the print, and the length and width of the heel should be conveyed over the air. Consider using descriptive terms rather than exact measurements for radio communication. Terms like "as wide as a pencil" might be understood better than "¼ inch".

  – Number or type of lugs (shape, measurements, etc.)

  – Number or spacing of any nail holes and/or stitches

  – Shape of the leading edge of the heel (i.e., straight, concave, "V" or "U" shaped, etc.)

  – Shape of the toe (sharply pointed, round, square, etc.)

  – Specific shape of marks in the pattern (i.e., circle, square, diamond, oval, line, thick line, broken line, wavy line, herringbone, etc.). Avoid using ambiguous terms such as "round" and "flat"; stick to picture terms.

  – Specific way of walking. Look for dragging of feet, scuffing, toes pointing out or in, wide straddle (feet placed widely apart), consistently shorter stride with one foot, long stride (runner or jogger), or anything that may make this track unique.

  – Look for tendencies or trends in where the subject walks and convey them. Does the subject always walk at the side of the road? Does the subject step over logs rather than on them? Does the subject tend to walk drainages rather than ridges? Does the subject avoid brush?

Does he or she walk in a straight line no matter what? If not, what tends to change the direction of travel (fences, wooded areas, water)?

- In sensitive situations where the details conveyed via radio are immediately important, have the receiving party confirm your description by repeating it back to you. In practice, this may be a good idea every time a print is described over the radio.

- Use a standardized track report to record your findings.

Strategy

If a SAR incident is managed properly, trackers will be called to participate early in the plan. Trackers need to know their place within the structured hierarchy and to whom they answer. These topics and others that are important to the tracker are covered in any of the fine educational programs dealing with search management. Only the considerations of approach and strategy that facilitate a tracking team's specific tasks will be discussed within this chapter.

Initially, after dealing with any administrative details, a tracking team called to a SAR incident should attempt to determine where the lost subject was last seen or known to have been. This information may be conveyed or it may have to be determined by the trackers themselves. Where was the person last seen? Where did he or she pass or what did he or she do? The area where the victim was last known to have been has the highest chance of containing tracks or other evidence that can be used by a tracker to determine a direction of travel. It takes only three prints to determine direction of travel, and if you can accomplish just this much, you will have contributed more to the search than most could ever hope.

From a subject profile, a tracker should be able to guess at what size print is being sought (small child, small adult, large adult, etc.) and the approximate length of the stride. The subject profile may even include a specific, complete print. When you have an idea of what is being sought, and once an area is identified as "hot" for sign, other people should be kept away to avoid confusion or destruction of the evidence. This cannot be overemphasized. Next, cut sign around the area (perimeter cut), trying to determine a direction of travel, and note any specific additional evidence such as a complete print. Better yet, carefully approach the last known point and examine the entire area without moving around unnecessarily. If a scuff, track, or other sign is visible, stand behind it and scrutinize the area in front of it for additional evidence that might suggest a general direction of travel. Look beneath your own feet to see

how they impact the area and look for this specific type of sign. Once the direction of travel has been determined from the last known point, another tracking team could cut an intersecting line. Be extremely careful not to damage any existing sign, as it may be all anyone has to go on. Take every precaution necessary to preserve any prints found, and see that they are documented and communicated to others involved in the search.

Once a direction of travel is determined, one tracking team always stays on the trail, following it "step-by-step" (Figure 13–10). That is, they never go beyond the last conclusive sign. This will mean that there is always someone on the trail. Other strategy can be applied to speed up the process, some of which will be discussed; however, the importance of keeping someone on the last track cannot be overemphasized.

The most time-consuming project is usually finding the first track. This is why it is important at the onset to keep everyone (non-trackers) away until sign can be cut and certain basic information gathered (print specifics, will tracking work, etc.). It is important to be able to find a track and be reasonably sure that it belongs to the lost subject. Accuracy is more important here than speed. Once the track is positively identified and a direction of travel is determined, then the pace can pick up quite a bit in most situations.

If following the trail from the last known point is not possible, another method of speeding up the pace is to employ "perimeter cutting" (similar to sign cutting). When initially cutting sign in an area, or when tracking becomes particularly slow, trackers can cut sign in a perimeter around an area where there is a good chance the subject has been. The purpose of such an effort is simply to discover sign at a farther distance from the last sign. If this perimeter team can positively identify the

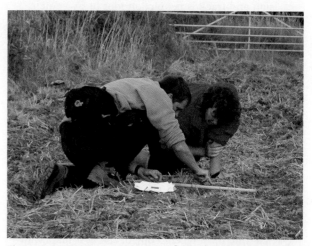

Figure 13–10 Once a direction of travel is determined, one tracking team always stays on the trail, following it "step-by-step."

track and direction of travel, they can become the step-by-step team and allow the rear team to perimeter cut around them. The perimeter cut can range from several yards to several miles, depending on the terrain and how long the victim has been missing.

The shape of the perimeter can be square, triangular, circular, or any shape. It can even follow compass headings. The only requirement is that, no matter which shape is chosen, the loop must be completed. Even if sign is found, the perimeter must be completed. Two trackers can cut sign in opposite directions, meeting to close the perimeter, or one team can cut sign continuously until they reach their starting point again. If no sign is found, consideration should be given to the fact that no one has entered the area.

If careful thought is put into where to cut a perimeter, much time and energy can be saved. Use natural barriers such as cliffs, large rivers, and thick brush, where a person would not likely pass, to limit the perimeter. Use areas where track and sign is easily seen to complete the perimeter (i.e., riverbanks, dry streambeds, plowed fields, tall grass, steep banks, trails, road edges, etc.). Pick areas that would allow you to be certain if someone passed. Now, the entire perimeter will be either easy to cut or impossible to pass through.

The same rules that apply for sign cutting, apply for perimeter cutting with the following additions:

1. Do not allow anyone to walk or drive within the perimeter being cut. This includes the trackers on Step-by-Step. They must stay with the track they are working. The most common destroyer of sign and track is people, on foot or by vehicle.

2. Each successive perimeter cut should be made just as carefully as the first.

If a perimeter cut is unsuccessful, it can mean that the cutting team missed something or that the subject has been passed and is between the two teams. In either case, it is extremely important that once a team gets on a track, they stay there until another positive ID is made. Close is not good enough. Someone must *always* be on the last track after a positive ID has been made.

To improve the "quality of service" trackers can offer when involved in a search effort, it is worth referring to the following guidelines. After all, it is far better to learn from mistakes of others than from your own!

1. Get the most recent copy of the best map available for your area. A USGS 7.5-minute topographical map is best for foot travel.

2. Make sure that both vehicular and foot traffic is kept to a minimum for the best sign cutting results within the high probability area(s).

3. Check for sign and track along trails and roads on the approach to the search area. Be track aware.

4. Get as much information as possible about the lost subject(s) before going into the field. Try to obtain a detailed subject profile.

5. Only one or two of the most experienced trackers should investigate the area (cut sign) initially. This minimizes conflicting sign.

6. Preserve evidence found at all cost. Document and catalog all likely tracks and sign while traveling into the search area, and be particularly aware of tracks that travel in unusual or erratic patterns. Establish a system for sorting and discarding prints, and make sure the tracking team's prints can be easily distinguished from any others. One way to accomplish this is to put an identifying mark on the footgear of every member of the tracking team.

7. Since hazards in an area are likely spots to find the subject, they are also good areas to look for sign. Look first in caves, mines, over cliffs, in holes, in ponds, etc., within the search area.

8. Make sure that a perimeter has been established beyond which a person could not pass without being noticed. In search management lingo, this is known as "confinement" or "containment".

9. Cut the perimeter within the confined area, but beware of presuming that no sign on a perimeter cut means that a sector can be ruled out. The subject may have traveled into the sector after the cut.

10. Talk to everyone confronted while traveling within the search area. Presume that everyone is suspect (e.g., the missing person) until proven otherwise.

11. Look for clues, not the lost subject, but do call out the subject's name at regular intervals, and then listen for a response. Bear in mind that, depending on the individual and the situation, some people may not answer. Children as well as escaped felons tend to act alike in that they both seem to hide when their name is called.

12. Use the Step-by-Step method of tracking.

Further Considerations

Now that tracking has been reduced to simple terms, it is time for an injection of reality (Figure 13–11). Tracking, although constructed of simple components, can involve some of the most complex issues in life. It deals with mysteries, grief, death, love, loss, and so much more. No dealings with such emotion-wrought topics could possibly be simple. Tracking works because it is a logical, analytical process that deals only with facts and not conjecture, hearsay, or emotion.

When a tracker is confronted with influences that do not contribute to the factual, logical input required, then confusion occurs. Tracking is not gauged by miles per hour; when a tracker is rushed, effectiveness suffers. Tracking is very "sense-intensive," so when a tracker is overwhelmed with sounds, sights, and unrelated thoughts, effectiveness suffers. As a tracker, try to concentrate on what you can control. Deal with the facts. Deal with them logically, and take your time.

Where tracking is required during an incident, situations will certainly arise that have not been addressed in this chapter. Incident Commanders will not call out trackers because they believe—often without a working knowledge of tracking—that tracking will not work in this particular situation. Good trackers will not be able to get to the subject in time to find them alive. External influences will apply undue pressure, most without an understanding of the tracker's art. Lost subjects may not be found. Clues may be misinterpreted. Lives may be lost.

Before you become totally disillusioned, however, remember that the same things occur in searches every day where tracking is not employed. Lives are lost and problems arise even when tracking plays no part. Tracking is only one set of tools that may be used to reach an objective. It is not the panacea nor is it a "silver bullet." However, when used properly, it may offer an effective option. Without tracking and its associated skills, the questions include: Are we really doing all we can as SAR personnel? Are we missing something? Could we do better?

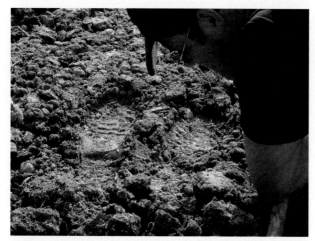

Figure 13-11 Tracking is not an equipment-intensive pursuit. Sight, patience, perseverance, and determination are requirements.

Tracking Fundamentals

Keep these thoughts or tracking "fundamentals" in mind when you are confronted with situations that cause you to hurry or improvise:

1. Only a tracker can determine whether or not tracking can be effective in any given situation. A jump-tracking Incident Commander is not a tracker.

2. Only trackers can decide when, how, and how thoroughly to search for subtle sign and track. Do not be pushed into hurrying. It does not work. Don't be stampeded into making mistakes.

3. Tracking is most effective when applied within an effective management scheme. Organization and leadership are always important.

4. Always be track aware. Be aware that for every mile that a person walks, there are thousands of clues.

5. Do not concentrate on determining if and when tracking will NOT work. Rather, concentrate on how tracking can work every time. Make it happen. Believed that it will work. Occasionally, you may be wrong.

6. Deal only with the facts. When inundated with theories, write down the facts and use them to develop a theory rather than searching for facts to substantiate one.

SAR Terms

Sign Discoverable evidence located in an area where a subject would likely have passed.

Sign cutting The process of looking for the first piece of evidence from which to track.

Track (also known as a print) A physical impression left from the passage of a person that can be positively identified as being human.

Tracking The process of following signs or tracks left by someone or something.

References

Carss, R. (2000). *The SAS Guide to Tracking.* Guilford, CT: The Lyons Press.

Cox, M., & Fulsass, K., eds. (2003). *Mountaineering: Freedom of the Hills,* 7th ed. New York, NY: Mountaineers Books.

Hill, K. (1997). *Managing Lost Person Incidents.* Chantilly, VA: National Association for Search and Rescue.

Taylor, A., & Cooper, D.C. (1990). *Fundamentals of Mantracking: The Step-by-Step Method,* 2nd ed. Olympia, WA: ERI, International.

Chapter 14

Search Background and Related Issues

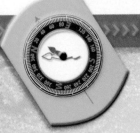

>>>> Objectives

Attitude and Philosophy

It is important that the motivation of the SAR personnel must be consistent with the search and rescue community's motto—"...these things we do, that others may live"—if satisfaction and any level of success is expected.

SAR exists for one reason only: to reduce suffering and pain for the missing or injured subject. There is little or no money in SAR, and there is rarely acclaim. It is tiring work that is often uncomfortable, unnerving, frustrating, smelly, hot, cold, sweaty, and rarely required when responders would find it convenient. Only on occasion is there is a "thank you," and injuries or even death are common. People involved in SAR must be focused, dedicated, skilled, confident, and thick-skinned.

That said, one can experience no greater satisfaction than is received from helping others. It is rare that a person accepts such a challenge, and rarer yet when a person who wants to help has the skill and knowledge necessary to offer assistance in a SAR situation.

Discipline is important in SAR because of the miserable conditions that often prevail when effective operations are so important. Bad weather, cold, heat, fatigue, lack of success, etc., are all conditions that can erode one's attitude. If a proper attitude cannot be maintained in less than ideal conditions, perhaps the searcher should reconsider his/her position in the organization.

SAR is hard work. Without discipline, SAR personnel may not only be ineffective, but also dangerous. Worse than not being sufficiently disciplined to handle difficulties encountered during a SAR incident, is not recognizing that problems exist. SAR personnel must be able to recognize when their own limits have been reached, whether they be physical, mental, or both. Physical limitations involve fatigue, pain, injury, etc., and mental

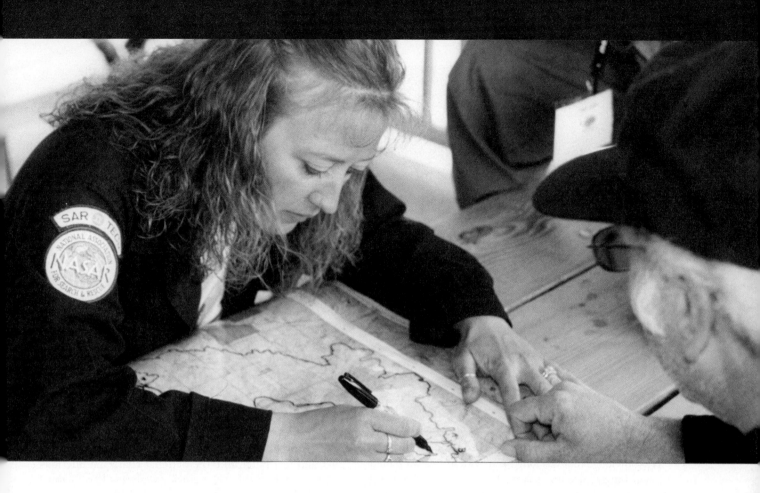

limitations can range from fear to mental fatigue, and may include boredom, apathy, and a lack of motivation.

Very often, coping with a physical or mental limitation means removing oneself from the environment that is causing the problem. Quitting or changing one's involvement in the search effort is much preferred to continuing in a useless—or worse, detrimental—role. Acting as though you can "handle it" not only wastes the time of supervisory personnel, it also wastes the time of other SAR personnel, the family, and may be dangerous to everyone involved. No one will ever fault a searcher for admitting that he or she has reached a personal limit. However, there may be grave consequences for ignoring the same.

Four to six hours of actual searching (excluding travel and rest time) is generally considered the average usefulness of a field searcher per operational period, although the time may vary depending on the situation. Effective searching is strenuous and sensory abusive. The senses that are required to search effectively need rest if they are expected to be useful. Effective searching requires an alert mind, an able body, and acute senses. A searcher must be rested, conditioned, and nourished. All of the senses are required for effective searching: sight (eyes), hearing

(ears), smell (nose), and "common" (your mind). Effectiveness diminishes when a searcher works for long hours without relief or rest. Attention to detail is important. Just *looking*—passive vision without interpretation—isn't always enough when you need to *see*.

Aggressive searching requires a positive attitude about finding clues and the subject of the search (Figure 14–1). The searcher must believe that there is a clue behind every stump and pile of rocks. Optimism must be prevalent. "The subject needs our help and I'm the one who is going to find the clue that leads us to him!"

It is very easy to think negative thoughts during a search. Some inexperienced searchers think that their effort is unsuccessful or wasted if the subject is not found immediately. "After all, if we were successful, we would have found the subject, right?" This type of attitude is at best self-defeating; and at worst flat wrong. Not finding a clue or the subject can be very helpful to the skilled search manager. A search resulting in no clues can be as good as a pile of clues—they both have meaning. It is far more fruitful to maintain a positive outlook while dismissing negative thoughts as fantasies of an idle mind. A good searcher thinks positively and avoids the alternative.

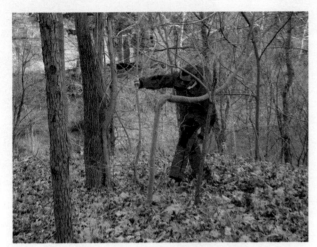

Figure 14–1 Aggressive searching requires a positive attitude about finding clues and the subject of the search.

Rudiments of Search Management: The "Crucials"

The principles of land search are based upon fundamental knowledge that has long been evident to search managers, but are also important to field searchers. This fundamental information, termed the "crucials," has been broken into seven statements that summarize management's minimum requirements for effective searching.

Search Is an Emergency

Search is an emergency because the subject may need emergency care, and the subject may need protection from himself or the environment. Time and weather destroy clues, and an urgent response lessens the search difficulty. Urgency is sometimes difficult to justify because left alone, lost people often will survive and walk out. Since the difficulty of a search is directly related to the size of the area to be searched, a fast response can minimize the travel time of the lost subject, keep the search area smaller, and more quickly lead to success. To respect the search subject's emergency (and that of the subject's family), searchers must respond urgently (search is an emergency until proven otherwise), search at night (the subject is probably immobile), maintain a visible effort (never quit), and create an atmosphere of positive urgency (everyone should act as if their actions will resolve the search). However, all SAR personnel must continue to approach the problem in an organized, disciplined manner. The sense of urgency should not be allowed to degenerate into disorganized, helter-skelter scrambling. In general, initial strategies that offer the maximum potential for locating a responsive, conscious subject should be used.

Maximize the Probability of Success in the Minimum Time With the Available Resources

The goal of search planning is to maximize the probability of successfully locating and assisting the subject in the minimum time with the available resources. Achieving this goal involves the complex balancing of many factors. These include: the probability that the subject is in one region versus another; how easy or hard it will be to detect the subject in each region; the search speed in each region; how long it will take and how difficult it will be to reach each region; the numbers and types of available search resources, etc. Very often the best distribution of search resources within the search area is not obvious or intuitive. In addition, searchers rarely have access to all the available information. Therefore, searchers should not try to second-guess the search manager, but instead concentrate on performing their assigned tasks to the best of their abilities. The number and type of resources assigned to each segment will be whatever is required to maximize the overall chances for success. A good search, from the searcher's perspective, is one where the search crew performed their assignment safely and precisely as instructed.

Search Is a Classic Mystery

Search is a classic mystery and, therefore, searchers must act and feel much like the fictional character, Sherlock Holmes, who said, "The clues are always here, I must simply have the skill and patience to discover them." Searchers and search managers must know what clues to look for and how to discover them.

Search for Clues and the Subject

Search for clues as well as the subject(s) because there are many more clues than subjects, and clue detection can substantially reduce search difficulty. Every person who travels on land leaves clues such as tracks, scent, and other discoverable evidence of his or her passing. Even not finding specific clues can be a clue in itself.

Focus on Aspects Important to Success

Concentrate on aspects that are important to search success and under your control. Doing otherwise is simply a waste of time, effort, and money. For example, thinking long and hard about the assignment given you by operations is much less productive than trusting him or her and simply accomplishing your assigned task.

Know if the Subject Leaves the Search Area

Know if the subject leaves the search area because a search without a subject is nonsense. Unless the subject is confined early, search difficulty increases rapidly.

Grid Search as a Last Resort

Use high coverage grid search as a last resort because the cost and risks are greater than many alternative techniques. Tight grid searching (line searching) takes many people, much organization, a great deal of support, and often too much time for the benefits derived. It is also extremely damaging to the environment and clues that were not detected, and may make subsequent searches almost impossible. Other techniques are frequently a better use of resources and should often be employed first before attempting to do a very thorough grid search.

Field personnel need to know something about what it is that compels those in charge to act in certain ways (e.g., acceptance of the "crucial" principles). Searchers need not possess all of the knowledge of the search manager, but they should understand the basic principles involved in managing and planning a search. With this basic knowledge, a field searcher can better understand why he or she is asked to perform certain tasks, and a searcher can better understand what is expected of them and why. This can also help the searcher to provide better feedback to the search management team.

Applying the principles dictated by the "crucials" allow for standardized thinking and a common approach to search problems. Ideally, field searchers should be thinking in the same way as search managers.

These crucials are based on the teachings of experienced search managers. Sound search operations should support these principles.

Clue Consciousness

Recall from the "crucials" that searchers must search for clues as well as lost subjects. There are more clues than subjects, the detection of clues reduces the search area, and the value gained from the detection of certain clues approaches that of the lost subject. In other words, be conscious of clues, not just the subject of the search.

Clue seeking is the major job of field personnel and following certain guidelines allows this job to get done more effectively. Clue seeking is an ongoing process that starts before callout and ends only after the final critique. Important clues can be found in the field as well as in the command post. Clues can be found, discovered, deduced, stumbled upon, assumed, etc., and there are as many ways to find clues as there are clues to be found.

Good clue seeking is learned. The art of clue seeking must be practiced frequently to develop and maintain a high level of skill. Experience is necessary to develop a sense of what information is important to the search (clues) and what is not (rubbish). Experience also makes it easier to recognize or discover clues.

Regarding the interpretation of a clue, an opinion should be formed based solely on the information avail-

able. Forming an opinion and then gathering information to support that opinion should be avoided. Do not immediately form an opinion about the value of a clue. Sometimes a clue, especially when clues are scarce, may seem more important than it actually is.

Clues should be gathered from all sources. Basing any theory or scenario on one source is, at best, questionable; and at worst, a mistake. Gather all information possible and assemble a complete subject profile on which to base further clue collection. Let the profile offer direction.

Clue Orientation

State-of-the-art search techniques are "clue orientated." That is, today's approach to search is dependent on the detection of clues. Any measure of clue detection is based on the unique combination of the characteristics of three things: the sensor (searcher), the search object (subject or clue generator), and the environment in which the detection opportunity will take place. Changing any one of these variables can significantly affect how easy or difficult an object is to detect. For example, a human searcher (sensor) looking for lime green golf balls (search object) on an open field with short, green grass on a bright, sunny day (environment) suggests some unique level of detectability. Changing the characteristics of any one of the three variables (sensor, object, or environment) could significantly change the detectability of the object sought.

For example, if the environment is changed to nighttime, or the search object is changed to something smaller and more difficult to see, or if the searcher is blind, the search becomes far more difficult. On the other hand, if the lime green golf balls were changed to beach balls, or if the grass were brown and contrasted with the lime green balls, detection may be easier.

> **INFO**
>
> **Clue Detection Is Based on the Unique Combination of the Characteristics of:**
> - The sensor
> - The search object
> - The environment
>
> SARTips

Although it will be discussed in more detail below, "effective sweep width" (also, "sweep width") is the term used to describe this measure of detectability. Sweep width is a function of a single, unique combination of the three described characteristics. It is a measure of the effectiveness with which a particular sensor can detect a particular object under specific environmental conditions. A specific combination of these three variables that would make detection easier suggests a larger sweep width. A specific combination of these three variables that would make detection difficult suggests a smaller sweep width.

Sweep width is a key element in the determination of the probability of detection (POD), which in turn is an important element in planning or evaluating a search (see section on Search Theory, page 228).

The "Sensor"

In the most general sense, the probability of detecting a clue (POD, see page 230) requires two things: (1) that the search object is in the area being searched, and (2) that the sensor is capable of detecting and recognizing the search object. The first is a search management concern regarding the deployment of resources and need not be discussed further in this context. The second is key to the detection process as carried out by field searchers.

To detect clues, searchers must be able to detect what they seek when given a detection opportunity. This requires that they know what to look for (e.g., potential clues) and know what to do when they find it. This is accomplished through training and practice. When a clue is discovered, searchers must know exactly what to do about it. Ideally, this should be determined during the assignment briefing prior to entering the field.

The characteristics of the "sensor" are important to detection. Untrained, fatigued, or distracted searchers are less likely to discover clues. The best search dog has only limited effectiveness if its handler cannot interpret the dog's signals. Certain sensors are better in certain environments, searching for certain search objects, than others. A skilled human searcher may be able to find a person lying in a field, but he or she may not be able to detect gasoline residue after a fire. In the latter situation, an arson dog may be the better "sensor."

How sensors are applied is also important. When looking for a lost person, the specific tactics chosen should be appropriate for the situation. For example, if the subject is likely to be responsive, attraction techniques may be productive. If the subject is not likely to be responsive, attraction techniques may be a waste of time. Search tactics should be carefully matched to the situation, because using an inappropriate tactic may not only miss a detection opportunity, it may destroy the evidence altogether.

The Search Object

The characteristics of the search object are important to detection. A large, brightly colored object that contrasts with its environment will be easy to detect visually. A small or camouflaged object will be hard to detect visually. Human subjects can do things that make them easier or harder to detect. They can start fires, deploy signals, discard rubbish, leave tracks, and wear brightly colored clothing. They can also evade detection, leave few tracks, discard nothing, and otherwise leave little evidence of their passing. The more a searcher knows about the subject (e.g., capabilities, equipment, etc.), the easier it will be to predict the type and quantity of clues the subject might leave. A comprehensive subject profile is essential to make this happen.

Human subjects leave predictable clues. Virtually every person who moves through an area leaves thousands of pieces of the evidence of his or her passing: tracks, scent, discarded material, etc. Thus, the most common problem is not a lack of clues, but too many of them and distinguishing between which are relevant and irrelevant. A detailed subject profile can enable both searchers and managers to either relate a particular clue to the subject or discount it altogether.

The five categories of search clues include *physical* (footprints, discarded material, etc.), *documentary* (summit log, trail register, etc.), *testimonial* (witnesses, family, friends, people in search area, etc.), *events* (flashing lights, whistle, yell, etc.), and *analytical* (the results of reasoning; e.g., if the subject wanted to get from A to B, he would have to go through location C). The key to effective clue-oriented search is to identify clues left by the lost subject and constantly monitor the search area for changes.

A good searcher must be able to distinguish between relevant and irrelevant clues, that is, those left by the subject versus those left by others (searchers, bystanders, etc.), and be able to interpret the numerous potential messages conveyed by them.

There are at least four pieces of information that human subjects may convey through the clues they leave:

1. The present location of the subject: a yell, a whistle, a flash of light, etc.
2. The previous location of the subject: evidence of where the subject was.
3. The destination of the subject: evidence of where the subject is going.
4. The subject was not here: a total lack of clues.

Searchers must be open to, and capable of, detecting clues that would lead to the discovery and development of this information.

All clues were generated at a specific point in time. If this exact time can be established, multiple clues can indicate direction of travel. This chronology or timeline of clues can be extremely helpful to search planners. Therefore, searchers should be sure to document exactly when their discovery was made (ICS 204, Unit Log, works well for this task; see Appendix 7) and determine as best they can exactly when the clue was generated.

The Environment

The characteristics of the environment are important to detection. Weather (wind, rain, snow, fog, etc.), light conditions, terrain, and obstructions can all conspire to either improve upon or detract from detection. In addition, difficult environmental conditions may have a detrimental effect on searchers (the sensor), thus reducing detection.

By definition, the search area is: "the smallest area, consistent with all available information, which contains all of the possible search object locations." Therefore, the search area should include all of the possible physical clues (possible search objects). To assure this, steps must be taken to assure that the subject does not leave the search area (containment) and that the search area includes all possible clue locations; both are concerns of search management and not field personnel. It is important, however, that field personnel remain confident that they will be provided numerous detection opportunities.

It is also important that searchers know what to do about the discovery of clues before the discovery is made. The best time to determine this is at the briefing when potential actions based on clue discovery can be agreed upon with management personnel.

Clue Specifics

There are several pieces of information that can help the searcher by providing hidden clues, and almost all of these can be supplied through the completion of a Missing Person Questionnaire. When the following information is used as a basis for ongoing clue detection, a sound foundation for discovery is laid.

1. What general category does the subject fit into (child, hunter, fisherman, hiker, climber, photographer, berry picker, despondent, etc.)?
   - What is the detectability of the particular category? Hunters wear bright colors while hikers may not, etc.
   - Does the category indicate whether the subject might be on or off the road? Hikers might be on a trail, whereas climbers will be on the rocks, etc.
   - Can the category indicate how far, or over what terrain, the subject may travel? Climbers may climb a cliff, but an elderly berry picker will probably not, etc.
   - Does the category of the subject indicate how far they might travel? Hikers may travel far, while elderly people may not, etc. How does the category of the subject affect their survivability? A hunter may be much better prepared for bad weather than a photographer, etc.
2. Identifying and studying the point last seen (PLS) or last known position (LKP) of the subject may uncover important clues.
   - What are the geographical restrictions encountered by the subject when he or she attempts to travel? Recreate the scene and, "put

yourself in their shoes." Identification of the LKP or PLS is important because it forms the starting point for all physical clue detection. Accuracy is important.

3. Investigating the circumstances of the loss of the subject can indicate where he or she started from, where he or she was going, and how he or she got there.
   - What was the subject supposed to be doing when the loss occurred?
   - Was the subject en route somewhere? To where? By what route?
   - Was the subject expected somewhere? Where? When? How prepared was the subject for the trip?
   - What was the attitude and personality of the subject(s) (aggressive, anxious, etc.)?
   - In the sequence of events, when did the searchers begin to search and where did they start?
4. The physical and mental health, as well as the general condition of the subject, can mandate urgency or offer other important guidance.
   - What is the subject's general capability? What can he or she do, and what can't he or she do?
   - What is the subject's state of health at the time of loss? Is he or she alcoholic, or a drug user or abuser? Does he or she have high blood pressure? Does the subject take any medications regularly? What will happen to him or her without the medications? What are the side effects of the medications? Are major medical problems involved, such as heart or lung problems, diabetes, etc. Does the subject have mental problems such as depression, phobias, or senility?
5. The subject's personality can be a factor in determining how he or she might handle certain situations and, therefore, can indicate how he or she acts and what he or she does.
   - Personality traits may include: aggressive or pondering; loner or gregarious; self-sufficient versus dependent; irritable or upset easily; despondent or depressed; independent, persevering, or realistic; neglectful; perfectionist.
6. Equipment that the subject was carrying not only can indicate his/her skill level, but can turn into a clue if dropped or lost by the lost subject. A complete subject profile indicating all equipment carried by the subject can be invaluable for related clue identification. It is also easy to assess preparedness of the subject by evaluating equipment carried. Footgear can be important in identifying tracks as those of the subject.

7. Terrain evaluation (in the search area) is important not only as an indicator of where and how the subject may travel, but also as an indicator of how long the subject(s) may survive.

   – Are there forks in the road or trail that may have confused the subject?

   – What sights or sounds might have been seen or heard (from the point last seen) that may have attracted the subject?

   – What barriers may limit the search area? These include rivers, natural routes that offer less resistance to travel, etc. Conversely, are there areas where the subject is not cut off by barriers?

8. The mission critique has much to offer in the way of identifying clues that were overlooked or overly emphasized. Many clues may be discovered after a mission when the scenario is fully disclosed. Analyzing these can offer information on how not to miss similar clues next time, and reasons for overlooking clues can be studied to identify better search methods or problems in the next search.

   – What was done wrong? What was done right?

   – Often, too much weight is put on a lone clue or group of clues, because there is little else to go on or the clue detector is not open-minded about his or her discovery. Recall that clues should never be considered simply at face value. Some thought should be put into whether or not any clue is relevant and then to its appropriate interpretation.

   – This new knowledge from the critique regarding clue detection, interpretation, and analysis should be cataloged and well documented so that lessons from them can be relayed to new generations of clue detectors.

9. Tracking is the art of following someone or something by stringing together a continuous chain of their sign. It can be quite effective when there is a positive last known point or point last seen. "Sign cutting" is defined as looking for sign in order to establish a starting point from which to track. "Sign" is any evidence of change from the natural state that is inflicted on an environment by a person's (or animal's) passage.

   – Tracking is a very intense, mental, analytical discipline that takes much practice. Tracking

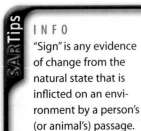

can be invaluable in a SAR incident when it is performed by skilled trackers, but it can also be a waste of time, and even harmful, if those practicing it are unfamiliar with its subtleties. The use of tracking in SAR has increased over past years, and the results have been quite remarkable.

– Sign cutting alone is worthy of study because its essence is the identification and analysis of discoverable evidence, which is an appropriate definition of clue consciousness (see Chapter 13, Tracking).

Search Theory

Operations Research (OR) is a professional scientific discipline that provides for a systematic approach to informed decision-making, especially in uncertain situations. Much of this work is done using specialized techniques to develop and manipulate mathematical and computer models of systems composed of people, machines, and procedures. "Search theory" is an applied mathematical subdiscipline of operations research that uses OR principles and methods to help resolve search problems. In short, search theory is a mathematical approach to determining how best to find that which we seek, and the principles of search theory apply to any situation where the objective is to find, in the most efficient manner, a person or object contained in some geographic region.

Search Theory in Use

Bernard O. Koopman (1900–1981), a Harvard educated scientist, established the basis for a rigorous study of search theory and practice with his pioneering work for the U.S. Navy during World War II. The work initially done by Koopman and colleagues was instrumental in the Allied approach to the Battle of the Atlantic and antisubmarine warfare. Although this application may seem far removed from searching for lost people on land, the basic theory of search established by Koopman applies to all types of searching, including that of inland search.

Search theory was applied to military SAR operations during and after World War II, but the U.S. Coast Guard provided the first comprehensive application to civil SAR in the 1950s. The methodology was incorporated into the first edition of the *U.S. National Search and Rescue Manual* in 1959, and it quickly gained acceptance by maritime SAR agencies worldwide and has remained in global use ever since. In addition, scientific research and development in search theory has progressed in fields as diverse as mining, mineral and oil exploration, and even archeology.

Although many of the principles of search theory are well beyond the scope of this text, comprehension of some key search theory concepts by field personnel can significantly improve communications between them and search planners.

Definitions

"Probability theory" is a branch of mathematics with which a person may systematically deal with uncertain events. Contemporary probability theory is well established and finds application in every area of scholarly activity from music to physics, and in daily experience from weather prediction to predicting the risks of new medical treatments. In a SAR event, uncertainties about events are prevalent, so a way to quantify these uncertainties and represent them more precisely with numbers is useful. Probability is often used to meet this need.

Some Search Theory Definitions

Area Effectively Swept (Z) – A measure of the area that can be (or was) effectively searched by searchers within the limits of search speed, endurance, and effective sweep width. The area effectively swept (Z) equals the effective sweep width (W) times search speed (V) times hours spent in the search area (T). That is, $Z = (W \times V) \times T$ for one searcher or one resource (such as a ground searcher, dog team, boat, or aircraft and its crew).

Coverage (C) – The ratio of the area effectively swept (Z) to the area searched (A), that is, $C = Z/A$. Coverage may be thought of as a measure of "thoroughness." The probability of detection (POD) of a search is determined by the coverage (discussed later in this section).

Effective Sweep Width (W) – A measure of the effectiveness with which a particular sensor can detect a particular object under specific environmental conditions; a measure of detectability. Effective sweep width depends on the search object, the sensor, and the environmental conditions prevailing at the time and place of the search. There is no simple or intuitive definition, although it is possible to illustrate the concept.

Figure 14–2 shows the effect of a clean sweep, where all of the objects within a swath are detected and no objects outside of the swath are detected. In this case the effective sweep width is literally the width of the swept swath. A total of 40 objects lay within the sweep width and all 40 were detected, as indicated by the white circles. A clean sweep where the searcher/sensor is 100% effective out to a defined range on either side of the track and completely ineffective at greater dis-

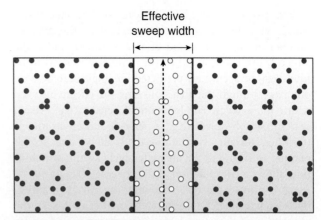

Figure 14–2 Effective sweep width for a clean sweep. The dotted line represents the searcher's track. Detected objects are denoted by white circles. The number missed within the sweep width is zero, and the number detected outside the sweep width is zero.

tances is unrealistic, but it serves to illustrate the sweep width principle.

Figure 14–3 represents a more realistic situation where objects are detected over a wider swath, but not all the objects within that swath are detected. In this case, the total number of objects detected was also 40 (like in Figure 14-2) but instead of making a clean sweep, the detections are more widely distributed. However, because in both cases 40 objects were detected over the same length of searcher track when the number of objects per unit of area was also the same, the effective sweep widths for both cases are equal.

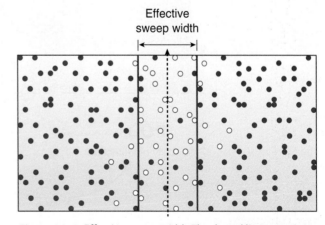

Figure 14–3 Effective sweep width. The dotted line represents the searcher's track; detected objects are denoted by white circles. The number missed within the sweep width is 11, and the number detected outside the sweep width is 11.

Effective sweep width is a measure of detectability because, in a hypothetical situation where the average number of objects per unit of area is known and if the sweep width is known, then the number of objects to be found can be accurately predicted for single searchers on one pass through the area. Knowing the effective sweep width for a given combination of sensor (e.g., visual search), search object (e.g., a person) and environment (weather, terrain, vegetation, etc.) allows the search planner to compute the area effectively swept, which in turn allows a computation of the coverage (Figure 14–4). As shown in Figure 14–5, knowing the coverage allows the search manager to accurately predict or assess the probability of detection for any search conducted under those or similar conditions.

An interesting property of effective sweep width is that it is defined as the width of the swath where the number of objects *missed inside* the swath equals the number of objects *detected outside* the swath.

Actual effective sweep width values for specific situations must be determined by rigorous scientific experiments. However, reasonably accurate estimates may be made from tables of effective sweep widths that have been determined by rigorous experiments for various typical search situations, by applying appropriate "correction factors" to accommodate other search situations.

A less accurate method of estimating sweep width for visual search is to assume the effective sweep width equals the "visibility distance," or the average maximum detection range. Both methods are different ways of thinking of the same value. Figure 15–5 (page 248) shows how to estimate an average maximum detection range. Since the relationship between effective sweep width and maximum detection range is not consistent across all search situa-

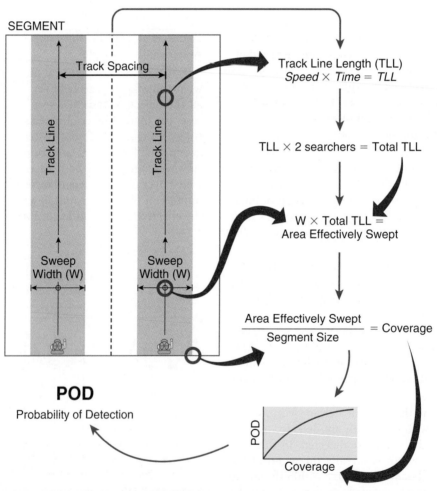

Figure 14–4 Detection elements of search theory. As searchers pass through a search segment, the amount of effort expended in the segment increases. Probability of detection (POD) is computed by multiplying the sweep width (W) by the total track line length (TLL; a measure of effort) and dividing the result, called the "area effectively swept," by the area of the segment. The final number is the "coverage" from which POD can be determined by using a "POD versus coverage" chart (see Figure 14–5). In the graph, the area effectively swept (orange area) equals one-half the size of the segment, so the coverage is 0.5. The POD for a coverage of 0.5 is 39%.

tions, this method may overestimate or underestimate the correct value. Therefore, it should be used only until more accurate effective sweep width data are available.

Effort (z or TLL) – a.k.a., track line length. The total distance traveled by all searchers (or a boat or aircraft and its crew) while searching in the assigned segment. Loosely speaking, the number of searcher-hours expended while searching can be called "effort," but without knowing the average search speed, it cannot be used to compute coverage.

Probability of Area (POA) – (also, Probability of Containment [POC]). The probability that the search object is contained within the boundaries of a region, segment, or other geographic area.

Probability of Detection (POD) – The probability of the search object being detected, assuming it was in the segment searched. POD measures sensor effectiveness, thoroughness, and quality. POD is a function of the coverage (C) achieved in the segment (see Figure 14–4).

Probability of Success (POS) – The probability of finding the search object with a particular search. POS measures search effectiveness. The accumulated probability of finding the search object with all the search effort expended over all searches to date is called "cumulative POS" (POScum).

Region – A subset of the search area based only on factors that affect POA; that is, regions may require segmentation prior to searching. Regions are based on probability of the search object's location, not on suitability for assigning search resources. A region may contain searchable segments, or a region itself may be a searchable segment. A searchable segment may also contain

one or more regions (based on probability), but rarely are the available data good enough to distinguish such small regions in ground search situations.

Search Area – The area determined by the search planner where SAR personnel will look for a search object. The search area includes the smallest area, consistent with all available information, which contains all of the possible search object locations, and therefore includes all regions and segments. The search area may be divided into regions based on the probable scenarios and into segments for the purpose of assigning specific tasks to the available search resources.

Search Object – A ship, aircraft, or other craft missing or in distress, or survivors, or related search objects, persons, or evidence for which a search is being conducted. A generic term used to indicate the lost person or evidence (clue) related to a lost subject. In the same segment, different search objects generally have different effective sweep widths (or "detectabilities"). This means that for any given search of a segment, different coverage areas, and hence different POD values, will be achieved for different search objects. A live, human search object is often referred to as a search subject.

Search Speed (V) – The average rate of travel (speed over the ground) of searchers while engaged in search operations within a segment.

Segment – A designated subarea (subset of the search area) to be searched by one or more specifically assigned search resources. The search planner determines the size of a segment. The boundaries of a segment are identifiable both in the field and on a map, and are based on suitability for assigning search resources, not probability of the search object's location.

Sensor – Human senses (sight, hearing, touch, etc.), those of specially trained animals (such as dogs), or electronic devices used to detect the object of a search. A human, multi-sensor platform is often referred to as a "searcher."

Sweep Width (W) – See "Effective Sweep Width."

Track Line Length (TLL) – (a.k.a. effort). Total distance traveled by searchers or boats or aircraft while searching (see also "Effort").

The probability that the subject of a search is contained in a particular segment is uncertain before and after the segment is searched (if the person was not found). However, this uncertainty can be described as a probability and estimated as a percentage (e.g., there is a 50% probability that the subject is contained in segment A1). An estimate of the probability of the subject being contained in a land segment is referred to as "POA" (Probability of Area). Maritime search planners refer to POA as "POC" (Probability of Containment). Although it is an important element of search planning, POA is rarely of concern to searchers.

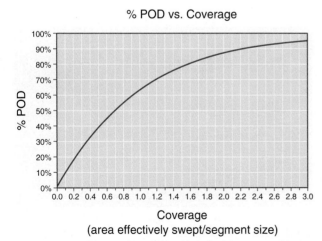

% POD vs. Coverage

Coverage
(area effectively swept/segment size)

Figure 14–5 To calculate the probability of detection (POD), find the computed coverage across the bottom of the graph, move up to the curve, and then move horizontally to the associated POD value.

The probability that the subject will be detected by searchers is also uncertain before and after a search has been conducted. This uncertainty can be described as a probability, estimated, and represented as a percentage; for example, there is a 50% probability that your search team will detect the subject, if indeed the subject is in the segment. The probability of the subject, or clues, being detected by searchers is referred to as POD, and assumes that the clues or subject is in the area being searched. If certain information about what searchers expect to observe, or actually observe, during a search can be provided to search planners, POD can be computed before a search is conducted (to plan an overall search strategy) and after a search is conducted (to evaluate the effectiveness of a search).

Success is seemingly easy to represent: either the searchers find something or they don't. However, to benefit from search theory, the chances of being successful (POS) can be estimated before a search is conducted, and then used as a planning tool by a skilled search planner. The probability of being successful is a function of both the probability that the subject is in the area (POA) and the probability that searchers will find the subject (POD). The probability of being successful is referred to as "POS" (probability of success). Once POD and POA are estimated, POS can be derived through this simple equation,

$$POS = POA \times POD$$

The objective of all search planning is to maximize the increase in overall cumulative POS with every search. When one or more lives are at stake, time is also an issue and the objective of all search planning becomes to maximize the overall cumulative POS in the shortest possible time. In other words, the driving concept of the application of search theory is to search in such a way as to maximize the chances of finding what you seek as fast as possible, that is, "Success Fast," a very sensible and intuitive goal.

While these calculations may have little value to the field searcher, they are used by search planners to numerically represent intangible possibilities that can be very useful for planning purposes. Quantifying probabilities allows a planner to better plan or evaluate a search. In short, POS in particular can help the search planner to make very important decisions that often would be significantly more difficult without the tools search theory provides.

Specifically, search planners will use probabilities and search theory to help them do the following:

1. Allocate resources so that:
   - The maximum overall POS possible is achieved with the available resources.
   - This maximum overall POS is achieved in the shortest possible time.
2. Decide when and how to search or re-search a segment.
3. Decide when to increase or decrease the search area.
4. Decide when to suspend an unsuccessful search or move the search area.
5. Rationalize actions to family and media.
6. Justify actions to others or in court.

The percentages themselves (30%, 40%, etc.) are meaningless unless they are used in a comprehensive system to apply the science of search theory. This system is developed and applied by search planners and managers. However, input from field searchers is vitally important if the values used by planners are to be truly useful.

Handling External Influences

When a person is reported missing and a search ensues, there is often great interest shown by news agencies (television, radio, print news, etc.), friends, family, and political entities (sometimes local but also state, federal, and international, depending on the situation and individuals involved). Thus, it is likely that during a search someone who is a journalist, a friend, a member of the subject's family, or someone with interest and influence beyond the scope of the search operation will eventually confront field SAR personnel (**Figure 14–6**). When this

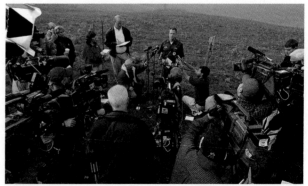

Figure 14–6 When media representatives inquire about search details, the potential for significant problems, and at least embarrassment, exists and field personnel must have a plan to handle the situation. A polite referral to the Incident Commander or Information Officer is best.

happens, the potential for significant problems and/or embarrassment exists, and field personnel must have a plan to handle the situation.

In most SAR incidents, the Incident Commander usually designates someone to deal with external influences. Typically in ICS, the Information Officer communicates with the news media, the Liaison Officer deals with external organizations, and a family liaison is assigned to deal with and manage family issues. The important point is that someone (or group) is specifically assigned to these duties and only the individuals assigned to these duties should be carrying them out. Before journalists, family members, and other interested parties are made aware of the proper channels for inquiries and information retrieval, they may approach anyone involved in the incident for information. Because of the potential for incomplete, uninformed, and/or inappropriate information to be disseminated, only those authorized by the Incident Commander should respond to these inquires. All others must be gently and courteously referred to the proper SAR personnel: the Incident Commander, Information Officer, Liaison Officer, etc. Direct the media and other, non-SAR people to someone who can talk to them, because most likely you are not authorized to do so.

Lost or Missing Person Behavior

Understanding and predicting the behavior of a lost or missing person can greatly enhance the chances for a successful search. Search managers especially need to know what to expect from a lost or missing person, but information regarding how this person might act can also be helpful to field personnel.

In this context, subjects who have been reported missing and subjects who are believed to be lost shall both be referred to as "lost persons."

Lost Person Behavior as Analyzed by the SAR Manager

Search managers, by analyzing the behavior of past lost persons, might be able to predict what the subject of the current incident might do, where he or she might go, and where he or she might end up under similar circumstances. A skilled search manager asks the following questions:

- What is the subject's state of health?
- What is his or her experience base? What has he or she experienced before?
- How does he or she handle being lost or confronting the environment in which he or she is lost?
- What could a lost subject do to affect the strategy of the search?

- What category does the subject fall into?
- How have other lost subjects behaved in similar circumstances?
- What does history indicate? Are there statistics?

Statistics compiled from past incidents indicate that members of a specific predetermined category of lost persons (i.e., children, teens, elderly folks, hunters, hikers, etc.) tend to act like others in the same category. If a search manager understands how members of the category that the lost subject fits into will act, the actions of the lost subject can be better anticipated.

Studies of hundreds of past searches indicate several trends in the way most people act. These historical trends often are utilized to aid in determining how present situations might be handled.

Lost Person Behavior in the Field

Knowledge of lost person behavior can also be advantageous to field personnel. It can help a searcher to understand where to look and what to look for. Basically, the advantages of applying lost person behavior in the field are rooted in three concepts:

1. An understanding of the behavior of past lost subjects can be applied in present situations to help predict actions.
2. An understanding of how the present lost subject has acted in the past might help predict future actions.
3. A thorough knowledge of the present subject(s) can offer guidance to the searcher and might suggest trends or propensities.

In short, when possible, SAR personnel should at least know how others generally have acted in the past under the present circumstances as well as how the current lost subject has acted in previous situations.

What has been learned from analyzing past SAR incidents and their subjects is that lost people tend to travel the path of least resistance. Places like roads, paths, railroad tracks, power lines, game trails, streams, and clear cuts are much more likely to produce clues than thickets, the other side of wide rivers, deep woods, mountains, deep snow, and obvious paths of great resistance. There are some notable exceptions. For example, Alzheimer patients tend to go until they get stuck, and this is often in areas through which other people would not have attempted to travel.

Weather and visibility also seem to play an important role in determining actions of a lost person. For example: bad weather usually forces a person to take cover and stop; darkness tends to cause a person to sleep; fog and low visibility may limit a lost subject's random wandering, etc. These historical trends are based upon the examination of what others have done in the past, but do not always hold true.

Analyzing past situations also indicates that a subject might do certain things to affect their survivability and/or detectability. This information can be of great value to field personnel. For instance:

1. Can the subject build a fire or shelter?
   - Fire rings, shelters, fires, etc., might be clues.
   - The ability to perform these skills can suggest greater survivability.
2. What equipment is the lost subject carrying?
   - Discarded gear that is identified as the lost subject's is a clue.
   - Equipment available to the subject can directly affect survivability.
3. What is the subject's detectability?
   - Is the subject wearing bright colored clothes or camouflage?
   - Will the subject be easy or difficult to see?
   - Is the subject likely to be responsive?
4. Can the subject respond or not?
   - Does a searcher have to stumble over the subject or just get within earshot?
5. Will the subject hide or come running?
   - An evasive subject (one who does not want to be found and will avoid searchers) is always more difficult and may be dangerous.

Where knowledge of lost person behavior is most likely to affect a search is in the field when a searcher simply puts him- or herself in the "shoes" of the lost subject. Trying to think like the lost subject can enhance one's understanding of where to look and what to look for.

Anticipating how a subject might act requires that SAR personnel have a thorough understanding of the subject's personality, attitudes, and other personal characteristics. This understanding must come from a complete subject profile, which is compiled from facts collected by an effective search management team. Of course, a complete profile must also be available to field personnel. The management team should not hesitate to distribute a subject profile to field personnel to assure maximum effectiveness of the information. A complete subject profile can be invaluable to field personnel, but search managers actually compile the subject information.

A complete subject profile leaves nothing to the imagination and includes a complete list of all information related to the lost subject. The profile is compiled through systematic and thorough investigation, interrogation, and questioning by the management team and should include a complete Missing Person Questionnaire. All available information should be included in the subject profile. Nothing should be left out. As a minimum, it should include the following:

1. Physical description of subject, clothing, and all equipment carried
2. Point last seen or last known point
3. Activities the subject is most likely to engage in (includes interests, hobbies, friends, etc.)
4. Standard practices (what do they usually do, where they usually go, how they usually act, etc.)
5. Personality traits (aggressive, loner, despondent, dangerous, fearful, etc.)
6. Has this happened before and, if so, what did they do before? (Where did they go, who did they see, etc.)
7. Physical and mental condition. (Is the subject healthy or sick? Handle stress well or badly and how? Experienced at this type of thing or not?)

In summary, searchers should put themselves "in the shoes" of the lost person. This involves thinking of how they might be feeling; imagining what they might be thinking about; and asking "what would I do if I was this lost person?" Put yourself into their shoes and allow this to influence your thoughts and ideas while acting within the constraints of the search plan.

Lost persons are much more likely to follow a route of easy travel. Consider these paths as likely areas for evidence/clues and check them thoroughly. Most, but not all, lost subjects follow paths of least resistance. Know this but be mindful of the exceptions.

Many studies regarding lost person behavior have been undertaken over past years, and studying this information will enhance the knowledge of any member of the SAR community. Examining these documents as well as others that deal with the behavior of lost people is strongly encouraged, but is beyond the scope of this book. The list of references at the end of this chapter is a good starting point for educating yourself.

Handling Evidence

SAR personnel can be the first to find a lost subject or clue, and established procedures should be followed to minimize problems. Whether SAR personnel find a small clue or an injured subject, how the individual or team handles the situation may have a large effect on the outcome of the search and any potential investigation.

Proper processing of discovered evidence is essential for overall effectiveness within a SAR incident. As clues are discovered, they must be interpreted and acted upon. This often takes more than just the ability to search. It involves the ability to search combined with the knowledge of how to handle what is discovered. If a searcher expects to locate the subject or solve a mystery, clues must be handled in such a way so as to facilitate all search efforts and to preserve evidence for subsequent investigation.

Although scene and evidence protection are not necessarily a primary responsibility of SAR personnel, a thorough knowledge of essential guidelines will serve to build better relations with all authorities, get the most from all clues, and preserve evidence for further investigation.

Briefing

The best way to handle any clue or piece of evidence is to have planned for its discovery and processing. The place to do this is at the briefing (see Briefing Checklist in Appendix 4).

At most organized SAR incidents, before starting their assignment, SAR personnel going into the field will be briefed by a member of the incident management team. That is, information will be conveyed to field personnel concerning such things as situation status, subject information, terrain in the search area, hazards to expect, and much more. A lot of information can be conveyed at a proper briefing, but specific instructions regarding how to handle and act on clues can often be the most important briefing information to the searcher.

Since evidence can take so many forms, instructions on how to handle it should cover all the possibilities, leaving very little to chance. Handling clues and evidence can be the single most important part of the investigation of an incident, and, therefore, may weigh heavily on its outcome. Searchers are often confronted with situations not common to many other field personnel. Therefore, searchers need to ask all the standard questions at briefings with certain search-specific additions. If not told, searchers should ask, and get answers to, the following questions regarding the handling of evidence:

1. Exactly how should the evidence be recorded (sketch, photograph, narrative description in writing, all of the above)?
2. Exactly how, if at all, should a print or sign be protected (cordoned off, covered, plaster cast, guarded)? Should someone else be called to handle this?
3. Should I act upon my interpretation of a specific piece of evidence, or should I report my findings and wait for further instructions? To what extent can I act on what is found?
4. What should I do as a searcher if I am confronted with two trails? Should I act as I see fit, or report it and wait for instructions? Is splitting the team up a viable alternative?
5. If the clue is an item that may have been discarded by the subject, do I note the location,

mark the location in an obvious way, and leave the item in place? Do all the above except recover the item and bring the information to the command post (immediately or at the end of the search assignment)?

Very often, experienced search teams will suggest to the person briefing them how they will handle certain situations. This may be the best course of action, especially if those charged with managing the incident are not fully familiar with the capabilities of the search team.

Specific Situations

SAR personnel may encounter four primary situations involving evidence and clues:

1. Evidence – clues that are discovered and must be processed.
2. Crash scene – usually a vehicle, occasionally an aircraft, often involves injury and death, and always involves important evidence.
3. Human remains – may involve any number of situations that can cause harm to an individual or group. Bodies often involve injury and always involve important clues.
4. Injury – scenarios where deaths may be encountered. These situations may involve evidence as well.

At any one of these situations, SAR personnel may be confronted with evidence that might be critical to the efficient resolution of a SAR situation. Therefore, all evidence, no matter how seemingly insignificant, should be handled as if it were of extreme value.

Evidence

Generally, evidence can be categorized as either "physical" or "incorporeal." Physical evidence is something that can be touched and held. Tangible objects such as shoes or gum wrappers are examples, but prints and sign also fall into this category. Incorporeal evidence, on the other hand, is nonphysical information or knowledge; these are intangible items that cannot be touched or held. Examples include the subject's age, a whistle blowing, a flashing light, or a report from a witness. The effectiveness of this type of evidence ultimately depends solely on how well it was recorded. In fact, this type of evidence is usually converted to physical evidence by field personnel. Photos of an event and written records of what happened, for example, were all once incorporeal items turned into hard, reproducible evidence by field personnel.

Physical evidence is far more desirable in the long run because it is relatively easy to preserve and reproduce later. Intangible evidence, however, can also be important. It is just not as persuasive when its credibility rests solely on how well it was recorded. After all, which would you find more persuasive: a fisherman with a tale of the "big one" that got away, a fisherman with a photo of the fish, or a fisherman with a big fish in hand? Physical evidence is always preferred.

Ideally, the recording and documentation of a clue and its surroundings should be of such quality that the entire scene could be reenacted or reproduced. The scene should be recorded so well that what went on before, during, and after the discovery of a particular piece of evidence can be accurately relived. This can be difficult when evidence is intangible and difficult to preserve. The recording of the event (i.e., photo, notes, sketches, etc.) becomes the physical evidence, so the more thorough the recording of the evidence, the better the evidence.

The following actions taken by the searcher can help turn intangible clues into physical evidence:

1. Take notes – Document placement of clues, position of people or bodies, and pertinent facts surrounding the scene. Leave nothing to the imagination, but do not expound. Stick to the facts and be able to corroborate them, if possible. Basically, describe in prose everything that you know regarding the scene and the situation.

2. Sketch the scene – Draw diagrams and pictures of pertinent objects involved at the scene and their position relative to each other. Not everyone is an artist, but simple line drawings can be invaluable.

3. Photograph – Take photos, if possible. This is an excellent way to document a scene, but relies heavily on light and equipment availability. Make sure to include something in the photo that will indicate scale, time, and date, if possible (a ruler, coin, newspaper, etc). Attempt to photograph at least three sides (four is better) of any one object, and back off for a larger view of the location of the object or person in relation to the surrounding landscape.

4. Corroborating witnesses – Get information from any witnesses who saw what you saw or who saw anything at all. Write down at least their names, addresses, and phone numbers so that they can be contacted later, if necessary. Also, note what they saw and/or did at the scene.

5. Retrieve and preserve – Collect clues, if within the scope of the briefing. Evidence and clues should be the focus of all sketches, photographs, and documentation, but retrieving and preserving the evidence itself is the ultimate objective. Be mindful of the fact that notes, sketches, and photographs may themselves become evidence.

In tracking, evidence usually takes the form of a print or sign that, of course, cannot be directly retrieved.

More importantly, both sign and prints are usually time-sensitive. That is, because they tend to disappear with time, the sooner prints are discovered and recorded, the more valuable they are to an investigation. Tracks, like ice cream with children, tend to disappear quickly. This means that photographs, sketches, and other documentation will usually need to be carried out immediately upon discovery of such evidence. The tracker will need to record a print right away to maximize its usefulness.

Evidence should not be allowed out of your possession or protection until it can be conveyed to an equally responsible person. When evidence is considered for use in a case, opportunities for alteration of the evidence, by natural or man-made causes, can reduce its credibility. That is, the better the chances that a piece of evidence could have been changed or altered, the less its significance, particularly in court. This is referred to as maintaining the "chain of evidence" and may weigh heavily on a clue's acceptability in court, where it counts. The "chain" is probably more important to law enforcement personnel than it is to SAR personnel, but the need for an understanding and appreciation of its existence and purpose should be obvious to anyone involved in what could become issues before a court.

Any SAR scene where evidence is found should be considered the scene of a crime until proven otherwise. Just as in emergency medical treatment where we treat for the worst injury possible, to be safe: any situation where evidence is collected is considered a crime scene until a responsible authority proves otherwise. This allows us to consider everything as evidence until we know different, thereby protecting any possibility.

Crash Scene

A crash scene may involve an aircraft, automobile, or other vehicle or machinery. Crash scenes may include injury and death, but almost always involve evidence. Often the only way to find out exactly what happened is to piece together the clues. How these clues are handled and processed initially may mean the difference between knowing what occurred and guessing.

At a crash scene, there are many things that SAR personnel can do to help victims of the incident as well as the subsequent investigation (Figure 14–7). However, there are also actions that could hamper an investigation, further complicate the victim's situation, and even result in personal injury to SAR personnel.

In the United States, the National Transportation Safety Board (NTSB), the Federal Aviation Administration (FAA), and the military all have a responsibility to investigate aircraft accidents that involve serious injury or death. In general, all civil aircraft accidents are investigated by the NTSB. Some non-fatal accidents will be looked at by the FAA and all military crashes will be

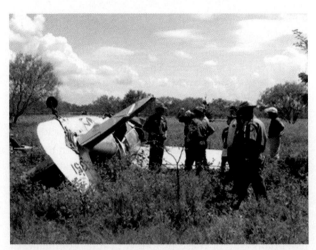

Figure 14–7 At a crash scene, there are many things that SAR personnel can do to help victims of the incident as well as the subsequent investigation.

handled by a respective branch investigating team. All of these agencies would like to see the site disturbed as little as possible. Notes, sketches, photographs, and relevant comments, such as body positions, locations of aircraft parts or pieces, and other pertinent observations, are all appreciated.

The NTSB will probably get involved with local agencies when modes of land transportation are involved in a crash. Some examples include crashes involving automobiles, trains, buses, and subways. The United States Coast Guard (USCG) might get involved in any crash that involves U.S. waterways, and state and local agencies may get involved when a crash involves a vessel (or vehicle) on state or locally governed waterways.

The most common crashes in the world involve automobiles and trucks. When this type of incident occurs, local law enforcement, fire service, and emergency medical services (EMS) may be involved, but one of these agencies usually has responsibility for the scene. Since SAR personnel may be members of any of these agencies, everyone involved should have a basic understanding of his or her role in this type of scenario.

In situations involving remote sites, SAR personnel may be asked to assist investigators in just getting to the site. In these cases, pointing out observations and subtle clues not readily apparent to the investigator could be very helpful. At sites that would be inaccessible to all but trained SAR personnel, team members may even be asked to conduct the entire on-scene investigation.

If wreckage must be disturbed to remove bodies, the coroner or medical examiner will need to coordinate with the responsible agency. If the investigator is not readily available, some other agencies can allow removal of bodies by the authority of the coroner. Any activity concerning

the dead should strictly follow guidelines established by the authority having jurisdiction over the situation.

A final step in the resolution of a crash site investigation is the disposition of the wreckage. In some cases, salvage will be by an insurance company or even private individuals. The removal of any wreckage must be coordinated with the investigating agencies and is usually performed in a specifically prescribed manner. If the wreckage of an aircraft is to be left at the site and it is visible from the air, it must be marked in an appropriate manner prescribed in that state. This is to preclude mistaking the site for a recent crash, if another search is initiated in the same area.

Guidelines for Handling Crash Scenes

1. Proceed with caution! Safety of SAR personnel is paramount. If the smell of spilled fuel is strong, approach from uphill and upwind.
   - With the presence of any fuel in the area, extreme caution should be used during any activities. Absolutely no smoking or use of fire or spark producing devices is allowed.
   - Absolutely assure the safety of personnel. Do whatever is necessary to see that everyone is prudently safe, and this may include leaving the scene altogether.
2. Prevent further injury to the patient or patients by stabilizing the scene. This usually involves minimizing hazards and should not be neglected.
3. Determine whether any subjects are alive or dead. If alive, begin emergency care to the best of your ability and training. If dead, secure the scene and notify a higher authority.
4. Establish a security perimeter for the site, but remember that SAR personnel, including trackers, usually have no legal authority to perform law enforcement functions and may not be able to forcibly prevent people from accessing the scene.
5. Handle any evidence such as baggage, personal effects, cargo, mail, tracks, etc., as specified in the briefing. If no such determinations have been made, protect and leave any evidence where it was found, unless it is in danger of obliteration or alteration by weather or environmental hazards.
6. Document, photograph, and/or sketch all pertinent evidence, especially if investigators will rely heavily on your observations (i.e., investigators cannot access scene or if evidence will be affected by weather or time).

Handling the Deceased at a SAR Scene

The discovery and investigation of serious injuries and accidental death can be one of the least enjoyable, but most important, aspects of SAR. As with most investigative cases, someone is stuck with the task of collecting clues, finding cause, and explaining a set of circumstances. The detailed study of the event and evidence of the situation is the legal responsibility of trained public officials such as coroners, medical examiners, or law enforcement officers, depending on the nature and location of the mishap. Frequently, however, evidence is produced or discovered by searchers who are obliged to help the responsible authorities as best they can.

While at times the circumstances or facts that lead up to a death may seem rather obvious, SAR personnel should understand that there are certain requirements and obligations, both to the state and family or friends. The inquiry process varies from jurisdiction to jurisdiction and state to state, but basic guidelines that apply to SAR team members have been established.

The first responsibility of someone arriving on the scene is to determine if the subject is, in fact, dead, alive, or critically injured. If this means moving or touching the individual, then go ahead and do whatever is necessary. Proper emergency care supersedes investigation at this point, and medical treatment is never interrupted, just supplemented, by evidence considerations. At the point that responders determine the subject is actually dead and medical treatment is deemed unnecessary by whatever means is generally accepted, every attempt should be made to preserve the surroundings and the exact position of the deceased and associated evidence.

Observe the scene and look for clues, evidence, or indications of what might have happened. If anything in the way of tracks, imprints, scuff marks, or possessions is in danger of being lost, preserve the information or scene description by writing it down or photographing objects before recovering them. Whichever approach to evidence handling is followed, it should coincide with the guidelines indicated in the briefing.

The area immediately surrounding a body or bodies should be secured with a rope, string, or tape after a subject(s) is (are) determined to be dead. This physical barrier insures that not only officials do not casually walk in and out of the area, but should also keep other curious onlookers out as well. Again, pay particular attention to any item within the cordoned area. In writing down whatever was observed, make sure that plenty of emphasis is placed on disturbances or movement made within the scene by SAR personnel, intentional or not. Failure to do this could result in being suspect of acting beyond one's authority or even destroying evidence. If at all possible, even if alone, remain at the scene until official help arrives. This could involve sending a passerby or another team member for help, if a radio is not available. Remember the "chain of evidence." Finding a clue and then abandoning it, for any length of time, could mean the dif-

ference between accepting and refuting certain evidence in court.

You or someone in your team may be required to make a written statement. This must be as accurate and detailed as possible, and involve only the facts, not conjecture. Ask for the advice of a knowledgeable person when considering what to include in an official statement. The advice of an attorney may also be prudent.

Unless specific instructions have been given to do so, do not search a deceased person for identification. That is an official function that must be carried out by responsible authorities. Depending on the state and local jurisdiction, a body may only be moved or pronounced dead by a coroner, deputy coroner, or medical examiner. Essentially one of these people is in total command of the site. Often, however, SAR personnel are called upon to assist in the investigation under the specific direction of one of these officials.

Always try to have a witness to any activity you are involved with around the scene of a death. Everyone becomes suspect when the ultimate tragedy becomes reality and a human dies. Nothing is protected and everything is possible. Most importantly, protect your own interests, have a reason for all that you do, and document everything well.

Handling Injuries at a SAR Scene

Considerations for handling injuries are similar to those for handling deaths. Protecting evidence is important, but falls second to proper emergency care. Treatment of injuries and alleviation of pain are major goals in SAR and should not be precluded by the collection of evidence. However, when the treatment is complete, the entire investigation may still hinge on any clues, observations, and recollections of those involved. Therefore, be mindful of investigative considerations while treating a patient in a SAR situation, and try to protect evidence while doing your best for the patient.

In summary, handle any clue as if it were the only piece of evidence, consider each and every discovery to be absolutely important until proven otherwise, and follow these simple guidelines:

1. Plan for the handling of evidence, including search-specific considerations, in the briefing. Do not wait until something is found.
2. Generate an accurate record of the evidence and its environment by taking notes, making sketches, photographing, or by retrieving the evidence.
3. Understand and maintain the "chain of evidence."
4. Treat injuries or assist the injured first, but be mindful of any evidence.

SAR Terms

Last Known Position (LKP) Last reported, estimated, or deduced position of the subject of a search.

Point Last Seen (PLS) Last position of the subject of a search as reported by a witness.

Search area The area, determined by the search planner, which is to be searched. The search area includes the smallest area, consistent with all available information, which contains all of the possible search object locations and, therefore, regions and segments.

Search object A ship, aircraft, or other craft missing or in distress, or survivors, or related search objects, persons, or evidence for which a search is being conducted. A generic term used to indicate evidence (clue) related to a lost subject or the lost subject. A live human search object is often referred to as a search subject.

Segment A designated subarea (subset of the search area) to be searched by a search resource.

References

Benkoski, S.J., Monticino, M.G., & Weisinger, J.R. (1991). A survey of the search theory literature. *Naval Research Logistics*, 38, 469–494.

Cooper, D.C., & Frost, J.R. (1999). *Selected Inland Search Definitions*. Cuyahoga Falls, OH: Private publication, 24 June 1999. (Available for sale by NASAR, 4500 Southgate Place, Chantilly, VA 20151, 703-222-6277.)

Cooper, D.C., Frost, J.R., & Robe, R.Q. (2004). *Compatibility of Land SAR Procedures with Search Theory*. Washington, D.C.: U.S. Department of Homeland Security, United States Coast Guard, Operations (G-OPR).

Cornell, E.H., & Heth, C.D. (1996). Distances traveled during urban and suburban walks led by 3- to 12-year olds: Tables for search managers. *Response*, 15, 6–9.

Frost, J.R. (1998). The theory of search: A simplified explanation. (Rev. ed.). Fairfax, Virginia: Soza and Company, Ltd. and U.S. Coast Guard.

Frost, J.R. (1999a). Principles of search theory, part I: Detection. *Response*, 17(2), 1–7.

Frost, J.R. (1999b). Principles of search theory, part II: Effort, coverage, and POD. *Response*, 17(2), 8–15.

Frost, J.R. (1999c). Principles of search theory, part III: Probability density distributions. *Response*, 17(3):1–10.

Frost, J.R. (1999d). Principles of search theory, part IV: Optimal effort allocation. *Response*, 17(3):11–23.

Heth, D.C., & Cornell, E.H. (1997). Characteristics of travel by persons lost in Albertan wilderness areas. *Journal of Environmental Psychology*, 18, 223–235.

Hill, K. (1997). *Managing Lost Person Incidents*. Chantilly, VA: National Association for Search and Rescue.

Hill, K. (1999). *Lost Person Behavior*. Ottawa, Ontario, Canada: The National Search and Rescue Secretariat.

Hill, K. (2001). *Distances Traveled and Probability Zones for Lost Persons in Nova Scotia*. (Unpublished data).

IMO/ICAO. (1999). *International Aeronautical and Maritime Search and Rescue Manual: Vols. I, II, & III*. London/Montreal: International Maritime Organization (IMO) and International Civil Aviation Organization (ICAO).

Koester, R.J., & Stooksbury, D.E. (1995). Behavioral profile of possible Alzheimer's disease patients in Virginia search and rescue incidents. In: *Wilderness and Environmental Medicine*, 6:34–43.

Koopman, B.O. (1946). *Search and Screening*. In: OEG Report No. 56, The Summary Reports Group of the Columbia University Division of War Research. Alexandria, VA: Center for Naval Analyses.

Koopman, B.O. (1980). *Search and Screening: General Principles with Historical Applications*, revised ed. New York, NY: Pergamon Press.

Mattson, R.J. (1975). *Establishing Search Priorities*. Private publication.

Mitchell, B.L. (1985). *A Summary of the National Association for Search and Rescue Data Collection and Analysis Program for 1980–1985*. Washington, DC: National Association for Search and Rescue.

National Search and Rescue Committee. (2000). *United States National Search and Rescue Supplement to the International Aeronautical and Maritime Search and Rescue Manual*. Washington, DC: U.S. Superintendent of Documents.

Robe, R.Q., & Frost, J.R. (2002). *A Method for Determining Effective Sweep Widths for Land Searches: Procedures for Conducting Detection Experiments*. Washington, DC: The National Search and Rescue Committee, USCG Contract Number DTCG39-00-D-R00009.

Stone, L.D. (1989). *Theory of Optimal Search*, 2nd ed. Military Applications Section, Operations Research Society of America. Arlington, VA: ORSA Books.

Syrotuck, W.G., ed. (1976). *Analysis of Lost Person Behavior: An Aid to Search Planning*. Westmoreland, NY: Arner Publications.

Washburn, A.R. (2002). *Search and Detection*, 4th ed. Linthicum, MD: Institute for Operations Research and the Management Sciences.

Chapter 15

Search Operations

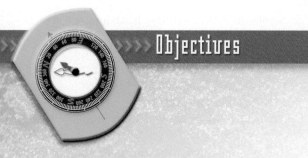

Objectives

Upon completion of this chapter and any course activities, the student will be able to meet the following objectives:

Describe the following processes:
  Checking in at the incident. (p. 254)
  Crew mission briefing. (p. 254)
  Crew mission debriefing. (p. 255)
  Checking out of the incident. (p. 256)

Describe the general functions of the various search crew positions. (p. 255)

Differentiate between indirect and direct search tactics (formerly referred to as "passive" and "active"). (p. 241-243)

Describe the following search tactics:
  Containment (confinement). (p. 242)
  Hasty search. (p. 242-243)
  Loose grid. (p. 243-245)
  Tight grid. (p. 245-247)
  Evidence search. (p. 247)

Define the following:
  Base line. (p. 243)
  Guide line. (p. 243)
  Guide person. (p. 243)
  Search lane. (p. 243)

Describe and demonstrate the use of the grid search naming system used by the Boy Scouts of America. (p. 250-251)

Describe how Average Maximum Detection Range (AMDR) is estimated in the field. (p. 248-250)

Describe at least five guidelines for skilled searching. (p. 251-252)

Describe two categories of what a searcher must prepare prior to call-out. (p. 252)

Tactics

Tactics are all techniques employed to actually find a lost subject or clues and are usually applied by the search manager immediately following first notice. Tactics are important to field personnel because they are the methods by which SAR team members get physically involved with the search function. Tactics usually involve a definite progression of techniques and generally fall into one of two classes, indirect or direct, although there may be some overlap between the two.

Indirect tactics are almost always the first to be employed, particularly with regards to fact finding or information gathering. It is through these tactics that the nature and seriousness of the incident are ascertained and a search area is established. Often indirect tactics themselves locate the subject or the subject is discovered by other means before direct search tactics can get underway.

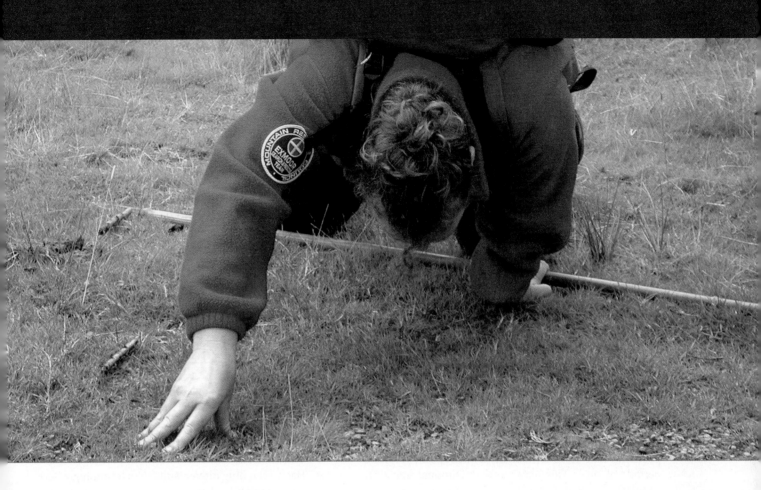

Although the use of indirect tactics should continue until the subject is located or search activities are suspended pending further developments, there usually comes a point when direct tactics should be employed and searchers sent into the search area to locate clues and the subject. Once started, direct tactics should continue until the subject is located or search activities are suspended pending further developments.

Indirect Tactics

Indirect tactics do not involve physically entering and moving through the search area to look for the subject or clues. Specific tactics used in this mode include fact finding (investigation), attraction, and containment. Fact finding is a process that continues from the first notice through the final critique. Attraction and containment can and should be used effectively together throughout the search, but their usefulness correspondingly declines as the chances of the subject being responsive diminish over time.

Fact Finding

Fact finding is performed by the search management team (those managing the search) often with the aid of other resources such as law enforcement entities, and includes collecting any information that can help focus or resolve the search. A Missing Person Questionnaire (see Appendix 5) can be used for this purpose, but any information relevant to the search contributes to the available collection of facts and the ability to develop an effective search plan. As in any investigation, leads must be followed until they generate no more leads, the subject is found, there is sufficient evidence that the incident is not of the type for which SAR resources and methods are appropriate, or search activities are suspended pending further developments.

A version of this type of indirect technique is the "continuous limited search." This approach is taken when most direct search techniques have not turned up clues or the subject and the search management team decides to continue the search on a limited basis only (e.g., no field deployment). It usually consists of continued investigation and/or using the area for regular training purposes, but nevertheless is considered an indirect search technique.

> **INFO**
> In the past, indirect and direct tactics were referred to as "passive" and "active." This nomenclature was changed because the land SAR definitions of the old terms conflicted with how they were used by military and some government SAR organizations.

SARTips

Attraction

Attraction techniques are efforts taken to cause the subject to be attracted to, and travel to, a desired location. This assumes a mobile/responsive subject. Specific attraction techniques include noise (sirens, whistles, yelling, PA systems, horns, etc.), lights (beacons, flares, fires, strobes, car or patrol lights, search lights, etc.), smoke, aircraft, balloons, skywriting, etc. When using noise, do not forget to have silent periods in which to listen and be aware that you might be hearing other teams or echoes. It is best if all teams agree to or are assigned the same specific silent periods, synchronize their watches and strictly observe these periods.

Containment

Containment techniques involve efforts taken to confine the movement of a lost subject in order to minimize the size of the search area. This type of approach is usually instituted by the search management team and is carried out as early as possible in a search. Specific types of containment include route blocks (trail, road, etc.), lookouts (a searcher in a high position overlooking the search area), track traps (looking for tracks in areas where tracking is very easy), patrols (roving searchers), and attractions. SAR personnel assigned to containment positions may have to remain at their posts for long periods of time. This may require additional logistical support (i.e., food, water, and other support materials), and searchers assigned to such posts should not hesitate to request it.

Direct Tactics

Direct tactics include all organized methods used in the search area to detect a lost subject or clues. Generally, there are three primary types of searches that can be employed by search managers and carried out by SAR personnel to find a lost subject: hasty searches; and two types of area searches, loose grid searches and tight grid searches. SAR personnel are also sometimes called upon for a fourth type of search, the evidence search. This is really just a special case of the tight grid search.

Hasty Search (Non-Area Search)

In general, a hasty search is a fast initial response of well-trained, self-sufficient, and very mobile searchers who check those places most likely to produce clues or the subject quickly. A hasty search also could be called a search of "points and lines." In geometry, points and lines have no area. Similarly, these types of search assignments do not have definable boundaries and therefore involve no measurable "area." Searching some place in a "hasty" fashion usually means that a defined search segment is not involved. Rather, hasty searches are meant as a means of discovering evidence and/or the subject quickly by visiting general locations where they are likely to be found.

Hasty search assignments might include likely spots (camps, abandoned vehicles, cabins, etc.), trails, tracks, paths, roads, and other features.

The criterion for hasty search is speed, as opposed to trying to achieve a certain level of coverage (high or low). The primary objective of hasty searches is to check specific places where the subject or evidence is likely to be discovered quickly and to obtain information about the search area (reconnaissance).

Features of hasty searches include:

- An immediate show of effort
- Requires few resources
- Frequently successful
- Helps define the search area by gathering intelligence or locating clues
- Clue consciousness is a critical success factor and teams used for hasty searches need to be track and sign aware (should have tracking skills) with a familiarity of the terrain being checked and its dangers.
- The subject is often assumed to be responsive at this phase.
- Hasty searching often results in determining where not to search further.
- Preplanning is crucial for the immediate availability and effective application of this type of resource.

Techniques used to accomplish hasty searches include:

- Thorough check of last known point (LKP) or point last seen (PLS) for clues, track, direction of travel, etc.
- Following known or suspected route
- Perimeter check—checking around the area where subject was known to have been; best used in concert with containment
- Sign cutting (looking for sign) all around a piece of evidence, abandoned vehicle, PLS, or LKP
- Checking of hazards, attractions, drainages, buildings, trails, roads, and any other places where the subject or evidence is likely to be discovered quickly if the subject is or has been there

A team that performs hasty searches usually comprises two to four searchers who are immediately available and very mobile. The team may spread out to look for clues around a trailhead, building, or other point of interest, but organized area searching is not usually involved. Literally running a trail, path, or track is a valid hasty search technique. This can be a fast way to determine that the subject is not currently on the trail.

Hasty teams also must be prepared to conduct effective area searches (see below) if the situation so indicates. For example, a hasty team locating a series of clues (e.g., discarded clothing, possibly indicating a severely hypothermic subject) must have the training and experience to recognize the meaning of these clues, determine the area into which the subject may have traveled, and quickly conduct an effective area search.

Hasty search techniques are usually used in the early stages of a search, but can be used anytime to check an unconfirmed sighting or to recheck specific, likely locations. The most effective hasty search resources include trained, clue conscious, hasty teams; trackers; dog teams; aircraft; and any very mobile, trained resource.

Other terms used to describe hasty searches include scratch, eyeball, quick-look, 360s, sign-cutting, ridge running, road/trail patrolling, and trail running. A hasty search has also been referred to as a "Type I" search, but this now conflicts with the NIMS resource typing system.

Some Grid Search Definitions

Base Line – A line, perpendicular to the direction of travel, on which the searchers line up.

Guide Line (a.k.a., control line) – The direction in which a searcher looks for guidance as to the status of the search line (control line).

Guide Person – The person who guides the search team. Always found at the end of the base line unless the guide is toward the center; then the guide person is in the center of the base line. On guide right situations, the guide person is on the right of the base line. On guide left situations, the guide person is on the left of the base line. On a guide right situation, the guide person guides on a feature to his or her right.

Search Lane – The area an individual searcher is assigned to scan.

Trail Tape/Ribbon/String Line – Material that can be used to indicate a line where no natural line exists. Toilet paper, surveyor's tape, string, and other similar material are tied so as to delineate an area. A definite line must be indicated by this material. One should be able to see at least the next marker when standing at a marker so that a line is discernible. The markers should be placed at eye level and doubled when indicating an end or turn in the line. The placement (how close together) of this material is dependent on the terrain and density of brush/vegetation.

Area Searches

When hasty searches alone do not resolve the search, expansion into "area searches" may be required. In an area search, a segment of the search area is searched in an or-ganized manner by a specific resource. The segment must have clearly defined boundaries that are identifiable on a map as well as in the field. Unlike a hasty search, an area search requires that the segment being searched have established boundaries. Each resource conducting an area search should seek to cover its assigned segment as uniformly as possible. That is, search teams and other resources should endeavor to spread their searching effort as evenly as possible over their assigned segments. The best way to do this is to organize the searchers in some type of line or grid search where individual searchers cover parallel lanes. Both loose and tight grid search tactics use search lanes, but they are scanned or covered in different ways as explained below.

If unlimited resources are available, they could and should be deployed to search everywhere there is some likelihood of the subject being. Unfortunately, resources are always limited and search planners must determine how best to use what is available to them. In the language of search theory, this is called "optimal effort allocation." The number and type of resources available as well as the type of object being sought will make a difference in the type of area search chosen for the situation at hand.

Loose Grid Search (Area Search)

In this type of search, search teams may consist of three to seven persons, but usually just three because of the ease of team coordination with fewer people. The goal of this technique is to cover larger geographic areas quickly and with fewer resources. The trade-off is lower overall coverage (less thoroughness), and the benefit is that it allows some reasonable level of coverage to be spread over a large area in a relatively short time. When a life depends on searching a very large area and there is no evidence strongly favoring one region over another, lower coverage in all segments may be better than no coverage in some to achieve higher coverage in others.

A team conducting a loose grid search would organize on a base line, usually at wide between searcher spacing, and proceed forward. Spacing between searchers is dependent on terrain and visibility. Generally with loose grid searches, the amount of overlapping area scanned by both searchers in adjacent search lanes should be minimal. The amount of area between adjacent search lanes that is scanned by neither searcher should likewise be minimal. As a rough guide, this can be achieved in the field by spacing searchers at a distance greater than the established average maximum detection range (AMDR; see Figure 15–5) for the environment being searched.

It is best if the members of the team can maintain an occasional visual and voice contact with one another, but this is not mandatory. Effective loose grid searching does not require all searchers to remain in line with each other. However, organizing the search pattern does help

Loose Grid

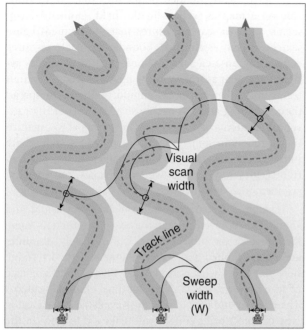

Figure 15–1 An example of a loose grid search showing a three-person search team. All searchers are free to purposely roam their respective search lanes, checking likely spots as they move forward. In this example, each searcher navigates on his or her own because each may not remain in visual contact with adjacent searchers. Because of the lack of organization between searchers, there may be areas of overlap and areas not scanned by any searcher. Overlap should be minimized when possible. With this technique, the distance between adjacent searchers on the base line should be more than the average maximum detection range (AMDR; or sweep width, if known), and searchers need not try to remain in constant visual contact with adjacent searchers.

avoid holes and overlaps in the coverage, keeping it more uniform.

Once the base line and guide for the search is established, the segment is divided into an appropriate number of search lanes based on the number of searchers, search speed (affected by terrain and vegetation), the amount of time assigned for the task (usually less than 6 hours), and the size of the segment. The goal of the team should be to finish their assigned task in the time allotted. If a loose grid search is assigned, it usually means that the team will have to move quickly over the segment. In carrying out a loose grid search, the team should not attempt to spend a great deal of time conducting a very thorough search. Thoroughness is not a characteristic of a loose grid search.

Loose Grid - Guide Center

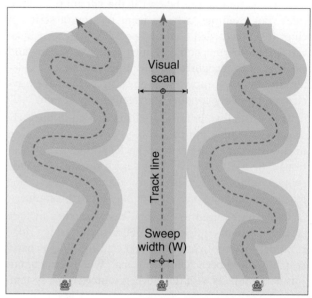

Figure 15–2 A more "organized" example of a loose grid search using a three-person search team. The lateral searchers are free to purposely roam their respective search lanes, checking likely spots as they move forward. Searchers may guide on one end (guide right, or guide left) or the center (as shown) and the navigator must guide on a compass heading or terrain feature. In this example, the navigator in the center serves as the guide for the team and travels a relatively straight course. The lateral searchers guide on, and remain in at least occasional visual contact with, the center searcher ("guide center"). Because they must stay close enough to see the "guide," and because this is a more organized search, coverage is generally higher than the example provided in Figure 15–1. More resources may be needed or it may take the same resources longer to complete a search using this method. Again, there may be areas of overlap and areas not scanned by any searcher, but overlap should be minimized when possible—otherwise it would not be a loose grid search. With this technique, distance between adjacent searchers on the base line should be more than the AMDR (or sweep width, if known).

One useful loose grid method is illustrated in Figure 15–1. Once the search lanes are established and their width determined, each member proceeds to search his or her assigned lane by weaving or roaming while moving forward across the segment. The searchers' movements should be purposeful; searchers should move to not only "cover" the area within the assigned lane as well as time permits, but should also roam laterally to look behind obstructions and investigate likely looking spots based on the information available. Figure 15–2 shows a variation of the loose grid method.

Loose grid searching requires more skill in navigation, clue detection, and "thinking like the subject" than the classical tight grid (high coverage) search described later. However, it also has a number of important characteristics:

- It is more flexible and requires much less coordination of individual searcher efforts than tight grid (high coverage) searching.
- Search lanes are relatively wide, often much wider than the average maximum detection range of the search object(s).
- Searchers can adjust and tailor their movements to the environment, thereby making more efficient use of their time and effort.
- It can be used in situations where more thorough search methods are difficult or impractical.
- Loose grid searches are generally less damaging to the environment and any evidence not found during the search than more thorough techniques.
- With trained, skilled, experienced searchers it generally takes less time to achieve a reasonable coverage than more thorough search methods.
- Often, the overall probability of success (POS) for the search effort as a whole can be increased more quickly with this technique than with more thorough search methods.
- Loose grid searches are often employed after hasty searches, especially if hasty searches found clues.
- This type of search should be used when subject responsiveness is assumed to be high.
- With appropriately skilled and alert searchers, this type of search may also locate clues.

Loose grid searching is the preferred method for achieving moderate (as opposed to very high) levels of coverage in reasonable amounts of time. In theory, it could be used to achieve high or very high coverages, but the tight grid search tactics are generally considered a better method when very thorough searching is required.

Techniques used to accomplish loose grid searches include:

- Relatively wide spacing between the centers of adjacent search lanes.
- Compass bearings or specific guides are often used to control search direction toward the opposite side of the assigned segment. Searchers can quickly move back and forth laterally while maintaining a net direction of movement across the segment.
- Often applied in a specifically defined area or segment of the search area to follow up where a clue has been found or to cover segments indicated by clues found elsewhere (such as those that establish a direction of travel).

Loose grid searches are usually used in the early stages of a search operation, especially if hasty searches have found clues and the time frame for subject survival is short. In some segments, particularly the heavily vegetated ones, loose grid searches may be the initial search tactic used. Loose grid searches also may be valuable in those situations where the search area is large, no particularly likely areas can be identified, and/or there are insufficient resources to achieve higher coverages in all segments.

The most effective resources for this type of search include clue conscious teams, dogs, sign-cutters, aircraft, and trained grid search teams. Other terms used to describe loose grid searches include open grid, low coverage searches, and the "3-compass-X" approach to search description (see Grid Naming System, page 250). In the past, loose grid searches also have been referred to as open grid, "Type II," and "critical separation" searches.

Many have experimented with, and taught, searchers to use sound, usually by means of yelling or the uncoordinated use of a whistle, to attract lost subjects. In 1992, Martin Colwell of Lion's Bay Search and Rescue in British Columbia, Canada, described a loose grid approach to using sound, whistles, and portable radios in a coordinated effort to attract a responsive subject. He called this technique, "sound sweeping."

In practical use, sound sweep searchers are lined up at very wide spacing along a boundary of the area to be searched. Colwell suggests that it is not necessary to coordinate a single start time for all searchers. Searchers simply walk into their search segment, usually guided by compass bearings or terrain (i.e., downhill), when they reach their starting locations. As they begin, a base or control station broadcasts over the radio a countdown call to all searchers at one- to two-minute intervals. For example, the base transmits, *Whistle blast, 5-4-3-2-1 BLAST."* On this command, all searchers stop, blow their whistles (ideally this would occur simultaneously) and then listen for a predetermined period of time for an audible response. If no response is heard, the searchers continue with their sweep. At the moment when searchers are blowing their whistles, it is recommended that they cover their own ears in order to maintain their sensitivity to faint responses.

Tight Grid Search (Area Search)

This type of search is a slow, highly systematic area search. It is generally used when a very thorough, high-coverage search of a segment is desired. In theory, it can be used to achieve any level of coverage from high to low. However, it is best suited for higher coverage searches.

A tight grid search is accomplished by searchers lining up on a baseline, usually at a relatively close spacing.

They then proceed along straight, parallel, equally spaced tracks—to the extent the terrain and vegetation will allow—scanning a swath that extends from themselves to at least halfway to the adjacent searchers, but ideally to the maximum detection range. Figure 15–3 illustrates a high coverage, tight grid search pattern.

Tight Grid

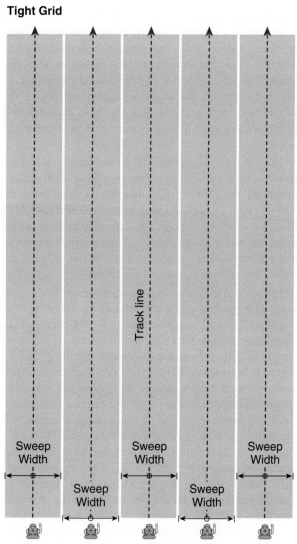

Figure 15–3 An example of a tight grid search with a five-person search team. Searchers may guide on one end (guide right, or guide left) or the center, and the navigator must guide on a compass heading or terrain feature. Note that the spacing between searchers is smaller than with the loose grid. This provides more opportunities for "visual overlap" between searchers and less opportunity for leaving areas unscanned, thus producing higher coverage. With this technique, the distance between adjacent searchers on the base line should be at, near, or less than the AMDR (or sweep width, if known).

A typical tight grid search might achieve a coverage between 1.0 and 2.0, and thus a probability of detection (POD) between 63% and 86% (see Figure 14–4, POD versus Coverage graph, for conversion). Even higher coverage is possible, but the amount of additional effort required to significantly improve the POD is usually considered excessive. For example, the 50% increase in effort needed to get from a coverage of 2.0 to a coverage of 3.0 would produce an increase in POD of less than 9% from 86% to 95%. Most often a search manager will find that the additional effort can be more effectively employed elsewhere in the search area.

The criterion for tight grid searching is generally thoroughness in a specific segment as opposed to rapid increase of overall POS. The main objective of thorough searching is to minimize the chances that a clue or the subject will remain undetected. This is basically the same as maximizing the POD by putting more effort (usually in the form of more searchers) into the segment.

Factors to consider in high-coverage, tight grid searching include:

- This type of searching can be extremely destructive to clues that are not detected, thereby ensuring they will *never* be found. Therefore, this type of search should be used *only as a last resort*.
- It is slow, taking a long time to cover the segment. If used in the early stages of a search, especially when resources are still scarce, the overall POS will generally grow very slowly.
- A great deal of effort is needed to coordinate searcher movement, maintain the line abreast formation, maintain searcher spacing, and keep all searchers on parallel tracks. This "overhead" represents time and effort that cannot be expended on searching.

Techniques used to accomplish thorough type searches include:

- Close-spaced or "tight grid" search with many searchers in a segment.
- Since marking the searched area is so important, trail tape, ribbons, string lines, or some similar method are frequently used for control.
- Areas scanned by adjacent searchers often overlap with an emphasis on thoroughness.

A team that performs high-coverage searches is usually made up of four to seven persons, rarely more. Unskilled searchers can be mixed with skilled searchers, but unskilled searchers should never attempt this type of search without skilled help. Overlap of search lanes is permissible and may be encouraged.

High-coverage searches are usually used when lower coverage searches have been tried with a resulting POD lower than desired, or when a thorough search of a segment is desired at the onset and the appropriate resources are plentiful. The most effective and thorough type of search resource is almost always trained grid search teams.

Other terms used to describe thorough type searches include: closed grid, sweep searches, "Type III" searches, saturation searching, and 7-guide-X (see Grid Naming System, page 250) approach to search description.

Evidence Search (Area Search)

SAR search teams are sometimes called upon to perform evidence searches, often at a crime scene (**Figure 15–4**). This type of search is a more thorough variation of the tight grid search. There are three differences between a tight grid search in a SAR situation and an evidence search: (1) an evidence search does not involve a live subject and, thus, time and urgency are less of an issue; (2) evidence searches often involve looking for small objects in limited areas; and (3) the rules of evidence (e.g., maintaining the chain of evidence, protection of the evidence, recording the evidence as it is found, etc.) will be strictly enforced on evidence searches. Nevertheless, the same techniques for organizing and employing searchers in a tight grid search apply.

Because an extremely high level of detection is often required in an evidence search (e.g., a high level of confidence that nothing was missed), more search effort is required in smaller areas. Because there is a direct relationship between search effort and coverage, doubling the search effort also doubles the coverage. In an evidence search, the amount of search effort employed is usually increased by searchers simply spending more time searching and taking their time to be very thorough. Twice the time at half the speed translates to a slightly higher coverage because of the marginal increase in the sweep width caused by slowing down. Search effort can also be increased by increasing the number of searchers; that is, twice the number of searchers at the same search speed translates to twice the coverage.

Important characteristics of evidence searches include:

- Time is not usually as important a factor as it is in SAR searches.
- Often there will be no second chance. Evidence not discovered on the first search may be destroyed, damaged, or modified by the search activity itself to the point where it cannot be used in court.
- Large amounts of effort must be concentrated in small areas to achieve high coverages for even very small objects. Hands and knees, shoulder to shoulder very tight grid, parallel sweeps are not uncommon.
- It is very important that each object found be left in place untouched and undisturbed by the searcher. When possible evidence is found, the searcher must immediately stop, announce the find so all other searchers stop as well, and call the object to the attention of a law enforcement official who will then decide what action to take. Often the actions taken will be to photograph the item in place, note exactly where, when, and by whom it was found, retrieve, mark and bag the item, and start a chain-of-custody record. Searchers may resume searching only when directed to do so by the appropriate official.

Evidence searches have also been referred to as "Type IV" searches, but this and similar older references to search "types" now conflict with the NIMS resource typing system.

Evidence Search

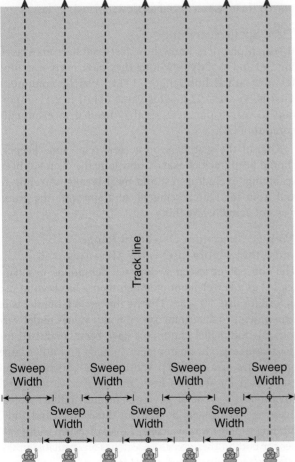

Track line

Sweep Width Sweep Width Sweep Width Sweep Width

Sweep Width Sweep Width Sweep Width

Figure 15–4 An example of an evidence (grid) search with a seven-person search team. Searchers may guide on one end (guide right, or guide left) or the center and the navigator must guide on a compass heading or terrain feature. Note that there is an overlapping area scanned by both searchers in adjacent search lanes. To accomplish this, the distance between adjacent searchers on the base line should be less than the AMDR (or sweep width, if known).

Information to Report to Planners After a Search

Several important pieces of information that affect search planning should be conveyed to search planners by field personnel after an area search is conducted:

1. Estimated forward search speed of the individual or team while searching
2. How long the individual or team searched (excluding rest breaks and such)
3. Field measurements of average maximum detection range (AMDR) or some similar field-observable measure
4. Other field-observable measures identified and requested by search planners prior to the assignment
5. A qualitative description of how well the team did with the search (e.g., excellent, good, fair, or poor)
6. A qualitative description of the search conditions (e.g., rough terrain that slowed and fatigued searchers, numerous thickets that could not be thoroughly investigated and still finish the assignment on time, etc.)

Forward Search Speed

An estimate of the average search speed is needed so the effort, or total distance traveled while searching, may be computed by search planners. Effort is needed along with sweep width to compute the area effectively swept by the searchers. Area effectively swept is needed to compute the coverage, before the POD can be objectively estimated. In addition, the search speed itself may affect the sweep width. If searchers move too quickly, they will not have as much time to scan their surroundings for the subject or clues. More rapid movement means they must devote more of their attention to the problems of navigating the terrain and less to searching. In short, too much speed could reduce the effective sweep width, coverage, and thus the POD. The opposite is true for much slower than normal search speeds. Therefore, it is essential that searchers provide an estimate of their average speed while searching, because it will affect the search planner's estimate of the POD and POS that were achieved.

One way to estimate forward search speed is to first measure search speeds during SAR exercises or on actual searches to determine the "normal" speed for you and your team. Using this measure as a reference, searchers then can describe their forward speed in comparison as either slow, normal, or fast. Values could then be assigned to each of these speed categories (e.g., slow = $0.5 \times$ normal search speed, normal = $1 \times$ normal search speed, and fast = $1.5 \times$ normal search speed) and used by search planners. Since differences of these magnitudes do not normally have a big effect on detectability for

ground searches, such general estimates are usually sufficiently accurate. However, to more accurately estimate their forward speed during a search, experiments could be conducted by field searchers. For example:

- It takes 30 minutes (0.5 hour) to search from point A to point B.
- The distance between point A and point B is 0.5 mile.
- Searchers describe their speed in this segment as "normal."
- 0.5 mile divided by 0.5 hours = 1.0 mile per hour.
- Normal speed = 1.0 mile per hour.

Similar "experiments" could be conducted in other environments to determine "normal" search speeds for that environment. Search planners could then use these experimentally-derived speeds when field personnel reported their search speed as slow, normal, or fast.

Time Spent Searching

If search planners know how fast searchers are traveling (V) and exactly how long they have been searching (t), the "track line length" (TLL) can be computed. That is, $V \times t = TLL$. This value (TLL) is very important to search planners, as they need it to eventually compute POD.

One of the searchers on a crew (e.g., time keeper) should keep track of exactly how long the team has been searching, excluding rest and meal breaks, traveling to and from the search segment, and any time the group was not actually searching.

Average Maximum Detection Range and Other Field-Observable Measures

The concept of sweep width (see definitions in Chapter 14) as a key element of search theory has been in use in SAR for over 50 years. During this period, hundreds of experiments to determine sweep width values under various environmental conditions have been conducted for the marine search environment (oceans and other large open water areas). Sweep width values also have been established for searches from aircraft over various land environments. Federal government and military objectives were the primary impetus for these efforts and, thus, funding support was available. Tables of sweep width values for both of these types of searches are available in the *International Aeronautical and Maritime Search and Rescue Manual* (*IAMSAR Manual*, 1999) published jointly by the International Maritime Organization and the International Civil Aviation Organization. This three-volume document is recognized globally as the standard text on aeronautical and maritime SAR operations and methods.

Unfortunately, prior to 2002 no such experiments had been conducted for ground searches, probably because land SAR is a local problem that is usually addressed by local, often volunteer, organizations and individuals with little or no funding. Recognizing this fact, the members of the National Search and Rescue Committee, a consortium of federal agencies, funded the development of an experimental model that could be used by land search teams to develop their own sweep width data. In addition, the committee also procured funding for a number of land sweep width experiments that were conducted in various eco-regions across the U.S. in 2003 and 2004. The report of the first project, titled "A Method for Determining Effective Sweep Widths for Land Searches: Procedures for Conducting Detection Experiments," is currently available at the U.S. National SAR Committee's web site. The report(s) from the sweep width experiments has not been completed as of this writing and will be available on the same web site in 2005. Both of these reports should be required reading for team leaders and search planners.

Until experimentally determined sweep width data becomes widely available for land search, some method for estimating "detectability" would be helpful in the application of search theory. Until specific sweep width estimation methods have been developed and/or tested, search planners may be able to use certain measurable observations made by field personnel to help establish an estimate of sweep width in a particular segment. Average maximum detection range (AMDR) is one measure that may be helpful because it depends on the same variables as sweep width (e.g., the unique combination of search environment, search object, and search sensor). But, other field-measurable observations may also be helpful. These may include items such as meteorological visibility, amount and type of precipitation, percent of cloud cover, vegetation density, and other measurable quantities yet to be identified or developed. Measurement of any of these or similar field-observable variables may be asked of field personnel after a search (in their debriefing).

The AMDR (**Figure 15–5**) can be estimated in the environment in which the search will be conducted, using a search object representative of that which is being sought (e.g., back-pack, sleeping bag, etc). Other writers have called it the "visibility petal" and the "rain dance," but it is the same thing: a field measurement of the average maximum (visual) detection range (AMDR). The AMDR can be quickly measured and documented in the search segment, and then reported during debriefing to search planners.

To measure the AMDR, place an object (similar to the search object) at a location judged to be representative of the conditions in the search area as a whole, usually in the segment to be searched. Beginning at the object, walk away from the object until it is no longer visible. Keep track of the number of paces of known length (sometimes called a tally) and use these to estimate the distance. Note or record the distance to this point. Continue away from the object for another 50 to 100 meters. Travel clockwise around the object about 45 degrees and move toward the object until it is sighted. Record the distance from this point to the object by counting the paces to the object from the point of sighting while returning to it along a straight line. Then move away from the object at 90 degrees to the right of the initial departure, which should be about 45 degrees from the direction of approach just used. Again, measure the distance to the point at which the object disappears. Repeat this sequence until eight (or so) detection distances are established.

Four of the distances in Figure 15–5 will have been measured while moving away from the object and four measured while moving toward the object. These distances can be easily estimated by having calibrated the length of one's pace and knowing the number of paces traveled. The AMDR is the average of these eight distance values and should be measured as accurately as possible. The AMDR also should be reevaluated for each search object and whenever there is a change in the environment sufficient to affect searcher visibility.

The AMDR measurement process performs several important functions:

- It gives searchers the experience of seeing how an object similar to the search object appears in the

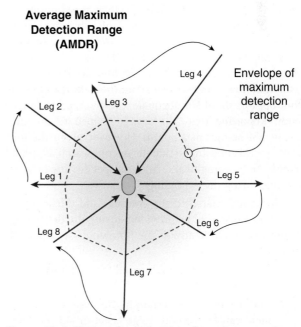

Figure 15–5 Method for estimating the average maximum detection range (AMDR).

environment where the search is to take place. (However, searchers must avoid becoming so fixated on this image that they overlook other items of importance that look differently, such as clues or even the subject.)

- Although AMDR, strictly speaking, is not a measure of detectability, it does give the search planner one quantitative measure of what search conditions were like.

- Having had the experience of performing an AMDR measurement, searchers may be in a better position to make other observations about their environment and search conditions.

Although skilled search managers will avoid such assignments, if a segment includes two or more significantly different environments (e.g., both open field and timbered forest), the AMDR—as well as any other observations made for the purpose of estimating sweep width—should be measured in each of the representative environments within the segment and reported accordingly. Search planners can then use these measurements to help compute coverage in each portion of the segment searched.

Qualitative Description of Completed Search

Fatigue, exhaustion, injuries, and other distractions that may not influence the field estimate of AMDR can reduce the effectiveness of a search crew during operations. Additional experiments in the land search environments using land search resources may eventually establish how sweep width is affected by each of these factors, but it is doubtful that all will ever be completely covered. Therefore, some method of subjectively estimating the overall quality of the search may be helpful. This can be as easy as subjectively reporting, during the debriefing, an assessment of how well the search went and how searchers feel about their efforts. Offering four options should be adequate: excellent, good, fair, or poor. Reporting that "the search seemed to go fine" might not be that meaningful. However, given the four choices and choosing to rate the overall search as "poor" should be meaningful and trigger a specific line of questioning during the debriefing.

All details related to the conduct and effectiveness of the search should be provided during the debriefing. These may include any of the following (see also Appendix 4):

1. The crew felt rushed/hurried (for whatever reason).

2. The size of, or the terrain in, the assigned segment caused the crew to go faster or slower than normal search speed for the conditions in the segment.

3. Prejudice – searchers complained of being assigned to a segment they thought would contain neither clues nor the subject.

4. Fatigue or exhaustion

5. Searcher boredom or other preoccupation

6. Anything that detrimentally affects any senses of the searcher

7. Non-uniform coverage – for example, difficult-to-search portions of the segment were avoided or a portion was not covered at all due to time and speed limitations.

8. Conditions (terrain, vegetation, weather, and/or lighting) were different from those described in the pre-search briefing.

The importance of accurately and completely reporting all observations made during a search cannot be overemphasized. When observations are reported by experienced search crew members, they are taken very seriously by search managers and planners. These observations will be used to evaluate sweep width estimates and coverage that ultimately factor into the estimation of search effectiveness in that segment. Erroneous, inaccurate, or vague information from field SAR teams can be devastating to an otherwise reasonable search plan.

Grid Naming System

A grid naming system has been developed by Explorer Search and Rescue (now called *Venturing*) teams in the Pacific Northwest to describe any specific grid (area) search pattern. The system consists of a *number–word–number* sequence that serves as the name of the pattern.

For example, 6–guide [right]–30, where the first number (on the left) describes the number of searchers on the grid or control line (6 searchers). The team leader is not included in this number if he/she is working behind the line (off of the base line). The word is either "compass" or "guide" and indicates what the team is using as the guide. The word is "compass" if the team is using a compass bearing for directional control and "guide" if the team is guiding on a string line, ribbon line, creek, road, ridge top, or virtually anything other than compass. "Left" or "right" can be added to the word "guide" to indicate which direction the base line should guide. The second number in the system describes the average between-searcher distance in feet or meters. Note that this is to indicate the *average* distance between searchers. Before the search is conducted, this number can be an estimate. However, after the search is conducted, the search team should accurately describe the distance, especially if it is different than the earlier estimate. Since the between-searcher distance is generally dependent on the type of search (loose or tight grid), the terrain, and the density of underbrush, the between-searcher distance estimated before the search can easily vary after the team is actually in the search area.

The above example (6–guide [right]–30) describes a search with six searchers on the guide line (and there may be one team leader behind the line), guiding right on something (as opposed to using a compass), with an average between searcher distance (or track space) of 30 feet.

This grid naming system has several advantages. It offers an easily recognized method of communicating the details of a search pattern so that the search management team and the field search team can assure mutual understanding. Also, it allows an opportunity to estimate a search team's base line width.

When search teams are assigned search segments using this terminology, the search management team must assure that the field team understands which type of area search (loose or tight grid) to perform. This assures that the team in the field understands how to configure themselves properly to achieve the desired results. Loose grid searches usually have little or no overlap in search lanes. High-coverage, tight grid searches may allow or require considerable overlap in search lanes.

Guidelines for Skilled Searching

Experienced SAR personnel have developed certain practical techniques and guidelines that have been found to be useful over the years. These guidelines include:

1. Stay alert and maintain the proper attitude for effective searching. Searching is hard work and can be boring, tedious, and extremely fatiguing. *You must be able to stay alert and maintain your usefulness during a search if you expect to be of any help at all.* The only thing worse than not keeping alert is not keeping alert and doing nothing about it. Many find it useful to mentally talk to themselves, "telling" themselves what to do, as an effective way to maintain focus and alertness. ("Look behind that log. What's in that creek bed?") This also helps preclude the, "I'm cold; it's wet; how much longer?" type of thought patterns. You must be able to recognize at what point you stop being an effective searcher. Furthermore, you must assert yourself when this occurs, so that you can be replaced and given a chance to correct the problem. If you cannot discipline yourself to search effectively in less than ideal condi-

tions (i.e., bad weather, cold, hot, tired, lack of success, etc.), then you should not participate in the search at all or at least reconsider your position in the command structure.

2. Use all of your senses for searching. Use your eyes, your nose, your ears, and most importantly, your head.

3. Scan the "searcher cube" while searching and while approaching the search area. That is, look up and down, look left and right, and look forward and behind. This approach to searching can allow one to see things that might not be visible when merely looking forward. While approaching a search area, searching the "searcher cube" also allows the searcher to become familiar with the surrounding terrain so the return journey is easier.

4. Yell and make noise occasionally and intermix regular moments of silence. Noise may attract or cause a response from a lost subject, and the silence permits you to hear the response. This can be particularly effective when the subject is thought to be only lost, uninjured, and responsive, which often occurs early in a search.

5. Always take the Boy Scout Motto to heart and "be prepared." Have the proper equipment and clothing with you, so that you can be an asset rather than a detriment. Have a ready pack, know what is in it, and how to use what it contains.

6. Learn the names of the searchers on either side of you in a line search and remember what color and type of clothing he/she is wearing. Know if those people change their outer layer of clothing and inform them if you change yours. Searchers wearing bright colored clothing are important during searches. Camouflage is unacceptable.

7. At night, never shine your flashlight or headlamp into your eyes or those of other searchers. It takes quite awhile for them to adjust their eyes to the dark again. Sometimes not using lights at all is preferred if safety and effectiveness can be maintained.

8. Always check the obvious. Use common sense and talk to hikers, check buildings and caves, and ask people in the area if they have seen anything. More than one search has ended when the subject was found helping in the search.

9. A field searcher has no reason to be talking with family of the subject or the media unless he/she has been assigned to do so. The proper way to handle the inquiry is to refer the individual to

the incident commander or the appropriate responsible personnel. For the same reasons, there should be no loose talk in or around the incident site. Think what you want, but speak only after thinking. Complaints about the mission should be made in private to one's supervisor, or saved for the postmission critique.

10. Search for clues as well as the subject. There are many more clues than subjects. Clues can substantially decrease the search area and indicate where not to search further. A lack of clues can be just as important as a great number of them. Do not be discouraged if you know you are searching effectively, yet you have turned up nothing. This negative information is very important to search planning.

11. The safety of the searchers is more important than the mission itself. YOU are more important than your partners, your PARTNERS are more important than the subject, and the subject is the reason why the search is happening. It may seem arrogant, but the above is always true. However, the searchers should be so confident in their own skills and those of their partners that they can concentrate solely on the needs of the subject. When this confidence is lacking, the searchers may be in jeopardy and something needs to be done.

Anatomy of a SAR Incident

The SAR Incident Cycle was described in Chapter 1. The elements of this cycle (Preplanning, Notification, Planning and Strategy, Tactics and Operations, Suspension, and Critique) are used to illustrate what SAR personnel should be doing at these various benchmarks. The details of this process are extremely important to the searcher, because no one will explain the process at the scene of a SAR incident. Arriving with an understanding of how the overall process works, from before the call-out to the postmission critique, is a distinct advantage for everyone involved.

Preplanning and Preparation

The concept of preplanning to SAR personnel is far different than it is to a search manager. Preplanning to a searcher means having the skill, knowledge, and equipment ready to perform in a SAR incident as well as being physically and mentally prepared. SAR personnel must know before an incident what may be expected of them. They must understand the standards by which they will be measured.

Equipment

Proper equipment must be ready for use at the first notice of an incident. Different areas and environments require different equipment. Knowledge of what is generally needed as well as what is specifically needed is imperative. Equipment must be ready for use and not require collection or repair at the time of call-out.

Self

Through study and experience, SAR personnel must possess an understanding of the fundamental information that will be necessary to perform safely, efficiently, and effectively at an incident. Everyone must be fully prepared educationally, emotionally, physically, and mentally for the rigors of a SAR incident. One's attitude is the capstone on the well-rounded field operator.

The searcher must be physically up to the challenges presented by most SAR incidents. Anything else shows a lack of planning and preparedness. The searcher must be mentally prepared to endure the strain of boredom, fatigue, and discomfort while maintaining an attitude of urgency and optimism for the cause. A searcher who responds to an incident in which he/she does not want to be involved should stay home. A searcher must want to search and be ready to do so at any time. The credo for SAR personnel should be, "Be Prepared," before a call-out occurs.

First Notice

First notice is the initial notification of responders to a SAR incident. First notice should really be broken into two distinct parts: (1) first notice of incident and (2) first personnel notice (call-out).

First notice of incident usually involves an individual in some official capacity (but not necessarily) to whom a lost or missing person(s) is reported. The report could be from relatives or friends, from a member of a party that recognizes a person is missing, by the discovery of evidence or clues (i.e., abandoned vehicle, registration system, deserted camp or equipment, etc.), distress signals, Emergency Locator Transmitter, etc. This type of notification usually involves some organization that the public believes has the authority and/or responsibility for SAR by way of an individual who represents that authority.

First personnel notice involves the calling of SAR resources to initiate a search and/or rescue. If further assistance is required, the one who takes the initial report must contact the appropriate personnel to affect further action. An individual SAR resource (searcher, rescuer, etc.) will be notified if he/she is needed, and this is termed "call-out."

Both of these types of first notice can be important to SAR personnel because any one person might be called upon to take the initial report or to respond to help.

When an initial report of a problem is received, a chain of events begins that can determine the entire course of the SAR event.

Notice of Incident

Initial contact (whether by phone, radio, or in person) is made by the person or persons who are reporting a problem. The impression that the report taker gives the reporting party and the initial actions that are taken often set the tone for the rest of the mission. If the report comes into an agency (such as a Sheriff's office, Park Service, Fire Service, etc.), the degree of professionalism and responsiveness may affect future missions as well. The most important initial considerations by the initial report taker should include the following:

1. The attitude of the report taker. The report taker should remain calm, professional, be inquisitive, have a tone of concern, and express a willingness to help.

2. The name and call-back telephone number and location of the reporting party. The reporting party should be told to remain there until told to do otherwise.

3. Urgency. This is not disorganized haste, but directed, efficient, planned, and coordinated action.

The report taker must sort out the initial information offered by the reporting party for importance and relevance while also attempting to acquire specific information that must be known immediately for effective decision making. Formats for the specific information required can be found on the Urgency Determination Form in Appendix 2 and the first two pages of the Missing Person Questionnaire in Appendix 5 (first notice information).

Once this information is collected, it can be entered into an Urgency Determination Form (see Appendix 2) and the relative urgency can be determined.

The initial report taker must now evaluate the information received in a calm, intelligent manner for subsequent action. This is also the time when a trained search manager must be involved. A trained search manager will want to talk to the reporting party in person, evaluate the initial information, determine the reliability of the sources, consider the facts, consider the probabilities, consider the possibilities, and then combine the information objectively before acting further. This might also be where a search manager begins to call-out initial resources.

One of the first actions of a trained search manager will be to request more information about the lost subject(s), and this is where the initial report taker (management trained or not) can begin filling out the Missing Person Questionnaire (MPQ; see Appendix 5). All questions on the MPQ should be filled in, if possible, leaving no blank spots for someone later to have to guess whether the question was ever asked.

The following is a general summary of what should be determined during the initial reporting of an incident:

1. Is there a problem?
2. How serious is it or could it get?
3. Where is the problem?
4. Who is involved?
5. How did it happen?
6. When did it happen?

Information should be compiled, so it can be used to make decisions about what is to be subsequently done.

Personnel Call-Out

For searchers, the initial call-out is the process by which they are notified that their services are needed. Certain information must be acquired from the notifying source so that an efficient and effective response can be made by the individual whose services have been requested. This checklist identifies what information should be available to the resource being requested:

1. Description of the situation (abbreviated), who is in charge (individual or organization), and who is making the call-out (name of person you are talking to and call-back number).

2. Description of terrain, weather, weather forecast, and elevation range where you will be involved.

3. Length of time needed (best guess will do) and length of time available should be conveyed.

4. Special equipment (personal or team) needed.

5. Map? Of where? What type, scale, etc.

6. Meeting place (check-in) as well as detailed directions (signs, suggested route, markers, how long should it take, etc.).

7. The name of the person to whom they should report upon arrival.

8. Any other pertinent information.

Certain information must be offered to the notifying source, so that they know what advantages or limitations an individual's (or organization's) involvement may carry. For example:

1. How long are you available (minutes, hours, days, or months)?

2. What equipment do you (or don't you) have?

3. What are your physical limitations (handicaps, conditioning, injuries, etc.)?

4. Do you need transportation or can you supply?

5. Describe training limitations (especially if your training differs from what is expected).

6. Any other pertinent information that is requested of you.

Check-In

Once the call-out procedures have taken place, all SAR personnel must travel to the incident site and check in with the appropriate person. The type of check-in required (formal versus informal) varies depending on the complexity and size of the incident; it may be verbal or may require actually filling out a form. Regardless of the method, check-in is an essential element of an accountability program that is necessary to maintain a safe working environment. Insist that your presence be documented and tracked, even if that service is not offered.

Briefing

After check-in and general assignments have been made, briefing will take place so that specific task assignments can be made. The briefing is a summary of the situation, past and present, conveyed by those who know to those who need to know and that provides information that will help orient personnel to all facets of the problem (safety, strategic, environmental, and tactical). A general briefing usually occurs initially when an individual is first indoctrinated at an incident and may be repeated when the overhead team changes shift. The purpose of a briefing is simply to convey necessary information to the personnel who need it.

Another type of briefing is assignment specific; that is, it involves the description of a particular task assignment. This assignment briefing takes place prior to every assignment that is made.

The term "briefing" is used whenever information is conveyed from the top of a hierarchy down to the ranks. Getting "briefed" basically means learning from superiors the details of the tasks you are expected to do. Briefing is just the information that searchers need to know.

The Planning Section Chief (ICS function) or a member of his/her staff is responsible for briefing. Team leaders are usually briefed, but entire teams may be briefed together in certain situations. Where team leaders are briefed, they in turn brief their teams. In large scale incidents, the Planning Section Chief may delegate briefing to a subordinate.

All SAR personnel should be aware of certain details of a briefing:

1. A briefing should be performed prior to a search shift (operational period) rather than during it.
2. A briefing should last less than 30 minutes and should be in both oral and written formats, if possible.
3. Short, as opposed to lengthy, briefings maintain a high morale, the credibility of SAR personnel, and ensure a timely response to the field.

4. Notes should be taken to assure accuracy. Assuring that the information conveyed and understood is very important.
5. Briefings should take place in a designated area, with plenty of room. That is, the area should be sheltered, quiet, and free from interruptions.

Ideally, much of the specific information needed in a briefing is included on an incident briefing form (ICS 201) or an assignment form (ICS 204), and is provided to search crew leaders (see Appendix 7 for ICS forms). It can also be helpful for an individual or team to design or procure a briefing checklist (see Appendix 4) to assure that at least the important issues are covered in a briefing. As a minimum, such a checklist should be based on the following information:

1. Situation status, objectives, strategies, and predictions. This includes what is happening now, what will happen later, and what we want to happen. A copy of any management briefing statement could be passed out as well.
2. Subject information. This includes a complete physical description, clothing and equipment description (carried and worn), physical and mental condition, behavioral traits, circumstances surrounding the search, medical/health problems of the subject, etc. Photos are helpful.
3. Clue considerations. The sole pattern of footwear, items carried, how to report clues, how to handle clues (logging, retrieve, mark, etc.), clue follow up, etc., is useful. A sketch of sole pattern is good.
4. Subject's trip plans.
5. Terrain, hazards, etc. in the assigned search area. A map helps.
6. Current and forecast weather in the assigned search area.
7. Equipment needed by searchers such as specific clothing, safety equipment, food and water, camera, medical gear, climbing gear, radios, etc.
8. Communication details. These include frequencies to be used, designators and codes, contact person and times, etc.
9. Reporting details. These include reporting locations, times, and to whom, where, and when to report.
10. Transportation details. How to get to where you are supposed to be, who will take you, and how, etc.
11. How to handle external influences such as family, media, subject's friends, etc., should they be encountered. Identify who is family, friends, and media as well as where to refer them.

12. Tactical assignments with explicit instructions. Know exactly where and how to search.
    - Specific area, where to start, and how to get there (copy of map helps).
    - Configurations, tactics, etc.
    - Procedures for handling discovered clues.
    - Adjacent teams and their location(s).
    - Have other teams searched the area?
    - When to start and stop. What if area is not finished when you are supposed to return?
    - Instructions for subject contact. What to do if the subject(s) is found dead, injured, or well? (Make sure rescue/evacuation plan is understood.)
    - Instructions for protecting scene.
13. Organization overview. To whom do you answer, and who answers to me?
14. Precise debriefing procedures.
    - Where, when, and with whom to debrief?
    - What information will be required and in what format?
15. Safety instructions. These include dealing with man-made hazards (helo, aircraft, fuels, etc.), terrain hazards, natural hazards (snakes, dogs, poisonous plants, other animals, etc.), etc.
    - What to watch out for?
    - What to do if ...?
16. What to do if member of team is injured. Stay with them, get help, or use the radio?

Assignment

Once the briefing has been completed, it is time to carry out the assignment described in the briefing.

Individual Responsibilities

While on assignment, an individual has certain responsibilities that bear on the effectiveness and safety of him/herself and his/her team. Teams for searching can vary in size, but should meet ICS doctrine for span of control that dictates that five be the general guideline for unit size. Within that unit, certain obligations must be met, and it should be the job of all team members to see that their responsibilities are carried out.

1. All members of the team must have their own personal gear and should not be dependent on anyone else for equipment. "Have your own and carry your own" should be the credo.
2. All team members should be dressed properly for the terrain and environment in which they will be involved. Everyone should have appropriate back-up clothing where necessary.

3. All team members should be physically and mentally prepared to perform difficult search and rescue operations, and not depend on it being an easy day.
4. Skills and skill limitations should be immediately relayed to the team leader. Nothing should be assumed.

Team Responsibilities

Every team should immediately assign, before deployment into the field, at least one member to the following responsibilities: navigator, tally, time keeper, and team leader. A team leader will probably be assigned before the group is put together, because every team must have a leader and the position is never assumed.

Even though every member of a team should always know where they are (geographically and with respect to the search area), one member should be assigned as team navigator so that each individual can check his or her accuracy.

A "tally" (distance measurer) is one who, by some method (usually stride), keeps track of distance traveled with relationship to the search area and search base.

The time keeper maintains a chronology, in writing, of what goes on and when it happens during the assignment period. Documenting everything is always a good idea. A team may assign one individual to do all of the writing, especially if someone takes shorthand or finds it easier than others to write while on the move.

Any job that the team leader deems necessary should be assigned before going into the field, because an individual may need time to prepare for his/her job responsibilities. Remember that, in addition to everything else, a searcher must search, and search well. If you have a problem with anything to which you have been assigned, speak up. Perhaps you can be reassigned.

Debriefing

After a field assignment is completed, debriefing is necessary for the extraction of relevant and pertinent information from field SAR personnel (Figure 15–6). Debriefing is the transfer of information from field personnel to the search management team after an assignment has been completed. The purpose of debriefing is to convey as much of the relevant information as possible to the search management team. Management's purpose is to extract the information from the field personnel. Without thorough information, subsequent planning can be misdirected, improper, inadequate, and incomplete. The term "debriefing" is used whenever information is conveyed from subordinates to supervisors in a hierarchy. Simply put, debriefing is the acquisition of information that management needs from field personnel.

The following are general guidelines regarding debriefing:

1. The Planning Section Chief (ICS function), or his/her equivalent, is responsible for seeing that an adequate debriefing is performed, but coordination of the debriefing is usually handled by a member of the Plans Section.

2. The team leader may debrief his/her team and then, in turn, be debriefed; however, eventually, all field personnel should be debriefed.

3. The debriefing of field personnel should be done on an individual basis, rather than two or three at a time, and it should take place as soon as possible after an individual (or team) exits the field.

4. Debriefing should be done in writing, if possible. Written information reduces confusion and misunderstanding, and can easily become part of the final documentation of the incident.

Any and all pertinent information should be solicited, and conveyed, during a debriefing, including the following list. Refer also to the briefing and debriefing checklists in Appendix 4.

1. Explicit and complete descriptions of the areas covered (and not covered) and activities carried out during search.

2. Estimate of the average maximum detection range for each specific sub-area of the assigned segment (see Figure 15–5).

3. Report any other observations made and measured for each specific sub-area of the assigned segment. These should have been described and requested by search planners prior to the assignment.

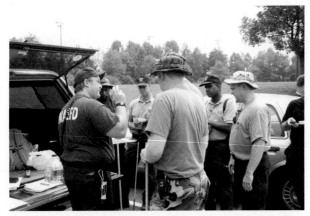

Figure 15–6 After a field assignment is completed, debriefing is necessary for the extraction of relevant information from field SAR personnel.

4. Qualitative description of search (excellent, good, fair, or poor)

5. Estimate of forward speed of the search unit (fast, normal, or slow)

6. Exact amount (in minutes) of time spent searching, excluding rest breaks, traveling to and from the segment, and the like

7. The exact location of any clues located, regardless of how insignificant they may seem (use maps, sketches, etc., to convey location)

8. A qualitative description of the search conditions (e.g., rough terrain that slowed and fatigued searchers, numerous thickets that could not be thoroughly investigated and still finish the assignment on time, etc.)

9. Specific difficulties encountered (such as gaps in coverage, terrain problems, communication problems, weather difficulties, physical fitness or illness, injuries, etc.)

10. Hazards encountered in the area. Be specific with respect to the location and description.

11. Suggestions, recommendations, and ideas for further activity in the area searched.

SAR personnel should use any and every method of conveying information. Sketches, maps, photos, briefing reports (assignment forms), notes, etc., may all be of value. Proper information conveyed to the "debriefer" is absolutely essential for an effective search and can be the most important part of a search.

Check-Out

Once the call-out, check-in, briefing, assignments, and debriefings have taken place, SAR personnel eventually get to check-out of the incident. This is part of the management function called "demobilization" and may be as simple as a verbal, "I'll see you later," or it may require a formal procedure such as completing and/or signing a form. The level of formality varies depending on the complexity and size of the incident, but precise check-out and demobilization details should be acquired at the incident briefing or debriefing. At check-out, a final accounting is made of all field personnel. If a formal critique is planned, details (such as when and where) can be relayed at this time.

The responsibility for the safety of SAR personnel does not end at check-out. It ends when all SAR personnel have safely arrived at their intended destinations. SAR personnel should not hesitate to request assistance or transportation if they are too tired to drive home on their own. Numerous injuries and notable deaths have occurred when fatigued SAR personnel have attempted to return home on their own after many hours of rigorous operations.

Return to Service

It is useful to begin mentally preparing for returning to response-ready status even before checking out of the current incident. This usually involves two steps: finishing up current involvement with the incident, and returning everything to full mission ready status.

First, make sure all of the paperwork and physical work is done for the present mission. Consider the following:

1. Debriefing forms finished?
2. Check-out?
3. Injury claim forms to fill out?
4. Expendable supplies used?
5. Personal supplies that need to be reimbursed?
6. Can you do anything to help others get back into service?
7. Do the search managers need any help demobilizing?
8. Can you help in any way at all?

Replace, replenish, and clean all gear and equipment so it will be ready for its next use (which could be anytime).

1. What expendable gear needs to be replaced?
2. What food and/or water must be replaced?
3. Batteries?
4. Medical supplies?
5. Does gear need to be cleaned?
6. Do clothing need cleaning?
7. Did you lose anything?
8. Did you break anything?
9. Did anyone borrow anything from you?
10. Did you borrow anything that needs to be returned?

Rest, eat, drink, and return your body to full mission ready status.

Maintaining a Personal Mission Log

SAR personnel should maintain a personal "mission log." This log should, as a minimum, contain the date and time of your involvement in a SAR mission, and a description of the details of your involvement (e.g., functions performed, positions held, etc). It is also a good idea to have your mission supervisor sign the log to validate your documented actions during the mission. Not only can such a log help track your experience, it can also help document your actions should questions later arise.

Some SAR organizations require the maintenance of such logs. For example, The SAR Program of the Commonwealth of Virginia Department of Emergency Services requires documentation of a certain amount of experience before becoming certified as a ground SAR Incident Command. A mission log validated by your team leader is permitted to satisfy this requirement.

Mission Critique

Participating in the mission critique, also called the incident debriefing or after action review, is an opportunity to help assure that mistakes made are not repeated and that things that were done right are noted. Make sure that you have made your ideas and problems known before you leave and offer a constructive critique rather than a destructive one. Be aware that some management teams will include a brief critique at the end of each assignment. In these cases, no incident critique may be performed.

A formal critique of any SAR incident, no matter how large or small, should always be attempted as soon as possible after the situation, before all those involved go home. A critique is a process intended to identify the lessons learned from an exercise or actual event and is not for placing blame, pointing fingers, or allowing adversaries to embarrass each other.

It is the responsibility of the SAR manager to provide for an effective critique of the entire search operation, but many times an individual must make the right noises to provoke action. It is especially important to hold a critique when a subject was not found. For a team or organization, a critique can help to review, revise, and improve the preplan. For the individual, it can help one to realize how to improve.

An individual's critique of him- or herself should include the following:

1. What gear did I need that I did not have (personal, team)?
2. How long did it take for me to mobilize? Could it be done better next time?
3. What particular skills do I need to work on (navigation, search technique, wilderness travel, physical condition, etc.)?
4. How can I improve myself?

The purpose of a mission critique should be to identify why and how the search occurred, how it could have been prevented, and to assess the effectiveness and efficiency of one's involvement in the operation. The questions are: what went right, what went wrong, and why?

What can you, as an individual resource involved in the operation, do to improve not only your response and actions, but also those of the entire operation? If you see something that would have made the operation run better, do something about it and mention it to someone who can affect change.

SAR Terms

Area search When a bounded segment of the search area is searched in an organized manner by a specific resource.

Briefing A summary of the situation, past and present, conveyed by those who know to those who need to know and that provides information that will help orient personnel to all facets of the problem.

Debriefing The transfer of information to the search management team from field personnel after an assignment has been completed, with the purpose of conveying as much of the relevant information as possible.

Direct tactics Tactics that include all organized methods used in the search area to detect a lost subject or clues.

First notice The initial notification of responders to a SAR incident.

Indirect tactics Tactics that do not involve physically moving through the search area to detect lost subjects or clues.

Loose grid search A systematic area search, accomplished by searchers lining up on a baseline, usually at relatively wide spacing, with the goal of covering larger geographic areas with fewer resources quickly.

Search lane The area an individual searcher is assigned to scan.

Tactics Techniques employed to actually find a lost subject or clues.

Tight grid search A slow, systematic area search, accomplished by searchers lining up on a baseline, usually at a relatively close spacing.

References

Benkoski, S.J., Monticino, M.G., & Weisinger, J.R. (1991). A survey of the search theory literature. *Naval Research Logistics*, 38:469–494.

Cooper, D.C., & Frost, J.R. (1999). *Selected Inland Search Definitions*. Private publication, June 1999; Cuyahoga Falls, OH.

Cooper, D.C., Frost, J.R. & Robe, R.Q. (2004). *Compatibility of Land SAR Procedures with Search Theory*. Washington, D.C.: U.S. Department of Homeland Security, United States Coast Guard, Operations (G-OPR).

Frost, J.R. (1999). Principles of search theory, part I: detection. *Response*, 17(2):1–7.

Frost, J.R. (1999). Principles of search theory, part II: effort, coverage, and POD. *Response*, 17(2):8–15.

Frost, J.R. (1999). Principles of search theory, part III: probability density distributions. *Response*, 17(3):1–10.

Frost, J.R. (1999). Principles of search theory, part IV: optimal effort allocation. *Response*, 17(3):11–23.

Hill, K. (1997). *Managing Lost Person Incidents*. Chantilly, VA: National Association for Search and Rescue.

IMO/ICAO. (1999). *International Aeronautical and Maritime Search and Rescue Manual: Vols. I, II, & III*. London/Montreal: the International Maritime Organization (IMO) and the International Civil Aviation Organization (ICAO).

Koopman, B.O. (1946). *Search and Screening*. OEG Report No. 56, The Summary Reports Group of the Columbia University Division of War Research. Alexandria, VA: Center for Naval Analyses.

Koopman, B.O. (1980). *Search and Screening: General Principles with Historical Applications*, revised ed. New York, NY: Pergamon Press.

National Search and Rescue Committee. (2000). *United States National Search and Rescue Supplement to the International Aeronautical and Maritime Search and Rescue Manual*. Washington, D.C.: U.S. Superintendent of Documents.

Robe, R.Q., & Frost, J.R. (2002). *A Method for Determining Effective Sweep Widths for Land Searches: Procedures for Conducting Detection Experiments*. USCG Contract Number DTCG39-00-D-R00009. Washington, D.C.: The National Search and Rescue Committee.

Soza and Company, Ltd., & U.S. Coast Guard. (1998). *The Theory of Search: A Simplified Explanation*, revised ed. Fairfax, VA: U.S. Coast Guard.

Washburn, A.R. (2002). *Search and Detection*, 4th ed. Linthicum, MD: Institute for Operations Research and the Management Sciences.

Washington Explorer Search and Rescue. (1999). *Washington Explorer Search and Rescue Team Member Training Manual*, 4th ed. Tacoma, WA: Washington Explorer Search and Rescue.

Chapter 16

Rescue

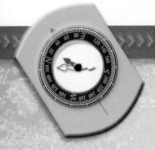

>>>>> Objectives

Upon completion of this chapter and any course activities, the student will be able to meet the following objectives:

List at least two types of materials and designs used in rope manufacture (p. 260-262)

Define and describe the following:
Dynamic rope. (p. 262)
Static rope. (p. 262)
Webbing. (p. 262)

List at least five rules of rope etiquette. (p. 264)

List three harness classifications. (p. 264-265)

Describe how to correctly tie these knots:
Figure 8 on a bight. (p. 266)
Figure 8 bend (follow through) around an object, joining two ropes together. (p. 267)
Water knot (overhand bend). (p. 268)

List the different advantages and disadvantages of materials used in carabiners. (p. 270)

List the functions of at least two different types of carabiners and describe procedures used in caring for them. (p. 270)

Describe the advantages and disadvantages of at least two types of stretchers or litters. (p. 270-274)

Describe how to tie an improvised harness. (p. 265)

Describe the procedures for packaging a patient and transporting him or her via litter. (p. 272)

Rescue Rope

In North America, the use of rope and rescue equipment by emergency services personnel has evolved to a very high level. The intent of this chapter is to convey the most basic rescue information SAR personnel will likely encounter on a mission. This introduction is not meant to serve as a complete or comprehensive training program in rescue of any type.

Even if proper equipment and techniques are used, the danger and harm that can occur to SAR personnel and patients cannot be overemphasized. Any activity that requires the use of a rope or rope rescue equipment to support a life is inherently dangerous. Proper and extensive training and experience should be gained from qualified sources if these skills are to be used in the field.

Rope is an important piece of SAR equipment. It may be used to secure SAR personnel in dangerous terrain, to assist transport of a victim, to access remote search areas and much more. The type of rope to use in any specific rescue situation is critical. So, a good place to start is a

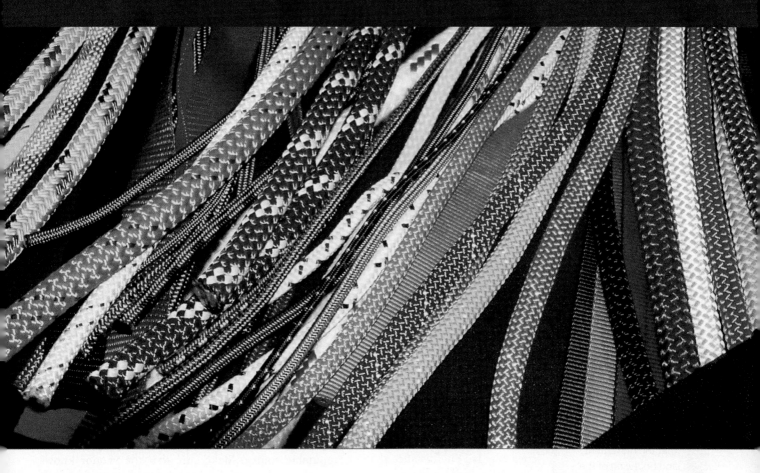

discussion of the way rescue rope is constructed and the material from which it is made.

Rope Construction

Since the discovery of nylon in 1938, synthetic fibers have proved indispensable in the construction of "life support" rescue rope. The most common materials now used to manufacture ropes used for climbing and rescue are polyester and nylon. These materials do not rot, are easily inspected for wear, and have a high strength-to-weight ratio. While they are not common in rescue work, natural fibers such as sisal, hemp, and manila are still used to make rope. However, natural fibers are recommended for utility purposes only, while synthetic fibers are exclusively and universally accepted as superior for supporting a human life (lifeline).

The type of construction or design of rope is critical to emergency service use, and today there are three main types of rope construction in use: laid, braided, and kernmantle. Of these, kernmantle is the most common in rescue rope.

Laid Rope

Laid rope is simply many small strands of twisted fibers that are combined with other strands to form the diameter of the rope. At one time, laid rope was the most common rope used for climbing, caving, and other similar activities. Unfortunately, it had the characteristic of "untwisting" when loaded with weight, spinning the rescuer during a rappel, and exposing all fibers throughout its length to dangerous abrasion. Thus, laid rope is not a good choice for a "lifeline".

Braided Rope

Braided ropes are woven by overlapping multiple strands much like one would braid hair. Much like laid rope, these ropes also allow the fibers of the rope to be exposed to abrasion and they stretch a great deal when loaded. One attempt to combat the abrasion and elongation problem led to so-called "braid-on-braid" construction, where a braided rope was woven over a smaller braided core. In practical application this did not solve either problem, as a failed outer braid severely diminished the strength of the overall rope. Braided ropes are not recommended for emergency use or as a lifeline. Braided ropes are commonly used for utility purposes and may be found in most hardware stores.

Kernmantle Rope

Kernmantle ropes are constructed using two parts, an outer sheath, and an inner core of strands (**Figure 16–1**). The outer sheath of kernmantle is a tightly woven tube that serves to support a load and also protect the inner core. The inner core consists of strands of fibers that are bundled together to provide the majority of the strength of the rope. These ropes are strong, fairly easy to tie knots in, and very abrasion resistant; failure of the sheath does not greatly affect the strength of the rope. This is the type of rope construction recommended for a lifeline in rescue work.

Kernmantle ropes come in two basic types, low-stretch (static) and high-stretch (dynamic), both of which may be used by rescuers and emergency personnel. In a low-stretch rope, the inner core is made of strands that are relatively straight and parallel to each other. When it is important that the movement and bouncing of the load be limited, static, low-stretch rope should be used. Static ropes are used for rappels, lowers, traverses, or crossings, and other situations where there will be little or no climbing required. Low-stretch rope is not used in situations where a rescuer may fall any distance that may shock-load a system.

SARTips

OPERATIONS
When it is important that the movement and bouncing of the load be limited, static, low-stretch rope should be used.

High-stretch rope consists of inner strands that are twisted or braided, thereby allowing them to elongate or stretch under load. This is an important consideration for any climbing activity, as the stretch of the rope will act as a "shock absorber" during a fall. This property benefits not only the climber, but also the rope itself. High-stretch ropes tend to be more pliable and easier to tie knots in. High-stretch ropes, however, are generally not as strong or as abrasion-resistant as their low-stretch brethren.

In the final analysis, most rope used on a search and rescue mission should be of low-stretch, kernmantle construction, and SAR personnel should not be ex-pected to perform rescues in a technical environment without extensive rope rescue training.

Webbing

Another type of rescue equipment often used with ropes is webbing. Webbing is light, easier to pack, and it can be used in a variety of situations. Webbing can be used to improvise a harness for a person to use when being attached to a rope, as an anchor component to attach the rope to an object, or to secure an injured victim to a litter. There are two main types of webbing construction: flat and tubular. Flat webbing is a single piece of material woven into a strip; it is inexpensive to manufacture, but tends to be stiff. The type of webbing commonly accepted as rescue webbing is tubular in cross-section (**Figure 16–2**). Tubular webbing is constructed in two very different ways: spiral (shuttle loom), and chain structure. The spiral construction method is the better choice for rescue work. The chain structure method is weaker and susceptible to abrasion that could cause it to unravel like a woven sweater. It is important to purchase tubular webbing intended for rescue from an appropriate and reputable source. Make sure that the vendor knows the intended use of the webbing and has worked with rescue organizations before.

Static Safety Factor

SAR personnel should be familiar with equipment standards that apply to rope used for rescue. One common standard for this purpose was developed by the National Fire Protection Association (NFPA) and is titled "NFPA 1983, Standard on Fire Service Life Safety Rope and System Components."

The latest version of NFPA 1983 requires a safety factor of 15:1 for all rope and components. This means

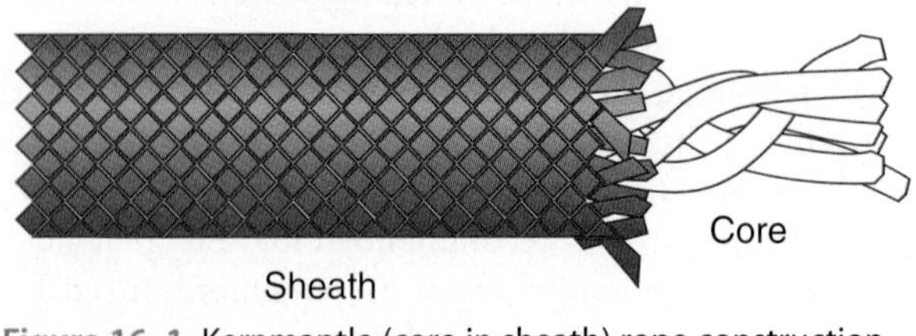

Kernmantle

Core

Sheath

Figure 16–1 Kernmantle (core in sheath) rope construction.

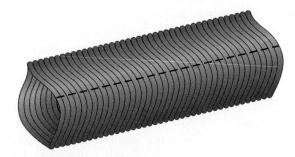

Figure 16–2 Tubular webbing.

that rope and rope rescue equipment should be able to withstand a load 15 times greater than a one- or two-person load (depending on the application). The standard defines a one-person load as 300 pounds, so a safety factor of 15:1 requires a 4500-pound breaking strength rating for rope. <u>Breaking strength</u> is defined as the point at which a rope fails under a load. A two-person load requires a safety factor or rating of 9000 pounds. Many rescue organizations have accepted this 15:1 safety factor.

In contrast, some wilderness SAR agencies rely on a safety factor of 10:1. This is done for several reasons, the most important of which is weight. Unlike in an urban/suburban setting where equipment weight is less important, in the wilderness, rescue equipment must be carried to where it is needed, sometimes involving great distances and rough terrain. Simply put, the 10:1 safety factor allows for lighter equipment; a definite benefit in the backcountry. Wilderness rescue groups also tend to be highly trained in the care and use of rope and related equipment, and are very much aware of its limitations.

Why is such a large safety factor required? These safety factors are <u>static safety factors</u> and are derived from the minimum breaking strength (MBS) calculations as supplied by the equipment's manufacturers (**Table 16–1**). Dynamic events—those that are the result of a shock load—put additional stress on rescue equipment. A 10:1 static safety factor gives a dynamic safety factor of 1.5 to 2:1, which is acceptable for most situations.

Another consideration in rope and webbing strength is the presence of knots. An accepted rule of thumb is that a knot in a rope will reduce its strength by 30%, and that certain knots (e.g., ring bend in webbing) may reduce its strength by as much as 50%. This reduction is not cumulative, so a single knot will have the same effect as two or three knots.

A kiloNewton (kN) is equivalent to 225 pounds (102 kilograms) and is a good estimate for the weight of one rescuer or patient. If you need to raise a two-person load and maintain a 10:1 safety factor, the rope should support 20 kN. If you have a three-person load, then use a 30 kN rope. Remember, you must consider the entire system. Do not use a single 20 kN carabiner in a system that is designed to support a 30 kN load.

SAR personnel should use rope systems that meet the requirements of their individual organization's guidelines and policies.

Software Care

Rope, webbing, harnesses, and other "soft" rescue equipment are collectively referred to as "software." This easily damaged gear must be used, monitored, and maintained carefully; thus, there are several special rules that apply to the use and care of this equipment.

Keep a Log
A detailed record must be kept of each piece of rescue equipment. This should include as a minimum its ID marking, size, type, manufacturer, date purchased, date in service, where purchased, and lot number. This information should be kept on file along with a detailed history of when and how the equipment was used over time. The use of any personal (non-team) equipment during a rescue should also be documented in this way.

Care
The first and cardinal rule of caring for software is never to step on or drag it. Doing so grinds tiny, sharp particles of sand into and between the fibers of the material. In kernmantle rope, these particles can work themselves through the sheath and into the core fibers, invisibly cutting and weakening the rope. The bottom line is to never step on or drag any rescue equipment, but especially rope and rescue software.

Storage
Software should be stored out of direct sunlight. Lengthy exposure to ultraviolet radiation is known to compromise the integrity of nylon fibers and will degrade its strength. Typical or even extended operational use should not cause a problem.

Table 16–1	Minimum and knotted breaking strengths for various sized ropes and webbing	
Rope Size	Typical Breaking Strength	Knotted Breaking Strength
8.0 mm (5/16 in)	15 kN (3500 lb)	10 kN
9.0 mm (3/8 in)	20 kN (4500 lb)	14 kN
11.1 mm (7/16 in)	30 kN (7000 lb)	20 kN
12.7 mm (1/2 in)	40 kN (9000 lb)	28 kN
25 mm (1 in) webbing	20 kN (4500 lb)	10 kN

A kiloNewton (kN) is equivalent to 225 pounds (102 kilograms).

Never expose rescue software to chemicals or petroleum by-products such as engine exhaust fumes and liquid petroleum vapors. Avoid exposure to batteries of any type as the associated acid and its vapors will attack and weaken most synthetic materials. Be especially cautious of this when storing software in a SAR ready pack. It is typically believed that a loss of approximately 2% of the breaking strength of software will occur when nylon is exposed to petroleum products, and immersing it in sulfuric acid causes a 30% reduction in breaking strength. Mildew and fungi also attack synthetic fibers, so rescue software should also be stored in a dry environment.

Keep rescue software away from high heat of any kind because it has the potential to melt and destroy synthetic materials. Also, avoid high friction and abrasion of the equipment. Do not allow nylon to run across nylon. That is, if a rope is in motion such as in a haul system it should not be allowed to contact a stationary length of rope or webbing. The heat generated from the friction can melt the webbing or rope and cause it to fail.

In general, keep rescue software as clean as possible. Storing all software in a rope or gear bag can do wonders for protecting it from outside dirt and chemicals.

Regular Inspections

All rescue software must be inspected before each use, or better yet, inspected before and after each use so it is ready for the next mission. Run the material through your hands slowly and carefully, feeling and checking for the following signs of wear:

- Discoloration – Indicates any one of many problems, including chemical damage, heat damage, or other abuses. A gray color on the exterior is not necessarily a problem as it may be caused by an aluminum descending device.
- Shiny areas – Indicates heat damage from friction.
- Fuzzy or torn exterior – Fibers may be worn or torn; on kernmantle this may also indicate damage to interior strands of the rope.
- Smaller or larger diameter areas – Indicates that the inner strands are damaged in some way, either cut or torn, or stressed and kinked upon themselves.
- Soft spots in rope – Places where rope is more flexible and soft also indicate interior damage.

Any significant wear and/or damage found in rescue software must be evaluated before use. Damage of the type indicated above should prompt the removal of the rope from lifeline status.

If rescue software becomes dirty, it can be cleaned. For rope, there are a number of specially made washing devices that can be attached to a hose. In a popular version of this device, the rope is pulled through a tube in

which jets of water, and in some cases brush bristles, scrub the rope as it passes. A washing machine may also be used to wash rope and rescue software. However, make sure to use a front-loading machine because the action of the agitator in top-loading machines can harm both the machine and the rope. When using a front-loading washing machine, it's best to place the rope in a mesh bag and use little or no detergent. The residual soap in a commercial machine is probably enough to clean it. If you must use soap, use the mildest type available; one safe for synthetic garments. Use cold water only when washing rescue software. Once washed, air-dry it in a clean dark place. NEVER dry a rope using heat or fire.

Ten Rules of Rope Etiquette

In summary, care of rope and rescue software is important. Thus, these ten rules should always be followed:

1. Never step on or drag a rope or rescue software.
2. Use software in a responsible manner, and keep a log of its storage and use.
3. Protect software from abrasion.
4. Do not leave rope under tension for any length of time and remove knots as soon as possible.
5. Store all software properly.
6. Soiled software should be gently and properly cleaned.
7. Avoid exposing software to sunlight (UV) and high temperatures.
8. Avoid nylon running across nylon (synthetic running across synthetic).
9. Avoid storing rope kinked; avoid kinking while coiling rope.
10. Check all software for damage often, at least before and after use.

Harnesses

In the field it may become necessary for SAR personnel to use rope to assist the search effort by allowing them to safely move through some type of hazardous terrain. This could be a steep slope, an icy area, slick rocky areas, or the area around a sinkhole or mine shaft. If technical rope rescue skills are required, training will be necessary that is beyond the scope of this book. During a SAR mission, personnel may need to be secured to a rope with a harness. Therefore, SAR personnel should be familiar with harnesses that may be used in rescue. Many types of commercial rescue harnesses are available. They are typically heavier than harnesses designed for rock climbing or caving. NFPA categorizes life safety harnesses into three classifications. A Class 1 harness is a common seat-harness that is designed for one-person loads. A Class 2 harness is designed for a two-person load, and a Class 3 harness is a full-body harness that not only fastens around the hips and waist, but also over the shoulders and around the chest. While a Class 3 harness may be the most secure, it is also the heaviest. Thus, it may not be the best choice for wilderness SAR.

In addition to a seat harness, a separate chest harness may be desired. However, when a chest harness is worn, a seat harness must be worn with it. One advantage of using a chest harness is to help the rescuer remain in an upright position. But, attaching a chest harness improperly may be worse than not having one at all.

"Ladder belts" or Pompier belts (simple belts designed to secure one to a ladder) are not appropriate for life-safety applications, and should not be used in lieu of an appropriate rescue harness.

For rescuers who (1) do not plan to be "on rope," (2) do not plan on spending long periods of time hanging from a rope, or (3) want to save weight, a commercial rescue harness may not be needed. In these cases, an improvised harness using one inch (1″) tubular webbing may work just fine. An improvised harness must fulfill two primary needs: it must keep the occupant securely attached to the rope, and the harness must stay securely attached to the rescuer even when inverted or in other unusual positions. Both are easily accomplished with a "Swiss Seat," which is a field-expedient, improvised harness (Figure 16–3).

Knots, Ties, Hitches, and Bends

A variety of knots may be required in rescue, but only a few are needed in most rescue situations. The key is to learn a few useful knots, and practice them often. The term "knot" refers to a broad class of rope attachments, but there are also other terms that can apply. For example, a **bend** is a knot used to join two pieces, or ends, of a rope. A **hitch** is used to attach a rope to a fixed object or fixed rope.

Knowing the parts of a length of rope may also be useful. A "bight" is a bend placed in a rope. The "standing end" of a knot is that portion of the rope that does not move in the knot creation. The "running end" of a knot is the end that is being moved about in the tying of a knot. The "tail" of a knot is the unused rope that is left over after the knot has been tied (Figure 16–4). A lengthy tail can be tied into a safety or backup knot, which is a secondary knot that prevents another knot from coming untied.

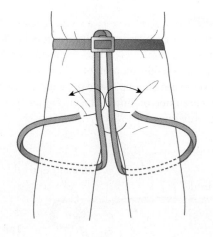

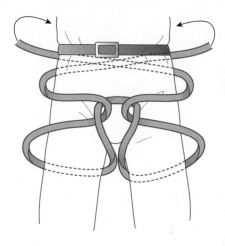

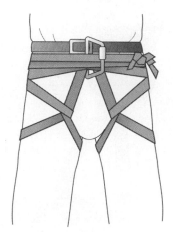

Figure 16–3 Tying a Swiss Seat.

Figure Eight

Possibly the most versatile family of knots is the figure eight family. The figure eight can be used as a bend or hitch. The figure eight on a bight (Figure 16–5) is a useful knot for creating a loop that can be used to attach the rope to a carabiner or other object. Figure 16–6 shows how to tie this knot.

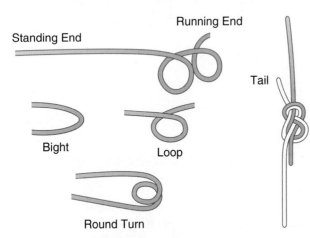

Figure 16–4 Parts of a rope and knot.

The figure eight follow-through (Figure 16–7) is similar to the figure eight on a bight, but it is used when a loop cannot be placed over an object. That is, it is used when the running end of the rope must be fed around an object like a pole or a tree. The figure eight follow-through is a common knot used by climbers to attach their harness to the belay rope.

It is important to keep rope usage to a minimum when tying knots. For example, there is no need to tie a one-foot diameter loop when you are only attaching it to a carabiner. Also, there is no reason to leave an excessive tail on a knot, as it could foul the rigging and it is a waste of rope.

The figure eight knots are generally used for tying rope and the square and water knots are generally used in webbing, although a square knot can certainly be used in rope. The versatile figure eight family of knots is a good

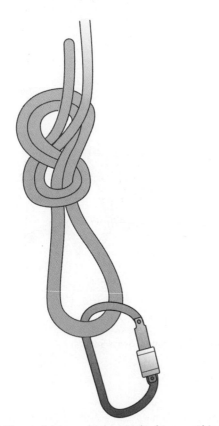

Figure 16–5 Figure eight on a bight attached to a carabiner.

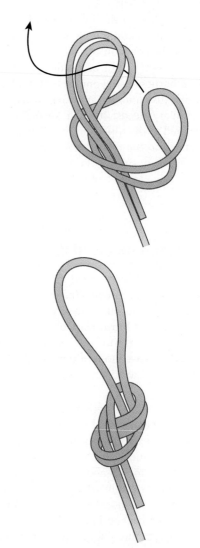

Figure 16–6 Tying a figure eight on a bight.

choice in many situations because they are easy to tie, easy to untie, easy to teach to others, easy to remember, and they hold fast—all characteristics of any good knot.

Square Knot or Reef Knot

The square knot is useful for joining two ends of webbing together in the creation of a field-expedient seat harness (Figure 16–8). However, this knot, also known as the "death knot," is not appropriate for use in bending rope ends together, because it is easily tied incorrectly and can untie itself when jostled. For tying a bend in a rope, use a figure eight bend (Figure 16–9).

Figure Eight Bend

When joining two ropes, use a figure eight bend (see Figure 16–9). Other commonly encountered bends are the ring bend (fisherman's bend, double fisherman's) and sheet bend. The ring bend is a compact and useful knot, but it is very difficult to untie after a rope has been loaded—more difficult than the figure eight bend. Again, the figure eight family will work well when bending two ropes.

The sheet bend is a good knot for attaching two ropes of different diameters. It has the additional advantages of not requiring much rope and being easy to untie after loading. A better variant is the double sheet bend, as this can be used for ropes that have the same diameter. One serious disadvantage, however, is that the tails of this rope will point perpendicularly to the line when the rope is loaded, which can cause the knot to more readily hang up in brush and rocks. Also, if this knot is worked back and forth it can be loosened. Because of these characteristics, the sheet bend and double sheet bend are not recommended for rescue applications.

Knots in Webbing

While many of the knots that work well in rope also work well in webbing, webbing is a bit slicker and may require specialized knots and bends. Webbing is generally used in the construction of anchors and field-expedient seat harnesses. As such, bends are more common in webbing than knots. To bend two ends of webbing into a loop or to join two pieces of webbing, use the overhand

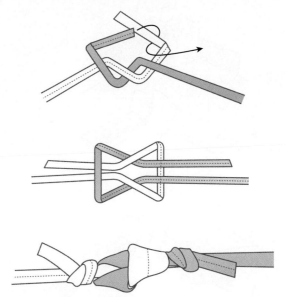

Figure 16–8 Tying a square knot in webbing. Note the safety knots in the tails.

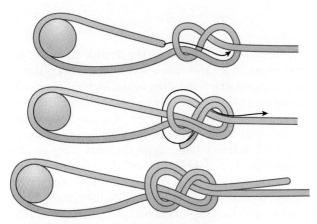

Figure 16–7 Figure eight follow-through.

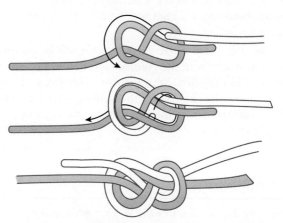

Figure 16–9 Tying a figure eight bend. This type of knot is used to attach the ends of two ropes.

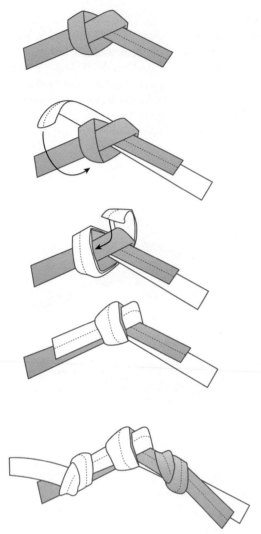

Figure 16–10 Tying an overhand bend, also known as a water knot.

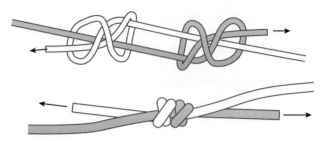

Figure 16–11 Tying a double fisherman's bend; used to join two ends of Prusik cord.

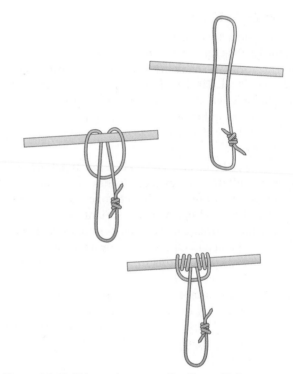

Figure 16–12 Tying a three-wrap Prusik to a lifeline.

bend, also known as the water knot (Figure 16–10). Be aware, however, this knot may be difficult to untie after being loaded.

The only place where a square knot will be encountered in rescue is in the construction of a Swiss Seat or other field-expedient seat harness. This knot can be used to join the two ends of the webbing in the last step of the construction of the seat harness (see Figures 16–3 and 16–8).

Prusik Slings

Another useful item to have in your SAR ready pack is a Prusik sling. This exotic sounding item is actually nothing more than a piece of accessory cord tied into a loop with a secure knot. The Prusik sling can be used to attach a harness to a lifeline. First use a three-loop wrap to attach the sling to the lifeline. Then, use a carabiner to attach the sling to the harness. The rope for the sling should be a piece of static kernmantle cord around 4 to 5 millimeters in diameter and about 6 feet (2 meters) long. Typically, this loop is tied together with a double fisherman's bend or "barrel knot." However, a figure eight bend is also acceptable. Figure 16–11 shows how the double fisherman's bend is tied, and Figure 16–12 shows how to tie a Prusik to a lifeline. When it is not loaded, the Prusik will move easily along the lifeline (Figure 16–13). When loaded,

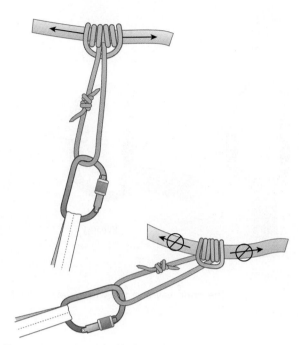

Figure 16–13 An unloaded Prusik attached to a lifeline (top), and the Prusik loaded (bottom).

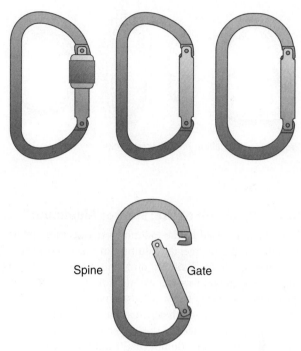

Spine   Gate

Figure 16–14 Types of carabiners and their parts. From top left to right: a "D" locking carabiner, a "D" non-locking carabiner, and an oval non-locking carabiner.

the Prusik grabs the lifeline and holds fast. It is important to receive proper instruction in the use of these slings before they are used.

Carabiners

In order to conveniently connect webbing and rope to harnesses, litters, and anchors, a carabiner, which is a metal link with a spring-loaded gate, is often used. **Figure 16–14** illustrates the parts of a carabiner, which come in many types, materials, and configurations.

Types of Carabiners

Carabiners come in both locking and non-locking varieties. A non-locking carabiner has a spring-loaded gate that closes over a pin, but there is nothing to keep the gate securely closed. Although they are not necessarily stronger, a locking carabiner has some means of preventing the gate from opening unintentionally, especially while under load. This is usually achieved by way of a screw-sliding barrel-type mechanism that slides over the gate latch. Locking carabiners are generally preferred for rescue operations.

Carabiners also come in a variety of shapes including oval, "D," and HMS (pear-shaped). The most common

carabiner shape used in rescue is the "D." This shape focuses the load along the spine, the strongest part of the carabiner. Oval carabiners are generally not as strong by design in that they distribute the load over the gate as well as the spine, but they are a bit more forgiving with respect to load angles as compared to a D-shaped carabiner.

Pear-shaped or HMS carabiners have a larger well, so that they are able to accommodate multiple ropes or other devices, and fit more easily through a seat harness. Pear-shaped carabiners are generally not as strong as D-shaped due to their geometry.

Mallion Rapide Screw Links

Another type of connecting device similar to a carabiner is the Mallion Rapide screw link (**Figure 16–15**). These devices are strong and generally made of steel. It is important to purchase the type that has been load tested with the strength stamped on the link. It is also important that these devices are only used with the gate closed. Unlike many carabiners, these devices must have a closed gate to achieve their rated breaking strength. Screw links are most useful for connections that don't require regular opening and closing. Aside from the common oval shape, screw links also come in triangular (delta or tri-link), square, and half-round configurations. These are useful when a multidirectional load is expected.

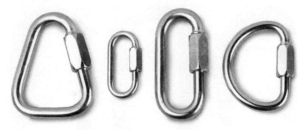

Figure 16–15 Mallion Rapide screw links.

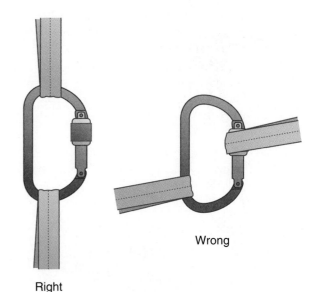

Right

Wrong

Figure 16–16 The right way and the wrong way to load a carabiner.

Which Carabiner to Use: Steel or Aluminum?

The materials used in the manufacture of carabiners are usually limited to steel and aluminum. Each has properties that are both desirable and undesirable. Steel has more strength and to some extent more durability; however, steel is heavy, tends to rust, and costs more than aluminum. Where very heavy loads are likely and weight is not a concern, steel is the better choice. Aluminum carabiners are lighter, do not rust (but they oxidize), and are generally cheaper than steel. The disadvantages of aluminum include that they may be more easily damaged by dropping or shock loading, the locking device is often easier to damage, and some sizes and designs are not as strong as steel.

Loading a Carabiner

Carabiners and screw links must always be loaded axially, and never across the gate (Figure 16–16). A carabiner's breaking strength is much lower when it is crossloaded. If loading at multiple angles is required, then a tri-link or half-round screw link is a better choice.

Carabiner Care

If they are to be used in rescue, carabiners must be properly stored and maintained. Each carabiner needs to be visually inspected before it is used. The gate needs to be tested to see if it will lock and examined for excessive wear or damage. The latching device and body also should be inspected for physical damage such as deep grooves and corrosion. Carabiners should be stored in a place where they will not be exposed to corrosion and/or damage.

Carabiners can be cleaned with soap and water if desired. It is not advisable to lubricate carabiners with any oil or similar lubricant, as this will collect dust and dirt. If slight lubrication is required, a small amount of dry graphite lubricant can be used.

Consider removing a carabiner from service if it has been shock loaded (application of a sudden, heavy load) or has fallen from height onto a hard surface (e.g., rock or concrete). Shock loading and falls onto hard surfaces

can cause small cracks to develop that can lead to weakness and premature failure. You should also remove a carabiner from service when the gate no longer closes on its own (e.g., stays in the open position).

Often the gate on a locking carabiner will become stuck in the closed position. This can happen when a carabiner with a locked gate is loaded. The stuck gate can often be loosened by re-loading the carabiner and slightly unscrewing the gate. If this does not work, you may choose to use pliers, but be sure to be careful and inspect the carabiner for damage after opening. Remember, finger-tight is just right. Locking the gate on a carabiner does nothing for its strength. The lock prevents the gate only from opening unintentionally.

For the purposes of searcher safety in a non-technical environment, an aluminum locking carabiner is adequate. It is recommended that SAR personnel should carry two of these in their SAR ready pack. At least one should reside on the outside of the pack as some helicopter crews may use this link to attach your pack to the floor of the helicopter.

Litters

Litters (also known as "stretchers") are devices used to transport an injured subject to a safe location. A litter may be hand carried or transported by any number of vehicles or aircraft. But, the specific type chosen must be dependent on the way in which it will be used. For example, any litter that will be used with a helicopter must be approved for use by the aircraft's crew. Many good litters will not be acceptable for use on aircraft.

There are a great number of litters available for use in SAR. The common types of litters that SAR personnel need to be familiar with include: improvised, basket, and flexible, wrap-around litters.

Improvised Litters

In most SAR work, a litter is available when it is needed. Should such a device not be accessible and moving a patient becomes necessary, a litter can be improvised from various materials.

Although their use in organized SAR should be rare, the simplest improvised litter can be made from a heavy plastic tarpaulin, tent material, or large polyethylene bag. By wrapping the material around a rock, wadded sock, or glove and securing it with rope or twine, the rescuer can fashion handles in the corners and sides to facilitate carrying. A coil of rope can also be fashioned into a litter—called a rope litter or clove hitch stretcher—but a 150- to 200-foot (46- to 61-meter) climbing or rescue rope is required. A sturdy blanket or tarp can be used in combination with ski poles or stout tree branches to construct a litter, or a similar device can be improvised by passing the poles through the sleeves of two heavy, zipped (closed) parkas. If long distances must be traveled or if pack animals are available, a litter may also be constructed so that it can be dragged or slid along the ground like a sled. None of these methods should be first choices when a patient needs to be moved, but any of them may be necessary when the right equipment is just not available.

Basket-Style Litters

The basket-style stretcher derives its name from its shape. The sides curve upward to protect the victim's sides and to prevent the victim from rolling out. Most basket-style litters combine a steel frame (solid, tubular, or both) with a shell of either steel wire netting ("chicken wire") or plastic. Although the traditional materials and design (i.e., tubular and flat, welded steel with a steel chicken wire covering) are still in use today (Figure 16–17), basket-style litters are more often constructed from tubular stainless steel or aluminum because of the added corrosion resistance, increased strength, and reduced weight. Because the wire mesh of the traditional Stokes litter is often uncomfortable for the patient, nylon "suspension" inserts are available as a replacement for the wire. A closed-cell foam sleeping pad can also be added to the bottom of the litter for added comfort and insulation.

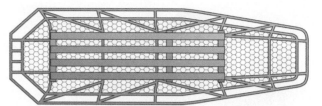

Figure 16–17 Conventional Stokes basket-style litter.

Taking advantage of substantial improvements in polymer research, some manufacturers began producing a stretcher shell composed of rigid plastic instead of steel mesh. This has the added advantage of sliding over ice, snow, scree, and mud more easily because of the smooth bottom. Ultraviolet (UV) light has been known to adversely affect the plastic. Older models in particular have been reported to become brittle upon extended exposure to UV light. Manufacturers of newer models claim this is no longer a significant problem, but it is still a good idea to protect all rescue equipment from sunlight and other elements. As an added safety measure, when rigging this type of litter it is important to tie into the metal rail and not just the plastic shell.

Some of these litters are manufactured in a break-apart design that facilitates backpacking it into a remote site. But, the overall strength of the device often suffers a bit with this design. All older-style break-apart litters that depend on pins should be backed up with 8mm rope or webbing, and they should be used with extreme caution in advanced technical rescue operations such as highlines (a technique where rope strung across a wide space fully supports the weight of a litter and patient). The structural weak point of many older basket-style litters, particularly with aluminum varieties, is the top rail. So, the U.S. Coast Guard recommends wrapping a piece of 1-inch tubular webbing around that rail for added security. Many companies have no data on the strength of this rail, and all rescue techniques that include attachments to this rail should have a backup method of attaching to, and supporting, the device and its occupant.

Flexible, Wrap-Around Litters

Although there are others available, the Skedco SKED® litter is the classic example of a flexible, wrap-around litter. It is essentially a drag sheet made from heavy duty,

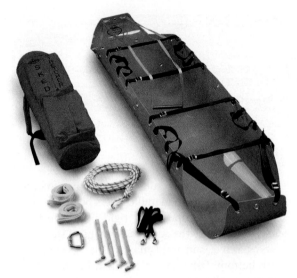

Figure 16–18 SKED® basic rescue system. Courtesy of CMC Rescue, Inc.

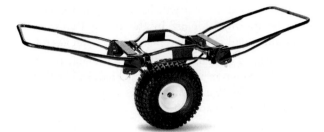

Figure 16–19 CMC Rescue Mule II Litter wheel with handles. Courtesy of CMC Rescue, Inc.

polyethylene plastic (Figure 16–18). It is designed to be used with a backboard (short or long) that helps immobilize the head and neck while keeping the SKED from collapsing around the patient.

Wrap-around litters like the SKED have proven to be excellent choices for use in caves and other confined space situations. In fact, the SKED was primarily designed as a confined space rescue litter. The litter ends fold over the head and feet to provide a secure, protective cocoon for the patient. There is a smaller version for children known as the Pediatric or "PED" SKED, and an "HMD" version designed for use in situations involving hazardous materials where decontamination may be necessary.

All attachments to the litter are made through built-in 3/4-inch brass grommets. The design incorporates systems for both horizontal and vertical evacuations. One of the best features of the SKED is that it rolls up into a Cordura backpack carrier, which makes the entire system extremely portable.

The SKED has some relative drawbacks. Since it is so flexible, it tends to bend at both ends. Thus, a backboard must be used to prevent the sides and ends from squeezing the patient. An extended carry may also be difficult with the SKED due to its flexibility. While basket or wire-frame litters have a handy rail to grasp, the litter carrier on a SKED must grasp a loop of webbing.

Patient Packaging

There are a variety of ways to "package" a patient in a litter. The manner in which the patient is packaged depends on his or her medical condition, the environment, and the manner in which he/she is to be evacuated.

Medical Condition
If the patient requires monitoring, will you be able to take the required readings with the method of packaging applied? Is the patient's airway clear? Will any injuries be exacerbated by the packaging?

Environment
Will the patient be warm enough? Remember, your patient is immobilized and can get very chilled even in relatively warm climates. Is there a chance of getting wet? If so, consider a vapor barrier and adequate shielding. Getting wet will not be comfortable. Remember to provide shade if the weather is hot and sunny. Don't leave a patient out in the open sun for very long, especially if it is hot. Find some shade, or at least provide some sunglasses for the carry-out where shade is not available.

Evacuation
Is the patient to be evacuated vertically? If so, then make sure that you provide some sort of foot-loops or stirrups so that they can bear some of their weight with their legs rather than hanging from a harness or other tie-in. Be sure to pad behind the knees (injuries permitting) and pack excess gear carefully around the patient. The less "slop" there is in the packaging, the more comfortable the ride. While there is some debate as to this practice, it may be a good idea to put a helmet on your patient. Some argue that a helmet is of minimal help when lying horizontal in a litter, and may cause airway issues. Consult your team policies and procedures for guidance.

Litter Accessories

There are a variety of accessories that can greatly help in litter evacuation. For long, relatively flat, or trail evacuations, a litter wheel may be helpful (Figure 16–19). The litter wheel bears the load of the litter, while the litter handlers provide balance. This does come with a price, however. The litter wheel must be carried to the patient.

Litter shields are more effective than helmets for protecting the heads of patients (Figure 16–20). A litter shield attaches to the head of the litter and covers the

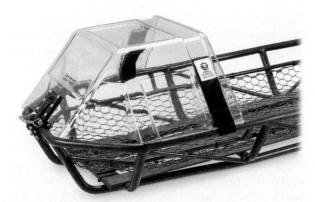

Figure 16–20 CMC Rescue Litter Shield. (Photo courtesy CMC Rescue, Inc.)

head and neck of the patient. Because nothing is on the patient's head, there is no problem with the airway and it protects the head, face, and neck of the patient, rather than just the top of the head as with a helmet. Also, the shield can be covered with a pad or duct tape to provide a sun, wind, or rain screen.

Also available are specialized sleeping bags that are designed with a litter-packaged patient in mind. These devices open like a clam shell, and have reinforced bottoms and loops on the sides to facilitate carrying. In addition, there are a variety of access openings that facilitate medical monitoring.

Litter Handling

Litters are used to facilitate moving patients to a place of safety and they can be used in a variety of situations. They can be lifted by rope, carried by vehicles, or, most commonly, hand-carried by rescuers. While handling your patient, be sure to communicate and keep him or her apprised of the situation and your progress. Include them in your conversation and remember to call them by name. Do not to refer to him or her as the "victim". Do not step over the patient if it can be avoided, and be careful with ends of webbing and other rescue hardware, as this can be very painful if dropped on a patient's face or body. Try not to shine a headlamp or flashlight into the patient's eyes, and be careful when using knives or scissors around the patient and rigging.

Standard Carry

The standard litter carry involves a team of six to eight rescuers distributed around the litter, three or four to a side. Normally, the person at the front of the left side is in charge and directs the activities of the others.

This method has the advantages of being fast, as little teamwork is required and it usually gives the patient a comfortable ride. Its disadvantages include that it is very

tiring for the handlers because it puts a constant strain on selected muscles, and ground vision is difficult, especially at night; a handler can easily trip over a rock and drop the litter.

If a litter handler starts to fall, he should call "Stop!" and let go of the litter. The "Stop" command is to prevent the litter team from running over the falling team member and injuring him or her needlessly.

More than one team will be needed if the distance to carry the litter is more than the team can cover in about 15 to 20 minutes. Team leapfrogging is a good method to use on long evacuations. One team will take the litter for a given distance while the other team goes ahead to rest and pre-plan the next stretch. At the pass off point, the first team will advance to the next point for rest and planning.

This can extend everyone's endurance quite a bit. Try to avoid making the distances too far. Extended rest periods can be harmful if people are allowed to cool off to the point of becoming chilled and then asked to carry a litter using cold muscles.

Caterpillar or Lap Pass

When footing is too unstable or there is an obstacle that prevents the litter team from progressing and falling becomes a possible hazard, the caterpillar (also called lap pass) becomes a useful option.

When the litter reaches the obstacle, the team pauses while every extra person lines up on the route ahead of the difficult terrain or obstacles. They form two lines facing each other about the width of the litter apart and alternate (in other words, they aren't all opposite each other). They usually sit down and try to make themselves as stable as possible. When everyone is set, you pass the litter down between the two lines. As the litter passes a person, he or she gets up and carefully but quickly moves around the line in the direction of travel, and gets set to pass the litter again. Done correctly, this provides a very stable and secure passage.

Turtle Carry

The turtle carry is most useful for negotiating very narrow passages, such as slot canyons or long spaces between two large boulders.

To accomplish the turtle carry, one hardy rescuer with gloves, kneepads, and a sense of humor gets on his hands and the litter is balanced on his back. Two other

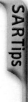

litter handlers are positioned at the head and the foot of the litter, where they mainly balance and guide the litter. They can take some of the weight of the liter, but the majority is carried by the "turtle" underneath. This is very slow and can be painful for the rescuer in the turtle role, but is sometimes the only option available.

Strap Carry

A strap carry is very useful to prolong one's endurance on long carry-outs. Construct a loop from webbing and girth hitch it to the litter rail. Bring the loop up and over your shoulder that is next to the litter, across your back and slip the loop over your other shoulder. If you start to fall, you can twist out of the loop by turning away from the litter.

Tag Lines

Once in awhile, you'll come upon a place where it is too low and narrow to do a standard carry, lap pass, or even a turtle carry. When this happens, you may have no option but to use tag lines (short pieces of rope or webbing) to drag the litter through.

After tying a piece of webbing or accessory rope (tag line) to the head and foot of the litter, crawl through the tight spot dragging the free end of the tag line. When one rescuer gets to the other end, pull the litter through with the tag line. The tag line tied to the other end of the litter is to help control it in case the ground is sloped or slippery. Tag lines may also be useful during low-angle and short, steep-angle maneuvers.

SAR Terms

Bend A knot used to join two pieces, or ends, of a rope.

Braided ropes Rope woven by overlapping multiple strands much like one would braid hair.

Breaking strength The point at which a rope fails under a load.

Hitch A knot used to attach a rope to a fixed object or fixed rope.

Kermantle rope Type of construction with two parts: a tightly woven outer sheath that serves to support a load and protects the inner core, and an inner core consisting of strands of fibers that are bundled together to provide the majority of the rope's strength. Kermantle is German for "core in sheath."

Laid rope Fibers are twisted into yarns which are in turn twisted into strands (usually three) to form a rope.

Static safety factor The ratio of breaking strength to load (e.g., 15:1) that allows an acceptable margin of safety for predicted loading of a rope rescue system.

References

Auerbach, P.S., ed. (2001). *Wilderness Medicine*, 4th ed. St. Louis, MO: Mosby, Inc.

Brown, M.G. (2000). *Engineering Practical Rope Rescue Systems*. Clifton Park, NY: Delmar Learning.

Cox, M., & Fulsass, K., eds. (2003). *Mountaineering: Freedom of the Hills*, 7th ed. New York, NY: Mountaineers Books.

Frank, J.A., ed. (1998). *CMC Rope Rescue Manual*, 3rd ed. Santa Barbara, CA: CMC Rescue.

Hudson, S. & Vines, T. (1999). High Angle Rescue Techniques, 2nd ed. Philadelphia: Mosby.

Roop, M., & Vines, T. (1998). *Confined Space and Structural Rope Rescue*. St. Louis, MO: Mosby.

Washington Explorer Search and Rescue. (1999). *Washington Explorer Search and Rescue Team Member Training Manual*, 4th printing. Tacoma, WA: Washington Explorer Search and Rescue.

APPENDIX 1

Task Force Structure Marking System

Structure Identification Within a Geographic Area

An important duty of a structure triage team is to clearly differentiate buildings in groupings such as by block(s) or jurisdictional areas/sectors. This geographic (area/sector) identification of buildings would be consolidated at the Command Post and used to deploy search and rescue personnel and/or track Structure/ Hazard Evaluation and Search Assessment information.

It is imperative that each structure within a geographic area is clearly defined. This identification will assist both in the specific ongoing search and rescue effort and in the long-term post-disaster identification of the site. This identification is important from a technical documentation perspective regarding the specific events that took place at a given site. Structure identification has a significant impact on overall scene safety and the safety of task force personnel.

It is important to clearly identify each separate structure within a geographic area when information is being disseminated to other operational entities. The primary method of identification should be the existing street name, hundred block, and building number. Obviously, such identification is not always possible due to post-disaster site conditions. In these situations, it is important that the task force personnel implement the following system for structure identification.

This system builds upon the normal pre-disaster street name, hundred block, and building number. As task force personnel establish a need to identify a structure within a given block they will:

1. Identify each structure by existing street name and building number.

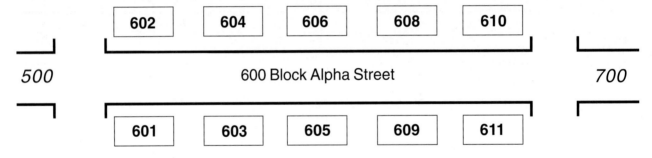

2. If some previously existing numbers have been obliterated, an attempt should be made to reestablish the numbering system based upon one or more structures that still display an existing number.

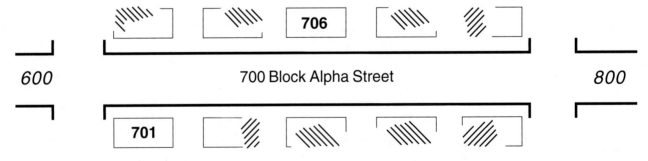

3. The damaged building(s) would be assigned numbers to separately identify them as indicated. The front of the structure(s) in question should be clearly marked using International Orange spray paint with the new number being assigned.

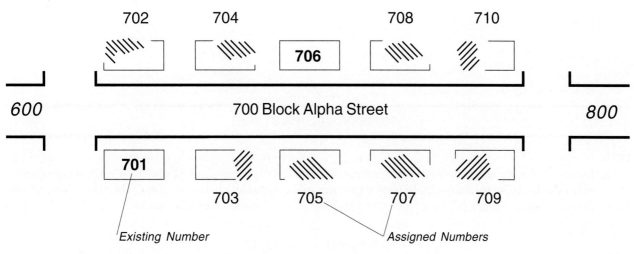

4. If no number is identifiable in a given block then task force personnel will identify the street name and the hundred block for the area in question on other structures in proximity to the site in question.

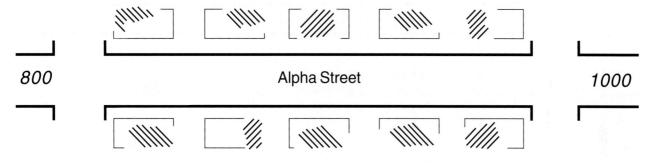

5. In this case, structures will be assigned the appropriate numbers to designate and differentiate them. The front of the structure(s) in question should be clearly marked using International Orange spray paint with the new number being assigned.

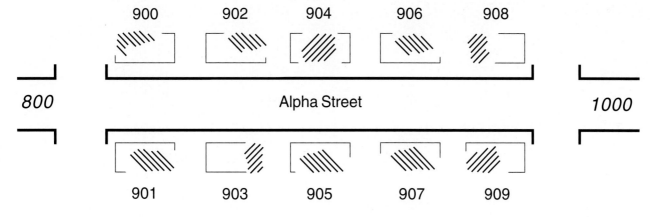

It is also important to identify locations within a single structure.

1. The address side of the structure shall be defined as SIDE 1. Other sides of the structure shall be assigned numerically in a clockwise manner from SIDE 1.

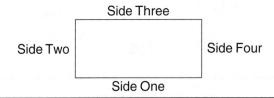

700 BLOCK ALPHA STREET

2. The interior of the structure will be divided into QUADRANTS. The quadrants shall be identified alphabetically in a clockwise manner starting from where the side 1 and side 2 perimeter meet. The center core, where all four quadrants meet will be identified as Quadrant E (i.e., central core lobby, etc.).

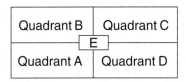

700 BLOCK ALPHA STREET

3. Multistory buildings must have each floor clearly identified. If not clearly discernible, the floors should be numbered as referenced from the exterior. The grade level floor would be designated floor 1 and, moving upward the second floor would be floor 2, etc. Conversely, the first floor below grade level would be B-1, the second B-2, etc.

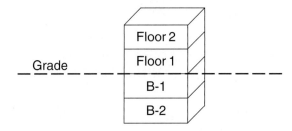

Urban SAR Victim Marking System

During the urban search function it is often necessary to identify the location of potential and known victims because debris in the area may completely cover, obstruct, or hide the location of any victims. When a known or potential victim is located and not immediately removed, victim location marking symbols are made by the search team or others aiding the search and rescue operation. These symbols should be made with orange spray paint or lumbar marker.

Figures 1 through 5 below illustrate examples of the marking system in use.

1 Initially, a large (approximately 2 feet or 0.6 meter across) "V" is painted near the location of a potential victim. Mark the name of the search team or crew identifier in the top part of the "V."

2 Paint a circle around the "V" when a potential victim is <u>confirmed</u> to be <u>alive</u> either visually, vocally, or by hearing specific sounds that would indicate a high probability of a live victim. If more than one confirmed live victim is discovered, mark the total number of victims under the "V."

3 Paint a horizontal line through the middle of the "V" when a <u>confirmed</u> victim is determined to be <u>deceased</u>. If more than one confirmed deceased victim exists, mark the total number of victims under the "V." Use both the live (circle) and deceased (horizontal line) victim marking symbols when a combination of live and deceased victims are determined to be in the same location.

4 If the victim's location is some distance from where the "V" symbol is painted, an arrow may be added next to the "V" pointing towards the victim. Show distance above the arrow.

5 Paint an "X" through the confirmed victim symbol after <u>all</u> victim(s) have been removed from the specific location identified by the marking.

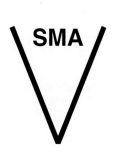

Figure 1 This example indicates a potential victim.

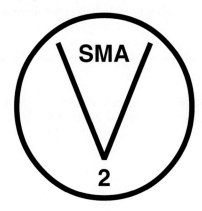

Figure 2 This example indicates two live victims have been confirmed to be alive.

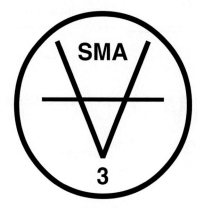

Figure 3 This example indicates three victims: a combination of confirmed alive and deceased in the same location.

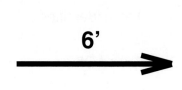

Figure 4 Arrow painted near the "V" points toward location of victim. Number above arrow indicates distance to victim from arrow.

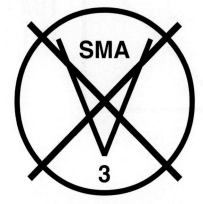

Figure 5 This example indicates that all three confirmed live victims have been removed from this location.

Building Marking System Structure/Hazards Evaluation

Structural specialist makes a 2′ × 2′ box on building adjacent to most accessible entry. This is done after doing hazards assessment and filling out hazards assessment form. Box is spray painted with International Orange and marked as follows:

 Structure is relatively safe for SAR operations. Damage is such that there is little danger of further collapse. (May be pancaked building.)

 Structure is significantly damaged. Some areas may be relatively safe, but other areas may need shoring, bracing, or removal of hazards.

 Structure is NOT safe for rescue operations and may be subject to sudden collapse. Remote search operations may proceed at significant risk. If rescue operations are undertaken, safe haven areas and rapid evacuations routes should be created.

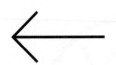 Arrow located next to the marking box indicates the direction of safest entry to the structure.

HM Indicates HazMat condition in or adjacent to structure. SAR operations normally will not be allowed until condition is better defined or eliminated.

EXAMPLE:

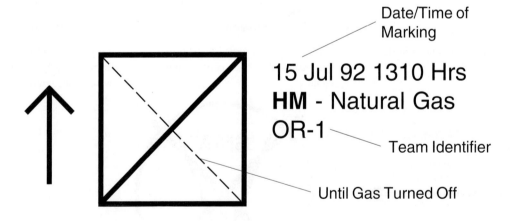

Date/Time of Marking

15 Jul 92 1310 Hrs
HM - Natural Gas
OR-1

Team Identifier

Until Gas Turned Off

Search Urgency

Remember the lower the number the more urgent the response!!!

Date Completed: _____
Time Completed: _____
Initials: _____

A. SUBJECT PROFILE .... _____

Age
Very Young 1
Very Old 1
Other 2-3
Medical Condition
Known or suspected injury or illness 1-2
Healthy 3
Known fatality 3
Number of Subjects
One alone 1
More than one (unless separation suspected) 2-3

B. WEATHER PROFILE .... _____

Existing hazardous weather 1
Predicted hazardous weather (8 hours or less) 1-2
Predicted hazardous weather (more than 8 hours) 2
No hazardous weather predicted 3

C. EQUIPMENT PROFILE .... _____

Inadequate for environment 1
Questionable for environment 1-2
Adequate for environment 3

D. SUBJECT EXPERIENCE PROFILE .... _____

Not experienced, not familiar with the area 1
Not experienced, knows the area 1-2
Experienced, not familiar with the area 2
Experienced, knows the area 3

E. TERRAIN & HAZARDS PROFILE .... _____

Known hazardous terrain or other hazards 1
Few or no hazards 2-3

TOTAL .... _____

If any of the seven categories above are rated as a one (1), regardless of the total, the search could require an emergency response.

••• THE TOTAL SHOULD RANGE FROM **7** TO **21** WITH **7** BEING THE MOST URGENT. •••

8-11 Emergency Response   *12-16 Measured Response*   *17-21 Evaluate & Investigate*

Track Identification Form

Date: _____ Time: _____ Location: _____

Mission Name: _____ Mission #: _____

Tracker: _____ Op. Period: _____

SUBJECT
Name: _____ Age: _____

Footwear Sample Available? YES   NO

Address: _____ Weight: _____

Height: _____ Sex: M   F

Physical Problems: _____

Physical Condition: _____

FOOTWEAR
Type: _____ Description: _____

Overall *Heel*
Length: _____ Width: _____ Length: _____ Width: _____

DISCARDABLES
Outer Wear: _____ Pants: _____

Shirt: _____

Inner Wear: _____ Rain Wear: _____

Head Wear: _____

Smoke: _____ Candy/Gum: _____

Other: _____

Track Identification Form

Location of Print: _____

SKETCH:
Date: _____ Time: _____ Heading: _____

Which measurement are you using for sketch? **INCHES** (Imperial) **CM** (Metric)

Sole Type: _____ Overall Pattern: _____

Ground Description: _____

Approx. Age of Print: _____

Stride: _____ Straddle: _____

Left **Right**

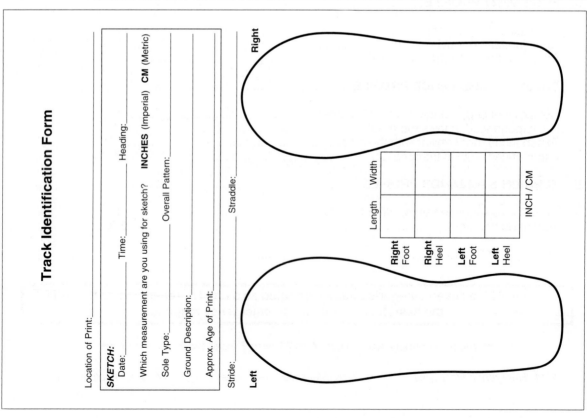

	Length	Width
Right Foot		
Right Heel		
Left Foot		
Left Heel		

INCH / CM

APPENDIX 4

Briefing and Debriefing Checklists

Briefing

1. Incident Action Plan - what is it and how I fit in.
2. Situation status and predictions.
3. Objectives and strategies (specific).
4. Tactical assignments with explicit instructions.
   - Hazards and safety instructions
5. Weather - present and forecast.
6. Specific equipment needs.
7. Communications details:
   - Frequencies or talk groups to be used
   - Designators and codes
   - Contact persons and times
   - What to do if communication problems arise
   - Emergency communications (whistle?)
8. Transportation details (if needed).
9. Reporting locations and times.
10. How to deal with media/family - where to refer.
11. Where to be at what times.
12. How to handle discovered evidence.
13. General hazards and safety instructions.
14. Debriefing procedures:
    - Where to debrief and with whom
    - When to debrief
    - What info will be expected, needed, or required
    - What format should the debrief be in (oral, written, sketches, maps, etc.)

Briefing should last less than 30 minutes and should be held before, not during, shift (operational period). A combination of written and oral briefings are most successful. **Take notes and ask questions.**

Debriefing

1. Explicit description of area covered and activities carried out.
2. Average maximum detection range (AMDR) for each sub-area of the assigned segment.
3. Report other field-observable measures identified and requested by search planners prior to assignment.
4. Qualitative description of search (poor, average, great).
5. Estimate of forward speed of search unit (fast, normal, slow).
6. Exact amount (in minutes) of time spent searching.
7. Location of any clues found, regardless of how insignificant they may seem (use map, sketches, etc.).
8. Gaps in area searched or any other problems with the search.
9. Specific difficulties encountered (communications, terrain, weather, fitness, injuries, etc.).
10. Hazards in the area - be specific with respect to location and description.
11. Suggestions, recommendations, and ideas for further search activity in the area searched.

Proper information conveyed in the debriefing is absolutely essential for an effective search. Use any means to convey what you want to say about the area searched (i.e., sketches, maps, briefing reports, notes, photos, videos, etc.).

Debriefing should be done in writing if possible, perhaps using an open-ended questionnaire for personnel coming out of the field. All debriefings should be performed one-at-a-time, on an individual basis, if possible. However, team leaders could debrief their team members and someone in turn debrief the team leader. The above list is a minimum.

Please feel free to copy this page (shrink it if necessary), laminate it, and carry it with you in your ready pack.

APPENDIX 5

Missing Person Questionnaire

NOTE: Use pencil/black ink, print clearly, avoid confusing phrases/words, unfamiliar abbreviations. Complete and detail answers for future use. Answer ALL questions, if possible.

FIRST NOTICE (Sections A - E only)

INCIDENT TITLE: _____ DATE: _____ TIME: _____

Person Taking Info: _____ Incident No:_____

A. SOURCE(S) OF INFORMATION – INFORMANT

Full Name: _____ DOB: _____ Sex: ☐M ☐F

Home Address (full): _____

_____

Phone: _____ 2nd Phone: _____ Relationship: _____

Where/How to Contact Now/Later: _____

_____

What Does Informant Believe Happened: _____

What Does Informant Want Done: _____

Instructions to Informant: _____

B. MISSING PERSON

Full Name: _____ DOB: _____ Sex: ☐M ☐F

Nickname(s)/Alias: _____ Birthplace: _____

Home Address (full): _____

_____

Local Address (full): _____

_____

Home Phone: _____ Local Phone: _____

Pager: _____ Cell Phone: _____ E-mail: _____

Category of Lost Subject: _____

General Experience and Familiarity With Area: _____

General Quality/Quantity of Equipment Carried & Preparedness For Environment: _____

COMMENTS: _____

_____

_____

C. ACTIONS TAKEN SO FAR

By: Family/Friends: _____ Results: _____

_____

Others: _____ Results: _____

_____

COMMENTS: _____

D. LAST SEEN

Date: _____ Time: _____ Where: _____

_____

Seen by Whom: _____ Location Now: _____

Who last talked at length with person: _____

Where: _____ Subject Matter: _____

Weather at Time: _____ Weather Since: _____

Seen Going Which Way: _____ When: _____

Circumstances of Loss (situation): _____

_____

Reason for Leaving: _____ Alone? ☐Y ☐N

Attitude (confident, confused, etc.): _____

Subject Complaining of Anything: _____

Subject Seem Tired: _____ Cold/Hot: _____ Other: _____

COMMENTS: _____

_____

E. PHYSICAL DESCRIPTION OF MISSING PERSON

Height: _____ Weight: _____ Age: _____ Build: _____ Eye Color: _____

Hair: Color: _____ Length: _____ Style: _____

Beard: _____ Moustache: _____ Sideburns: _____

Facial Features/Shape: _____ Complexion: _____

Distinguishing Marks (scars, moles): _____

Overall Appearance: _____

Photo Available? ☐Y ☐N Where: _____ Need to be Returned? ☐Y ☐N

Known or Suspected Significant Illness or Injury? ☐Y ☐N

Explain: _____

Comments: _____

_____

_____

_____

SUBSEQUENT INVESTIGATION

F. PLANS OF SUBJECT

Started From: _____ Day/Date: _____ Time: _____

Going to: _____ Via: _____

Purpose: _____

For How Long? _____ Return Date: _____ Alone? ☐Y ☐N Group Size: _____

Return Time: _____ From Where: _____

By Whom/What: _____

Done Trip Before? ☐Y ☐N Details: _____

Transported by Whom/Means: _____

Vehicle Now Located at: _____ Type: _____ Color: _____

License No: _____ Verified? ☐Y ☐N By Whom: _____

Additional Names, Cars, Licenses, etc. For Party: _____

Alternate Plans/Routes/Objectives Discussed: _____

Discussed With Whom: _____ When: _____

Comments: _____

_____

_____

G. CLOTHING WORN BY MISSING PERSON

	Style	Color	Size	Other

Shirt/Sweater: _____

Pants: _____

Outerwear: _____

Innerwear: _____

Head Wear: _____

Rain Wear: _____

Glasses: _____

Gloves: _____

Extra Clothing: _____

Other: _____

Footwear: _____

Sole Type: _____ Sample Available? ☐Y ☐N Where: _____

Scent Articles Available? ☐Y ☐N What _____ Secured? ☐Y ☐N

Where is the Scent Article Now? _____

Overall Coloration as Seen From Air: _____

H. OUTDOOR EXPERIENCE

Familiar with Area?: ☐Y ☐N How Recent: _____ Other: _____

Other Areas of Travel: _____

Formal Outdoor Training Qualification: _____

Where: _____ When: _____

Medical Training: _____ When: _____

Scouting Experience: _____ When: _____ Where: _____

How Much: _____ Scout Rank: _____ Scout Leader? ☐Y ☐N

Military Experience? ☐Y ☐N What: _____ When: _____ Where: _____

Rank: _____ Other: _____

Generalized Previous Experience: _____

How Much Overnight Experience: _____

Ever Been Lost Before? ☐Y ☐N Where: _____ When: _____

Ever Go Out Alone? ☐Y ☐N Where: _____

Stay on Paths or X-C: _____

How Fast Does Subject Hike: _____

Athletic/Other Interests: _____

Climbing Experience: _____

COMMENTS: _____

I. HABITS/PERSONALITY

Smoke? ☐Y ☐N How Often: _____ What: _____ Brand: _____

Alcohol? ☐Y ☐N How Often: _____ What: _____ Brand: _____

Recreational Drugs: ☐Y ☐N How Often: _____ What: _____

Gum Brand: _____ Candy Brand: _____ Other: _____

Hobbies/Interests: _____

Outgoing/Quiet: _____ Gregarious/Loner: _____

Evidence of Leadership: _____ Give Up Easy/Keep Going: _____

Legal Trouble (past/present): _____

Hitchhike? ☐Y ☐N Accepts Ride Easily: _____

Personal Problems: _____

Religious? ☐Y ☐N Faith: _____ To What Degree: _____

Personal Values: _____

Philosophy: _____

Person Closest To: _____ In Family: _____

Emotional History: _____

Education: Highest Grade Achieved: _____ Current Status: _____

College Education: _____

   School Name: _____

   Teacher(s): _____

   Subject/Degree: _____ Year: _____

Local/Fictional Hero: _____

COMMENTS: _____

_____

J. HEALTH/GENERAL CONDITION

Overall Health: _____

Overall Physical Condition: _____

Known Medical/Dental Problems: _____

Knowledgeable Doctor: _____ Phone: _____

Handicaps: _____

Known Psychological Problems: _____

Knowledgeable Person: _____ Phone: _____

Medication: _____ Dosages: _____

Knowledgeable Person: _____ Phone: _____

What Will Happen Without Meds: _____

Eyesight Without Glasses: _____ Spares? ☐Y ☐N Where Are Spares: _____

COMMENTS: _____

K. EQUIPMENT

	Style	Color	Brand	Size
Pack:				
Tent:				
Sleeping Bag:				
Ground Cloth/Pad:				
Fishing Equipment:				
Climbing Equipment:				
Light:				
Knife:				
Camera:				

Stove: Fuel: Fire Starter? ☐Y ☐N What:		
Liquid Container:	How Much Fluid:	What Kind Fluid:
Compass:	Map:	Of Where:
How Competent With Map/Compass:		

Food: _____ Brands: _____

_____

Skis: Type: _____ Brand: _____ Color: _____ Size: _____

Bindings: _____ Pole Type: _____ Length: _____

How Competent: _____

Snowshoes: Type: _____ Brand: _____ Color: _____ Size: _____

Bindings: _____ How Competent: _____

Money: Amount: _____ Credit Cards: _____

Other Documents: _____

COMMENTS: _____

_____

L. CONTACT PERSON WOULD MAKE UPON REACHING CIVILISATION

Full Name: _____ Relationship: _____

Address: _____

_____

Phone: _____ Anyone Home Now: _____

M. CHILDREN

Afraid of Dark? ☐ Y ☐ N Animals? ☐ Y ☐ N Afraid of: _____

Feeling Toward Adults: _____ Strangers: _____

Reactions When Hurt: _____ Cry: _____

Training When Lost: _____

Active/Lethargic/Antisocial: _____

COMMENTS: _____

_____

N. GROUPS OVERDUE

Name/Kind of Group: _____ Leader: _____

Experience of Group/Leader: _____

Address/Phone of Knowledgeable Person: _____

Personality Clashes Within Group: _____

Leader Types in Group Other Than Leader: _____

What Would Subject Do if Separated From Group: _____

Competitive Spirit of Group: _____

Intragroup Dynamics: _____

COMMENTS: _____

_____

O. PRESS/FAMILY RELATIONS

Next of Kin: _____ Relationship: _____

    Address: _____

    _____

    Phone: _____ Occupation: _____

Person to Notify When Subject Found: _____ Relationship: _____

    Address: _____

    _____

    Phone: _____ Occupation: _____

Significant Family Problems: _____

Family's Desire to Employ Special Assistance: _____

COMMENTS: _____

_____

_____

_____

P. ADDITIONAL SEARCH INFORMATION

Residence Checked By: _____ When: _____

Initial IC: _____ Second IC: _____

Missing Person's Employer: _____

    Employer's Address: _____

    Employer's Phone: _____ Sup's Name: _____

Missing Person's School: _____

    School's Address: _____

    School's Phone: _____ Teacher's Name: _____

Q. ADDITIONAL PERSONS HAVING INFO ABOUT MISSING PERSON

(1) Name: _____ Relationship: _____

Address (full): _____

Phone: _____ Other Contact Info: _____

Info Possessed: _____

Follow up: _____ By: _____

(2) Name: _____ Relationship: _____

Address (full): _____

Phone: _____ Other Contact Info: _____

Info Possessed: _____

Follow up: _____ By: _____

(3) Name: _____ Relationship: _____

Address (full): _____

Phone: _____ Other Contact Info: _____

Info Possessed: _____

Follow up: _____ By: _____

R. OTHER INFORMATION

_____

_____

_____

_____

_____

_____

_____

_____

_____

_____

_____

_____

APPENDIX 6

Equipment List

The following equipment is commonly compiled to form what is referred to as a "24-hour ready pack." Such a pack holds those items that will assist the holder in functioning safely and effectively during a SAR mission. Some items may be carried on a belt, in pockets, or strapped to the person. This is the minimum equipment recommended to be carried on all missions in non-urban or wilderness areas. Your local equipment requirements may vary. Consult a physician for recommendations about analgesics and other drugs that you may carry in the SAR pack.

Personal First Aid and Survival Kit
1 - Plastic bag, zip lock, qt. size, for kit
4 - Acetaminophen or aspirin tablets
4 - Antacid tablets
2 - Antiseptic cleansing pads
1 - Antiseptic ointment
6 - Band aids, various sizes
1 - Candle, long burning
2 - Cotton swabs, non sterile
1 - Duct tape, 5-10 ft.
1 - Leaf bag, large

8 - Matches in a waterproof container
1 - Moleskin
2 - Quarters for phone call
1 - Razor blade, single edge safety type
1 - Roller gauze bandage
2 - Safety pins, large
1 - Splinter forceps, tweezers
1- Space type blanket or space-type sleeping bag
1- Towelette, clean
1- Whistle

(Non-urban) Personal SAR Equipment
1 - Pack, 1800 cubic inch (minimum)
4 - Bags, various sizes, zip locked
1 - Bandanna, handkerchief
1 - Cap or other headgear
2 - Carabiners, locking gate
1 - Clothes bag, waterproof
1 - Clothing, adequate for climate
1 - Clothing, extra set, suitable for climate
1 - Compass, orienteering
1 - Flagging tape, roll
1 - Flashlight or lantern
1 - Flashlight extra, extra batteries and bulb
1 - Footwear, sturdy, adequate for climate
1 - Gloves, durable, even in summer
1 - Goggles, or eye protection, clear
1 - Insect repellent
1 - Knife, multi-purpose
1 - Lip balm, with sunscreen

1 - Measuring device, 18 in. minimum
1 - Metal cup or pot
1 - Mirror, small
1 - Nylon twine or small rope, 50 feet
1 - Pad and pencil
2 - Prusik cords (6mm – 8mm; 6 ft. length)
1 - Rainwear, durable
1 - SAR personal identification
1 - Shelter Material, 8x10 plastic or coated nylon
1 - Scissors, multi-purpose
1 - Socks, extra pair
1 - Sunscreen lotion
1 - Tissue paper or baby wipes (recommended)
1 - Tracking stick, 42" long
1 - Watch
2 - Water containers, at least liter size
1 - Webbing, 1" tubular - length suitable for harness
1 - Wire, 5-10 ft., woven steel
8 - Wire ties, plastic, self locking

Optional Personal Support Equipment Recommended But Not Required
2 - Antihistamine, 25mg Benadryl
2 - Extra leaf bags
1 - Extra water container
1 - Foam pad
2 - Food, nonperishable

1 - Gaiters
1 - Rain cover, pack
1 - Sterno or stove
1 - Sun glasses, 97% UV protection
1 - Trail snacks
1 - Water purification tabs

The following requirements are for an **urban SAR pack**. This should only be carried when its use is approved.

Personal First Aid and Survival Kit (Same as in the 24-hour ready pack.)

(Urban) Personal SAR Equipment	1 - Raincoat & pants durable
1 - Fanny pack, 600-1200 cubic inch	1 - SAR personal identification
4 - Bags, various sizes, zip locked	1 - Small pad and pencil
1 - Bandanna, handkerchief	1 - Sunglasses, 97% UV protection
1 - Cap or other headwear	1 - Sunscreen lotion
1 - Clothing, adequate for climate	1 - Tissue paper or baby wipes
1 - Compass, orienteering	1 - Tracking stick, 42" long
1 - Flagging tape, roll	1 - Watch
1 - Flashlight or lantern	1 - Water container, at least liter size
1 - Footwear, sturdy, adequate for climate	
1 - Knife, multi-purpose	
1 - Map	(Items **bolded** above are variances from the non-urban pack list)
1 - Mirror, small	

INCIDENT BRIEFING	1. INCIDENT NAME	2. DATE	3. TIME

4. MAP SKETCH

ICS-201 NFES 1325	PAGE 1	8. PREPARED BY (NAME & POSITION)

7. SUMMARY OF CURRENT ACTIONS

| ICS-201 NFES 1325 | PAGE 2 | |

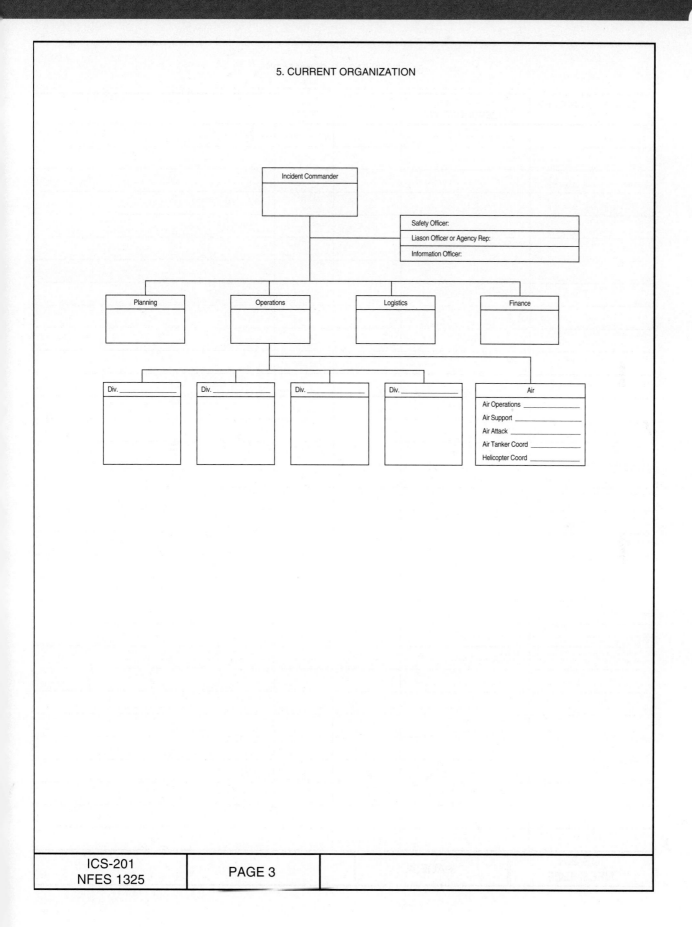

5. CURRENT ORGANIZATION

6. RESOURCES SUMMARY

RESOURCES ORDERED	RESOURCES IDENTIFICATION	ETA	ON SCENE	LOCATION / ASSIGNMENT

ICS-201 NFES 1325	PAGE 4	

INCIDENT OBJECTIVES	1. Incident Name	2. Date	3. Time

4. Operational Period

5. General Control Objectives for the Incident (include alternatives)

6. Weather Forecast for Period

7. General Safety Message

8. Attachments (mark if attached)

- ☐ Organization List - ICS 203
- ☐ Div. Assignment Lists - ICS 204
- ☐ Communications Plan - ICS 205
- ☐ Medical Plan - ICS 206
- ☐ Incident Map
- ☐ Traffic Plan
- ☐ (Other)
- ☐
- ☐

9. Prepared by (Planning Section Chief)	10. Approved by (Incident Commander)

ICS 202

ORGANIZATION ASSIGNMENT LIST

1. INCIDENT NAME	2. DATE PREPARED	3. TIME PREPARED

POSITION	NAME	4. OPERATIONAL PERIOD (DATE/TIME)

5. INCIDENT COMMANDER AND STAFF

Position	Name
INCIDENT COMMANDER	
DEPUTY	
SAFTEY OFFICER	
INFORMATION OFFICER	
LIAISON OFFICER	

6. AGENCY REPRESENTATIVES

AGENCY	NAME

7. PLANNING SECTION

Position	Name
CHIEF	
DEPUTY	
RESOURCES UNIT	
SITUATION UNIT	
DOCUMENTATION UNIT	
DEMOBILIZATION UNIT	
TECHNICAL SPECIALISTS	

8. LOGISTICS SECTION

Position	Name
CHIEF	
DEPUTY	

a. SUPPORT BRANCH

Position	Name
DIRECTOR	
SUPPLY UNIT	
FACILITIES UNIT	
GROUND SUPPORT UNIT	

b. SERVICE BRANCH

Position	Name
DIRECTOR	
COMMUNICATIONS UNIT	
MEDICAL UNIT	
FOOD UNIT	

9. OPERATIONS SECTION

Position	Name
CHIEF	
DEPUTY	

a. BRANCH I- DIVISION/GROUPS

Position	Name
BRANCH DIRECTOR	
DEPUTY	
DIVISION/GROUP	
DIVISION/GROUP	
DIVISION/GROUP	
DIVISION/GROUP	
DIVISION/GROUP	

b. BRANCH II- DIVISION/GROUPS

Position	Name
BRANCH DIRECTOR	
DEPUTY	
DIVISION/GROUP	
DIVISION/GROUP	
DIVISION/GROUP	
DIVISION/GROUP	
DIVISION/GROUP	

c. BRANCH III- DIVISION/GROUPS

Position	Name
BRANCH DIRECTOR	
DEPUTY	
DIVISION/GROUP	
DIVISION/GROUP	
DIVISION/GROUP	
DIVISION/GROUP	
DIVISION/GROUP	

d. AIR OPERATIONS BRANCH

Position	Name
AIR OPERATIONS BR. DIR.	
AIR TACTICAL GROUP SUP.	
AIR SUPPORT GROUP SUP.	
HELICOPTER COORDINATOR	
AIR TANKER/FIXED WING CRD.	

10. FINANCE/ADMINISTRATION SECTION

Position	Name
CHIEF	
DEPUTY	
TIME UNIT	
PROCUREMENT UNIT	
COMPENSATION/CLAIMS UNIT	
COST UNIT	

PREPARED BY(RESOURCES UNIT)

203 ICS (1/99)

NFES 1327

ASSIGNMENT LIST	1. Branch	2. Division/Group

3. Incident Name	4. Operational Period
	Date: Time:

5.   Operations Personnel

Operations Chief		Division/Group Supervisor	
Branch Director		Air Attack Supervisor No.	

6.   Resources Assigned this Period

Strike Team/Task Force/ Resource Designator	Leader	Number Persons	Trans. Needed	Drop Off PT./Time	Pick Up PT./Time

7. Control Operations

8. Special Instructions

9.   Division/Group Communication Summary

Function	Frequency	System	Channel	Function	Frequency	System	Channel
Command				Logistics			
Tactical Div/Group				Air to Ground			

Prepared by (Resource Unit Leader)	Approved by (Planning Section Chief)	Date	Time

ICS 204   NFES 1328

INCIDENT RADIO COMMUNICATIONS PLAN

1. Incident Name	2. Date/Time Prepared	3. Operational Period Date/Time

4. Basic Radio Channel Utilization

Radio Type/Cache	Channel	Function	Frequency/Tone	Assignment	Remarks

5. Prepared by (Communications Unit)

ICS 205

NFES 1330

MEDICAL PLAN	1. Incident Name	2. Date Prepared	3. Time Prepared	4. Operational Period

5. Incident Medical Aid Station			

Medical Aid Stations	Location	Paramedics Yes	No

6. Transportation

A. Ambulance Services

Name	Address	Phone	Paramedics Yes	No

B. Incident Ambulances

Name	Location	Paramedics Yes	No

7. Hospitals								

Name	Address	Travel Time Air	Ground	Phone	Helipad Yes	No	Burn Center Yes	No

8. Medical Emergency Procedures

Prepared by (Medical Unit Leader)	10. Reviewed by (Safety Officer)

ICS 206

303

APPENDIX 8

SAR RESOURCE TYPING

The selected documents that follow are derived from the U.S. Department of Homeland Security (DHS), Federal Emergency Management Agency (FEMA), National Mutual Aid and Resource Management Initiative. This initiative supports the National Incident Management System (NIMS) by establishing a comprehensive, integrated national mutual aid and resource management system that provides the basis to type, order, and track all (Federal, State, and local) response assets. Selected search and rescue resources have been included here for informational purposes only. They were published by FEMA in September 2004.

For more information, visit the National Mutual Aid and Resource Management web site.

Resource	Canine Search and Rescue Team— Avalanche Snow Air Scent					

Category: Search and Rescue (ESF #9) **Kind:** Team

Minimum Capabilities: Component	Metric	TYPE I	TYPE II	TYPE III	TYPE IV	OTHER
Dog Team: 1 Dog 1 Handler 1 Support Person	Search Capabilities	Capable of self-sustaining and searching for 24 hours in extreme weather and terrain conditions through avalanche debris fields	Capable of self-sustaining and searching for 24 hours in snow-covered environments in extreme weather conditions and moderate terrain			N/A
Knowledge and Equipment for Avalanche/ Snow Search Dog Teams		Personal snow travel equipment and gear to self-sustain for 24 hours; Equipped to include cross-country skis or snow shoes, poles, probe poles, snow shovel, and avalanche beacon; Training, including avalanche safety and winter survival, including building snow cave, First Aid for both human and dog, personal/dog safety, and radio communications	Personal snow travel equipment and gear to self-sustain for 24 hours; Equipped to include cross-country skis or snow shoes, poles, probe poles, snow shovel, and avalanche beacon; Training, including avalanche safety and winter survival, including building snow cave, First Aid for both human and dog, personal/ dog safety, and radio communications			N/A

Comments: Note: Many of these resources are capable of searching in a disaster environment, such as a wilderness team in outlying areas of a tornado zone, etc. It is critical that canine management personnel, knowledgeable in multi-use of canine resources, are available to Incident Command. This will not necessarily be reflected in this document.

Resource | Canine Search and Rescue Team— Disaster Response

Category: Search and Rescue (ESF #9)

Kind: Team

Minimum Capabilities: Component	Metric	TYPE I	TYPE II	TYPE III	TYPE IV	OTHER
Dog Team: 1 Dog 1 Handler 1 Support Person	Search Capabilities	A disaster search canine that has successfully completed the DHS/FEMA Disaster Search Canine Readiness Evaluation for both Type II; capable of national and international responses	A disaster search canine that has successfully completed the DHS/FEMA Disaster Search Canine Readiness Evaluation for Type II only; capable of national and international responses	A disaster search canine that has successfully completed Disaster Search Canine Readiness Evaluation through an organized disaster task force – non-FEMA; Capable of national and international responses	A search canine with minimal exposure to disaster search; Capable of local/regional response only; No task force participation	
Knowledge and Equipment for Search Dog Teams		All requirements as set forth by DHS/FEMA National US&R Response System	All requirements as set forth by DHS/FEMA National US&R Response System	All requirements as set forth by organized task force for availability for national/international response	Agility; Obedience; First Aid-Human/Dog; Haz-Mat; Disaster; Environment Exposure minimal; Initial responder readiness through local agency	

Comments: Please note that many of these resources are capable of searching in a disaster environment, such as a wilderness team in outlying areas of a tornado zone, etc. It is critical that canine management personnel, knowledgeable in multi-use of canine resources, are available to Incident Command. This will not necessarily be reflected in this document.

Resource — Canine Search and Rescue Team— Land Cadaver Air Scent

Category: Search and Rescue, Other

Kind: Team

Minimum Capabilities: Component	Metric	TYPE I	TYPE II	TYPE III	TYPE IV	OTHER
Dog Team: 1 Dog 1 Handler 1 Support Person	Search Capabilities	Capable of locating less than 15 grams of human remains during disaster ops; Capable of self-sustaining for 24 hours	Capable of locating deceased persons (greater than 15 grams) in disaster ops; Capable of self-sustaining for 24 hours	Capable of locating less than 15 grams of human remains buried, hanging, ground level, or in vehicles, nondisaster	Capable of locating less than 15 grams of human remains buried, hanging, ground level, nondisaster	Capable of locating deceased persons (greater than 15 grams) buried, hanging, ground level, nondisaster
Knowledge and Equipment for Land Cadaver Search Dog Teams		Training and equipment for biohazard environment, including OSHA guidelines, scene preservation, documentation, collection, chain of custody, and scene security; First Aid for both human and dog, personal/dog safety, and radio communications; Disaster ops training and capabilities	Training and equipment for biohazard environment, including OSHA guidelines, scene preservation, documentation, collection, chain of custody, and scene security; First Aid for both human and dog, personal/dog safety, and radio communications; Disaster ops training and capabilities	Training and equipment for biohazard environment, including OSHA guidelines, scene preservation, documentation, collection, chain of custody, and scene security; First Aid for both human and dog, personal/dog safety, and radio communications	Training and equipment for biohazard environment, including OSHA guidelines, scene preservation, documentation, collection, chain of custody, and scene security; First Aid for both human and dog, personal/dog safety, and radio communications	Training and equipment for biohazard environment, including OSHA guidelines, scene preservation, documentation, collection, chain of custody, and scene security; First Aid for both human and dog, personal/dog safety, and radio communications

Resource — Canine Search and Rescue Team—Water Air Scent

Category: Search and Rescue (ESF #9)

Kind: Team

Minimum Capabilities: Component	Metric	TYPE I	TYPE II	TYPE III	TYPE IV	OTHER
Dog Team: 1 Dog 1 Handler 1 Support Person	Search Capabilities	Capable of working swiftwater/stillwater environments; Trained and equipped to perform search ops on foot and from any type of watercraft Type VI Capable of working salt-water and very large fresh water environments from both boat and shore	Capable of working stillwater environments; Trained and equipped to perform search ops on foot and from any type of watercraft Type VII Capable of working salt-water and very large fresh water environments from shore only	Capable of working swiftwater and stillwater ops from shore only	Capable of working swiftwater ops from shore only	Capable of working stillwater ops from shore only
Knowledge and Equipment for Water Search Dog Teams		Type I, III, IV, VI, VII Water Helmet; Class V Water Vest; Throw Rope; Swiftwater lifesaving skills; Knowledge of water rescue and boat operations; First Aid for both human and dog; Personal/dog safety; Radio communications	Type II, V Water Helmet; Class III-V Water Vest; Throw Rope, Stillwater lifesaving skills; Knowledge of water rescue operations in stillwater environment; First Aid for both human and dog; Personal/dog safety, Radio communications equipment			

Comments: Note: Many of these resources are capable of searching in a disaster environment, such as a wilderness team in outlying areas of a tornado zone, etc. It is critical that canine management personnel, knowledgeable in multi-use of canine resources, are available to Incident Command. This will not necessarily be reflected in this document.

Resource: Canine Search and Rescue Team—Wilderness Air Scent

Category: Search and Rescue (ESF #9)

Kind: Team

Minimum Capabilities: Component	Metric	TYPE I	TYPE II	TYPE III	TYPE IV	OTHER
Single Resource	Search Capabilities	Capable of search and self-sustaining for 72 hours in all weather and low angle wilderness terrain or larger areas of 60+ acres	Capable of searching and self-sustaining for 48 hours in all weather and low angle wilderness terrain or larger areas of 60+ acres	Capable of searching high probability local wilderness terrain for short durations (24 hours or less) or small areas 40-60 acres	Capable of searching high probability local wilderness terrain for short durations (12 hours or less) or small areas 40-60 acres	Human discriminating (scent source necessary)
Single Resource	Search Capabilities	Capable of searching and self-sustaining for 72 hours in all weather and low angle wilderness terrain or larger areas of 120+ acres	Capable of searching and self-sustaining for 48 hours in all weather and low angle wilderness terrain or larger areas of 120+ acres	Capable of searching high probability local wilderness terrain for short durations (24 hours or less) or small areas of 60-120 acres	Capable of searching high probability local wilderness terrain for short durations (12 hours or less) or small areas of 40-60 acres	Nondiscriminating (locate all human indication in area)

Comments: There are significant differences in the training required for urban versus wilderness environments, both in air scent/area and trailing/tracking. Because of the vast differences, often a resource highly skilled in one environment may not function as well in the other environment because of a lack of continuous training in the environment. Teams may be cross-trained in both environments, depending on the team training criteria.

Note: Many of these resources are capable of searching in a disaster environment, such as a wilderness team in outlying areas of a tornado zone, etc. It is critical that canine management personnel, knowledgeable in multi-use of canine resources, are available to Incident Command. This will not necessarily be reflected in this document.

Resource

Canine Search and Rescue Team— Wilderness Tracking/Trailing

Category: Law Enforcement/Security, Search and Rescue (ESF #9)

Kind: Team

Minimum Capabilities: Component	Metric	TYPE I	TYPE II	TYPE III	TYPE IV	OTHER
Dog Team: 1 Dog 1 Handler 1 Support Person	Search Capabilities	Capable of trailing in wilderness terrain; Aged 24+ hours; 1 mile or longer; Heavy contamination	Capable of trailing in wilderness terrain; Aged 4-12 hours; 1 mile or longer; Heavy contamination	Capable of trailing in wilderness terrain, Aged 1.5-4 hours; .5-1 mile; Heavy contamination	Capable of trailing in wilderness terrain; Aged 0-1.5 hours; .25-.5 mile; Heavy contamination	Discriminating (scent source must be available)
Knowledge and Equipment for Search Dog Teams		Personally equipped for 24 hours for dog/handler; Wilderness survival skills; Capable of establishing and maintaining direction of travel; First Aid for both human and dog; Personal/ dog safety; Radio communications; Skill in collection of scent articles	Personally equipped for 24 hours for dog/handler; Wilderness survival skills; Capable of establishing and maintaining direction of travel; First Aid for both human and dog; Personal/ dog safety; Radio communications; Skill in collection of scent articles	Personally equipped for 24 hours for dog/handler; Wilderness survival skills; Capable of establishing and maintaining direction of travel; First Aid for both human and dog; Personal/ dog safety; Radio communications; Skill in collection of scent articles	Personally equipped for 24 hours for dog/handler; Wilderness survival skills; Capable of establishing and maintaining direction of travel; First Aid for both human and dog; Personal/ dog safety; Radio communications; Skill in collection of scent articles	N/A

Comments: As these dogs use scent articles, they are commonly referred to as trailing dogs. However, occasionally, a unit may refer to such dogs as tracking dogs. They do have the capability of human discrimination between sources with the aid of a provided scent source. Care should be taken to determine if a tracking dog requires the use of an article or not.

Note: Many of these resources are capable of searching in a disaster environment, such as a wilderness team in outlying areas of a tornado zone, etc. It is critical that canine management personnel, knowledgeable in multi-use of canine resources, are available to Incident Command. This will not necessarily be reflected in this document.

Resource — Mountain Search and Rescue Team

Category: Search and Rescue (ESF #9)

Kind: Team

Minimum Capabilities: Component	Metric	TYPE I	TYPE II	TYPE III	TYPE IV	OTHER
Team	Personnel	Field team leader; Field team members; Medical specialist	Field team leader; Field team members; Medical specialist	Field team leader; Field team members; Medical specialist	Field team leader; Field team members; Medical specialist	
Personnel Training	Navigation Training	Same as Type II	Same as Type III	Same as Type IV, plus proficiency in back country navigation including: The ability to triangulate a position, ascertain a UTM, utilize GPS, and follow a route to a new location using a topographical map and compass	Navigation (map and compass)	
Personnel Training	Survival Training	Operational and technical proficiency in personal survival in mountainous terrain and snow and ice environments	Operational and technical proficiency in personal survival in mountainous terrain and snow and ice environments	Technical proficiency in personal survival in mountainous terrain and snow and ice environments	Technical proficiency in personal survival in mountainous terrain	
Personnel Training	Technical Training	Same as Type II, plus proficient at estimating the mechanical forces involved in technical rescue systems and estimating factors of safety; Proficiency in the use, placement and analysis of mechanical anchors and anchor systems; Proficiency in the use of highlines; Proficiency in the use of slings, etriers, Prusik hitches and mechanical ascenders; Proficiency in the organization and direction of technical litter evacuation	Same as Type III, plus understanding of the mechanical forces involved in technical rescue systems; Proficiency in the selection and setup of rescue anchor systems; Proficiency in technical litter evacuation and transport; Litter descents (on steep, vertical, and overhanging rock, on scree and snow, and traversing); Lowering of a subject without a litter; Raising a subject or litter; Knowledge of procedures involved with helicopter transport	Proficiency in bagging, coiling, throwing and storing static and dynamic ropes; Proficiency in tying common knots, and knowledge of their applications and strength efficiencies; Proficiency in search techniques including in hasty and line search techniques, directing line searches, and probe lines		

(continued)

Resource: Mountain Search and Rescue Team (cont'd)

Category: Search and Rescue (ESF #9)

Kind: Team

Minimum Capabilities: Component	Metric	TYPE I	TYPE II	TYPE III	TYPE IV	OTHER
Personnel Training	Alpine Training	Proficiency in winter camping in any area, including above timberline; Proficiency in snow and ice climbing; Proficiency in avalanche search and rescue, including recognition of avalanche hazards, avalanche search and rescue organization and leadership, scuff searches, use of SAR dogs; Proficiency in high and low-angle, technical snow and ice rescues and evacuations	Ability to recognize avalanche hazards and to perform avalanche search and rescue including probe lines and avalanche; Avalanche awareness training	Understanding of the fundamentals of mountain weather; Avalanche awareness training	Basic understanding of mountain weather; Ability to walk in mountainous terrain; Ability to backpack personal equipment plus one rope at least four miles with an elevation gain of at least 2000 feet; Avalanche awareness training	
Personnel	Basic Training	Same as Type II, plus technical proficiency in one-person rescue and self-rescue techniques; Proficiency in mantracking; Ability to integrate into and operate using ICs; Ability to plan, organize and direct search and rescue missions	Same as Type III, plus ability to operate using ICS	Same as Type IV	Proficiency in search techniques; Awareness of mantracking and maintaining site integrity; Understanding of the ICS	
Medical Specialist	Training	National standard EMT curriculum; ACLS, BTLS	National standard EMT-B curriculum or advanced wilderness first responder; BTLS	Same as Type IV	National standard first responder or wilderness first responder curriculum; BTLS	
Team	Sustained Operations	60 hours	48 hours	24 hours	12 hours	

Resource	Mountain Search and Rescue Team

Category: Search and Rescue (ESF #9)

Kind: Team

Minimum Capabilities: Component	Metric	TYPE I	TYPE II	TYPE III	TYPE IV	OTHER
Team	Rescue Capabilities	Same as Type II, plus: Highly trained rescue personnel with multi-pitch, high-angle experience on vertical rock, ice, and steep snow	Same as Type III, plus single-pitch, high-angle rock rescue	Backcountry, low-angle scree evacuation	Trained rescue personnel with experience in non-technical back-country evacuation/carryouts	
Team	Search Capabilities	Capable of searching during the day or night; Capable of searching any terrain, including severe rock; Competent IC and section chief	Capable of searching steep, timbered terrain, excluding severe rock, day or night; Competent search team leaders/technicians	Self-sustaining for 48 hours in all weather/terrain, except severe winter/rock	Capable of searching moderate terrain; May be outdoorsmen with basic training	
Team Rescue Equipment		Same as Type II, plus 8-10 ropes of various lengths (200-400 ft)	Same as Type III, plus 6-8 ropes of various lengths and a full complement of rescue/climbing gear	Same as Type IV, plus 4-6 ropes of various lengths	Harnesses; Helmets; Basic hardware; Rope; Radio communications on a common frequency	
Search Equipment		Equipped to be self-sustaining for 60 hours in all environments; Radio communications on common frequency	Equipped to be self-sustaining for 48 hours in all environments; Radio communications on common frequency	Equipped to be self-sustaining for 24 hours in all weather/terrain, except severe winter/rock	Equipped to be self-sustaining for 12 hours in all weather/terrain, except severe winter/rock	

(continued)

Resource | Mountain Search and Rescue Team Resource (cont'd)

Category: Search and Rescue (ESF #9)

Kind: Team

Minimum Capabilities: Component	Metric	TYPE I	TYPE II	TYPE III	TYPE IV	OTHER
Personal Equipment	Supplies and Materials	Same as Type II, plus food for 60 hours	Same as Type III, plus water container of two-liter capacity and/or quantity of water appropriate for the conditions; Food for 48 hours; Second light source	Same as Type IV	Appropriate clothes and footgear for both fair and foul weather; Water container of 1-liter capacity and/or quantity of water appropriate for the conditions; Day pack; Five large, heavy-duty plastic trash bags; Food for 24 hours; Headlamp or flashlight; Lighter, matches and candle, or equivalent waterproof fire source; Knife; Compass; Personal First Aid Kit; Waterproof pen/pencil and paper; Whistle; Two pairs plastic or vinyl examination gloves	
Medical Equipment	Supplies and Materials	As appropriate for level of training, as applied in wilderness environment and meeting local protocols and requirements	As appropriate for level of training, as applied in wilderness environment and meeting local protocols and requirements	As appropriate for level of training, as applied in wilderness environment and meeting local protocols and requirements	As appropriate for level of training, as applied in wilderness environment and meeting local protocols and requirements	

Comments: Mountain Search and Rescue Team: Search for and rescue people in trouble either above the timberline or in high-angle areas below the timberline, which can include glacier, crevasse, backcountry and alpine search and rescue, and educate the population in safe activities so they will be able to avoid the dangers that result in the need for rescue.

Definitions

GPS	Global Positioning System
Navigation	The practice of charting a course for a group of people (team) using basic tools such as a map and compass.

Resource — U S & R Task Forces

Category: Search and Rescue (ESF #9)   Kind: Team

Minimum Capabilities: Component	Metric	TYPE I	TYPE II	TYPE III	TYPE IV	OTHER
Personnel	Number of People per Response	70-person response	28-person response			
Personnel	Training	NFPA 1670 Technician Level in area of specialty; Support personnel at Operations Level	NFPA 1670 Technician Level in area of specialty; Support personnel at Operations Level			
Personnel	Areas of Specialization	High angle rope rescue (including highline systems); Confined space rescue (permit required); Advanced Life Support (ALS) intervention; Communications; WMD/HM operations; Defensive water rescue	Light frame construction and basic rope rescue operations; ALS intervention; HazMat conditions; Communications; and trench and excavation rescue			
Personnel	Sustained Operations	24-hour S&R operations; Self-sufficient for first 72 hours	12-hour S&R operations; Self-sufficient for first 72 hours			
Personnel	Organization	Multidisciplinary organization of Command; Search; Rescue; Medical; HazMat; Logistics; Planning	Multidisciplinary organization of Command; Search; Rescue; Medical; HazMat; Logistics; Planning			

(continued)

Resource — U S & R Task Forces (cont'd)

Category: Search and Rescue (ESF #9)

Kind: Team

Minimum Capabilities: Component	Metric	TYPE I	TYPE II	TYPE III	TYPE IV	OTHER
Equipment	Sustained Operations	Potential mission duration of up to 10 days	Potential mission duration of up to 10 days			
Equipment	Rescue Equipment	Pneumatic Powered Tools; Electric Powered Tools; Hydraulic Powered Tools; Hand Tools; Electrical; Heavy Rigging; Technical Rope; Safety	Pneumatic Powered Tools; Electric Powered Tools; Hydraulic Powered Tools; Hand Tools; Electrical; Heavy Rigging; Technical Rope; Safety			
Equipment	Medical Equipment	Antibiotics/Antifungals; Patient Comfort Medication; Pain Medications; Sedatives/ Anesthetics/Paralytics; Steroids; IV Fluids/Volume; Immunizations/ Immune Globulin; Canine Treatment; Basic Airway; Intubation; Eye Care Supplies; IV Access/Administration; Patient Assessment Care; Patient Immobilization/Extrication; Patient/PPE; Skeletal Care; Wound Care; Patient Monitoring	Antibiotics/Antifungals; Patient Comfort Medication; Pain Medications; Sedatives/ Anesthetics/Paralytics; Steroids; IV Fluids/ Volume; Immunizations/ Immune Globulin; Canine Treatment; Basic Airway; Intubation; Eye Care Supplies; IV Access/ Administration; Patient Assessment Care; Patient Immobilization/Extrication; Patient/ PPE; Skeletal Care; Wound Care; Patient Monitoring			

Resource — U S & R Task Forces

Category: Search and Rescue (ESF #9)

Kind: Team

Minimum Capabilities: Component	Metric	TYPE I	TYPE II	TYPE III	TYPE IV	OTHER
Equipment	Technical Equipment	Structures Specialist Equip.; Technical Information Specialist Equip.; HazMat Specialist Equip.; Technical Search Specialist Equip.; Canine Search Specialist Equip.	Structures Specialist Equip.; Technical Information Specialist Equip.; HazMat Specialist Equip.; Technical Search Specialist Equip.; Canine Search Specialist Equip.			
Equipment	Communications Equipment	Portable Radios; Charging Units; Telecommunications; Repeaters; Accessories; Batteries; Power Sources; Small Tools; Computer	Portable Radios; Charging Units; Telecommunications; Repeaters; Accessories; Batteries; Power Sources; Small Tools; Computer			
Equipment	Logistics Equipment	Water/Fluids; Food; Shelter; Sanitation; Safety; Administrative Support; Personal Bag; Task Force Support; Cache Transportation/Support; Base of Operations; Equipment Maintenance	Water/Fluids; Food; Shelter; Sanitation; Safety; Administrative Support; Personal Bag; Task Force Support; Cache Transportation/Support; Base of Operations; Equipment Maintenance			

Comments: Federal asset. There are 28 FEMA US&R Task Forces, totally self-sufficient for the first 72 hours of a deployment, spread throughout the continental United States trained and equipped by FEMA to conduct physical search and rescue in collapsed buildings, provide emergency medical care to trapped victims, assess and control gas, electrical services and hazardous materials, and evaluate and stabilize damaged structures.

Resource — Wilderness Search and Rescue Team

Category: Search and Rescue (ESF #9)

Kind: Team

Minimum Capabilities: Component	Metric	TYPE I	TYPE II	TYPE III	TYPE IV	OTHER
Team	Rescue Capabilities	Same as Type II	Backcountry, low-angle evacuation	Same as Type IV	Trained rescue personnel with experience in nontechnical back-country evacuation/carryouts supported by local technical experts	
Team	Search Capabilities	Capable of conducting self-sustaining full search operations for 72 hours in all weather and low-angle wilderness terrain; Competent and experienced Incident Command staff	Capable of conducting self-sustaining full search operations for 48 hours in all weather and low-angle wilderness terrain; Competent and experienced Incident Command staff	Same as Type IV	Capable of searching high-probability local wilderness terrain for short durations (24 hours or less)	
Team	Personnel	At least 6 team leaders and 48 team members to support at least 6 operational field units (at least 1 member of each team must be a medical specialist – see below); Management staff following ICS model	At least 4 team leaders and 28 team members to support at least 4 operational field units (at least 1 member of each team must be a medical specialist – see below); Management staff following ICS model	At least 2 team leaders and 6 team members to support at least 2 operational field units; Must be supported by local EMS and technical rescue personnel	At least 1 team leader and 3 team members; Must be supported by local EMS and technical rescue personnel	
	Medical Specialist	National standard EMT curriculum; ACLS, BTLS	National standard EMT-B curriculum or wilderness first responder; BTLS	Not required – supported by local EMS	Not required – supported by local EMS	
	Overhead Incident Management	Incident staff capable of managing wilderness search operations	Incident staff capable of managing wilderness search operations	Unit level mission release; No search management capabilities	Unit level mission release; No search management capabilities	

Resource Wilderness Search and Rescue Team

Category: Search and Rescue (ESF #9)

Kind: Team

Minimum Capabilities: Component	Metric	TYPE I	TYPE II	TYPE III	TYPE IV	OTHER
	Crew Availability	Available for more than 1 full day of operations	Available for more than 1 full day of operations	Available for at least 1 full day of operations	Available for at least 1 full day of operations	
	Sustained Operations	72 hours	48 hours	24 hours	24 hours	
	Training	Same as Type II, plus: Personnel demonstrate proficiency in mantracking and working with expert mantrackers	Same as Type III, plus: 1 member of each team must be current to the requirements of the medical specialist (see above); Must also be knowledgeable of procedures involved with helicopter transport and coordination with search crews, both ground and air; Must have the ability to operate in an ICS structure, and be able to plan, organize, and direct search and rescue missions; Team members must have training for operations in remote locations for extended periods	Same as Type IV, plus: Proficiency in back-country navigation (including the ability to triangulate a position, ascertain a UTM, use GPS, and follow a route to a new location using a topographical map and compass); Must be proficient at conducting and directing search lines	Must be able to operate the team's equipment; Team members are not expected to operate in remote field locations for extended periods; Must have basic navigation training using a map and compass; Must have technical proficiency in personal survival in local wilderness terrain; Must have awareness of mantracking and maintaining site integrity; Must have a basic understanding of the ICS; Must have proficiency in hasty search techniques	
	Transportation	4x4 vehicles that can transport each team throughout or to the search area	Vehicles that can transport each team throughout or at least to the search area; 4x4s are not required, but recommended	1 vehicle that can transport each team throughout or at least to the search area; 4x4s are not required, but recommended	1 vehicle that can transport the team throughout or at least to the search area; 4x4s are not required, but recommended	

(continued)

Resource · Wilderness Search and Rescue Team (cont'd)

Category: Search and Rescue (ESF #9)   Kind: Team

Minimum Capabilities: Component	Metric	TYPE I	TYPE II	TYPE III	TYPE IV	OTHER
Equipment	Clothing	Same as Type II	Same as Type III	Same as Type IV	Appropriate level of PPE for working environment	
	Communications	Same as Type II	Same as Type III, plus VHF capability to communicate with aircraft	Same as Type IV, plus VHF communications capability with other teams	VHF Radios for team communications; Cell Phone	
	Search & Rescue	Same as Type II	Equipment to support remote extrication and field transport of survivors	None required	None required	
	Supplies	Equipped to be self-sustaining for 72 hours in local wilderness environments	Equipped to be self-sustaining for 48 hours in local wilderness environments	Same as Type IV	Equipped to be self-sustaining for 24 hours in local wilderness environments	
	Medical	Same as Type II	Same as Type III, plus ability to support survivors	Same as Type IV	As appropriate for level of training, as applied in wilderness environment and meeting local protocols and requirements for support of the team	

Comments: Team members will usually only work a maximum of 12-hour shifts, depending on individual unit policies and procedures. Crew availability does not require continuous availability of specific personnel, only that crews are available to those specifications, though some personnel may have extended assignments in the field. Medical support and technical rescue equipment is expected to be provided by local EMS and other technical rescue personnel for Type III and IV teams.

APPENDIX 9

ICS Glossary

This glossary contains definitions of terms used in the Incident Command System (ICS) National Training Curriculum. It does not contain terms or definitions related to specific resources for particular application areas. Users should supplement this glossary with agency-specific terms and definitions as appropriate.

– A –

Action Plan See Incident Action Plan.

Agency An agency is a division of government with a specific function, or a non-governmental organization (e.g., private contractor, business, etc.) that offers a particular kind of assistance. In ICS, agencies are defined as jurisdictional (having statutory responsibility for incident mitigation) or assisting and/or cooperating (providing resources and/or assistance). (See Assisting Agency, Cooperating Agency, and Multi-agency.)

Agency Executive or Administrator Chief executive officer (or designee) of the agency or jurisdiction that has responsibility for the incident.

Agency Dispatch The agency or jurisdictional facility from which resources are allocated to incidents.

Agency Representative An individual assigned to an incident from an assisting or cooperating agency who has been delegated authority to make decisions on matters affecting that agency's participation at the incident. Agency Representatives report to the Incident Liaison Officer.

Air Operations Branch Director The person primarily responsible for preparing and implementing the air operations portion of the Incident Action Plan. Also responsible for providing logistical support to helicopters operating on the incident.

Allocated Resources Resources dispatched to an incident.

Area Command An organization established to: 1) oversee the management of multiple incidents that are each being handled by an Incident Command System organization; or 2) to oversee the management of a very large incident that has multiple Incident Management Teams assigned to it. Area Command has the responsibility to set overall strategy and priorities, allocate critical resources based on priorities, ensure that incidents are properly managed, and ensure that objectives are met and strategies followed.

Assigned Resources Resources checked in and assigned work tasks on an incident.

Assignments Tasks given to resources to perform within a given operational period, based upon tactical objectives in the Incident Action Plan.

Assistant Title for subordinates of the Command Staff positions. The title indicates a level of technical capability, qualifications, and responsibility subordinate to the primary positions. Assistants may also be used to supervise unit activities at camps.

Assisting Agency An agency directly contributing tactical or service resources to another agency.

Available Resources Incident-based resources which are ready for deployment.

– B –

Base The location at which primary logistics functions for an incident are coordinated and administered. There is only one Base per incident. (Incident name or other designator will be added to the term Base.) The Incident Command Post may be collocated with the Base.

Branch The organizational level having functional or geographic responsibility for major parts of incident operations. The Branch level is organizationally between Section and Division/Group in the Operations Section, and between Section and Units in the Logistics Section. Branches are identified by the use of Roman Numerals or by functional name (e.g., medical, security, etc.).

– C –

Cache A pre-determined complement of tools, equipment, and/or supplies stored in a designated location, available for incident use.

Camp A geographical site, within the general incident area, separate from the Incident Base, equipped and staffed to provide sleeping, food, water, and sanitary services to incident personnel.

Check-in The process whereby resources first report to an incident. Check-in locations include: Incident Command Post (Resources Unit), Incident Base, Camps, Staging Areas, Helibases, Helispots, and Division Supervisors (for direct line assignments).

Chain of Command A series of management positions in order of authority.

Chief The ICS title for individuals responsible for command of functional sections: Operations, Planning, Logistics, and Finance/Administration.

Clear Text The use of plain English in radio communications transmissions. No Ten Codes or agency-specific codes are used when utilizing Clear Text.

Command The act of directing and/or controlling resources by virtue of explicit legal, agency, or delegated authority. May also refer to the Incident Commander.

Command Post (See Incident Command Post.)

Command Staff The Command Staff consists of the Information Officer, Safety Officer, and Liaison Officer. They report directly to the Incident Commander. They may have an assistant or assistants, as needed.

Communications Unit An organizational unit in the Logistics Section responsible for providing communication services at an incident. A Communications Unit may also be a facility (e.g., a trailer or mobile van) used to provide the major part of an Incident Communications Center.

Compacts Formal working agreements among agencies to obtain mutual aid.

Compensation Unit/Claims Unit Functional unit within the Finance/Administration Section responsible for financial concerns resulting from property damage, injuries, or fatalities at the incident.

Complex Two or more individual incidents located in the same general area which are assigned to a single Incident Commander or to Unified Command.

Cooperating Agency An agency supplying assistance other than direct tactical or support functions or resources to the incident control effort (e.g., Red Cross, telephone company, etc.).

Coordination The process of systematically analyzing a situation, developing relevant information, and informing appropriate command authority of viable alternatives for selection of the most effective combination of available resources to meet specific objectives. The coordination process (which can be either intra- or inter-agency) does not involve dispatch actions. However, personnel responsible for coordination may perform command or dispatch functions within the limits established by specific agency delegations, procedures, legal authority, etc.

Coordination Center Term used to describe any facility that is used for the coordination of agency or jurisdictional resources in support of one or more incidents.

Cost Sharing Agreements Agreements between agencies or jurisdictions to share designated costs re-

lated to incidents. Cost sharing agreements are normally written but may also be oral between authorized agency or jurisdictional representatives at the incident.

Cost Unit Functional unit within the Finance/Administration Section responsible for tracking costs, analyzing cost data, making cost estimates, and recommending cost-saving measures.

Crew (See Single Resource.)

– D –

Delegation of Authority A statement provided to the Incident Commander by the Agency Executive delegating authority and assigning responsibility. The Delegation of Authority can include objectives, priorities, expectations, constraints, and other considerations or guidelines as needed. Many agencies require written Delegation of Authority to be given to Incident Commanders prior to their assuming command on larger incidents.

Deputy A fully qualified individual who, in the absence of a superior, could be delegated the authority to manage a functional operation or perform a specific task. In some cases, a Deputy could act as relief for a superior and therefore must be fully qualified in the position. Deputies can be assigned to the Incident Commander, General Staff, and Branch Directors.

Demobilization Unit Functional unit within the Planning Section responsible for assuring orderly, safe, and efficient demobilization of incident resources.

Director The ICS title for individuals responsible for supervision of a Branch.

Dispatch The implementation of a command decision to move a resource or resources from one place to another.

Dispatch Center A facility from which resources are assigned to an incident.

Division Divisions are used to divide an incident into geographical areas of operation. A Division is located within the ICS organization between the Branch and the Task Force/Strike Team. (See Group.) Divisions are identified by alphabetic characters for horizontal applications and, often, by floor numbers when used in buildings.

Documentation Unit Functional unit within the Planning Section responsible for collecting, recording, and safeguarding all documents relevant to the incident.

– E –

Emergency Management Coordinator/Director The individual within each political subdivision that has coordination responsibility for jurisdictional emergency management.

Emergency Medical Technician (EMT) A health-care specialist with particular skills and knowledge in pre-hospital emergency medicine.

Emergency Operations Center (EOC) A pre-designated facility established by an agency or jurisdiction to coordinate the overall agency or jurisdictional response and support to an emergency.

Emergency Operations Plan The plan that each jurisdiction has and maintains for responding to appropriate hazards.

Event A planned, non-emergency activity. ICS can be used as the management system for a wide range of events, e.g., parades, concerts, or sporting events.

– F –

Facilities Unit Functional unit within the Support Branch of the Logistics Section that provides fixed facilities for the incident. These facilities may include the Incident Base, feeding areas, sleeping areas, sanitary facilities, etc.

Field Operations Guide A pocket-size manual of instructions on the application of the Incident Command System.

Finance/Administration Section The Section responsible for all incident costs and financial considerations. Includes the Time Unit, Procurement Unit, Compensation/Claims Unit, and Cost Unit.

Food Unit Functional unit within the Service Branch of the Logistics Section responsible for providing meals for incident personnel.

Function In ICS, function refers to the five major activities in the ICS, i.e., Command, Operations, Planning, Logistics, and Finance/Administration. The term function is also used when describing the activity involved, e.g., the planning function.

– G –

General Staff The group of incident management personnel reporting to the Incident Commander. They may each have a deputy, as needed. The General Staff consists of -
Operations Section Chief
Planning Section Chief
Logistics Section Chief
Finance/Administration Section Chief

Generic ICS Refers to the description of ICS that is generally applicable to any kind of incident or event.

Ground Support Unit Functional unit within the Support Branch of the Logistics Section responsible for the fueling, maintaining, and repairing of vehicles, and the transportation of personnel and supplies.

Group Groups are established to divide the incident into functional areas of operation. Groups are composed of resources assembled to perform a special function not necessarily within a single geographic division. (See Division) Groups are located between Branches (when activated) and Resources in the Operations Section.

– H –

Helibase The main location for parking, fueling, maintenance, and loading of helicopters operating in support of an incident. It is usually located at or near the incident base.

Helispot Any designated location where a helicopter can safely take off and land. Some helispots may be used for loading of supplies, equipment, or personnel.

Hierarchy of Command (See Chain of Command.)

– I –

ICS National Training Curriculum A series of 17 training modules consisting of instructor guides, visuals, tests, and student materials. The modules cover all aspects of ICS operations. The modules can be intermixed to meet specific training needs.

Incident An occurrence either human caused or by natural phenomena, that requires action by emergency service personnel to prevent or minimize loss of life or damage to property and/or natural resources.

Incident Action Plan Contains objectives reflecting the overall incident strategy and specific tactical actions and supporting information for the next operational period. The Plan may be oral or written. When written, the Plan may have a number of forms as attachments (e.g., traffic plan, safety plan, communications plan, map, etc.).

Incident Base Location at the incident where the primary logistics functions are coordinated and administered. (Incident name or other designator will be added to the term Base.) The Incident Command Post may be collocated with the Base. There is only one Base per incident.

Incident Commander The individual responsible for the management of all incident operations at the incident site.

Incident Command Post (ICP) The location at which the primary command functions are executed. The ICP may be collocated with the incident base or other incident facilities.

Incident Command System (ICS) A standardized on-scene emergency management concept specifically designed to allow its user(s) to adopt an integrated organizational structure equal to the complexity and demands of single or multiple incidents, without being hindered by jurisdictional boundaries.

Incident Communications Center The location of the Communications Unit and the Message Center.

Incident Management Team The Incident Commander and appropriate Command and General Staff personnel assigned to an incident.

Incident Objectives Statements of guidance and direction necessary for the selection of appropriate strategy(s), and the tactical direction of resources. Incident objectives are based on realistic expectations of what can be accomplished when all allocated resources have been effectively deployed. Incident objectives must be achievable and measurable, yet flexible enough to allow for strategic and tactical alternatives.

Information Officer A member of the Command Staff responsible for interfacing with the public and media or with other agencies requiring information directly from the incident. There is only one Information Officer per incident. The Information Officer may have assistants.

Initial Action The actions taken by resources which are the first to arrive at an incident.

Initial Response Resources initially committed to an incident.

Incident Support Organization Includes any off-incident support provided to an incident. Examples would be Agency Dispatch centers, Airports, Mobilization Centers, etc.

– J –

Jurisdiction The range or sphere of authority. Public agencies have jurisdiction at an incident related to their legal responsibilities and authority for incident mitigation. Jurisdictional authority at an incident can be political/geographical (e.g., city, county, state, or federal boundary lines) or functional (e.g., police department, health department, etc.). (See Multijurisdiction.)

Jurisdictional Agency The agency having jurisdiction and responsibility for a specific geographical area, or a mandated function.

– L –

Landing Zone (See Helispot)

Leader The ICS title for an individual responsible for a Task Force, Strike Team, or functional unit.

Liaison Officer A member of the Command Staff responsible for coordinating with representatives from cooperating and assisting agencies.

Logistics Section The Section responsible for providing facilities, services, and materials for the incident.

Life-Safety Refers to the joint consideration of both the life and physical well being of individuals.

– M –

Managers Individuals within ICS organizational units that are assigned specific managerial responsibilities, e.g., Staging Area Manager or Camp Manager.

Management by Objectives In ICS, this is a top-down management activity which involves a three-step process to achieve the incident goal. The steps are: establishing the incident objectives, selection of appropriate strategy(s) to achieve the objectives, and the tactical direction associated with the selected strategy. Tactical direction includes: selection of tactics, selection of resources, resource assignments, and performance monitoring.

Medical Unit Functional unit within the Service Branch of the Logistics Section responsible for the development of the Medical Emergency Plan, and for providing emergency medical treatment of incident personnel.

Message Center The Message Center is part of the Incident Communications Center and is collocated or placed adjacent to it. It receives, records, and routes information about resources reporting to the incident, resource status, and administrative and tactical traffic.

Mobilization The process and procedures used by all organizations federal, state, and local for activating, assembling, and transporting all resources that have been requested to respond to or support an incident.

Mobilization Center An off-incident location at which emergency service personnel and equipment are temporarily located pending assignment, release, or reassignment.

Multi-agency Incident An incident where one or more agencies assist a jurisdictional agency or agencies. May be single or unified command.

Multi-agency Coordination (MAC) A generalized term which describes the functions and activities of representatives of involved agencies and/or jurisdictions who come together to make decisions regarding the prioritizing of incidents, and the sharing and use of critical resources. The MAC organization is not a part of the on-scene ICS and is not involved in developing incident strategy or tactics.

Multi-agency Coordination System (MACS) The combination of personnel, facilities, equipment, procedures, and communications integrated into a common system. When activated, MACS has the responsibility for coordination of assisting agency resources and support in a multi-agency or multijurisdictional environment. A MAC Group functions within the MACS.

Multijurisdiction Incident An incident requiring action from multiple agencies that have a statutory responsibility for incident mitigation. In ICS these incidents will be managed under Unified Command.

Mutual Aid Agreement Written agreement between agencies and/or jurisdictions in which they agree to assist one another upon request, by furnishing personnel and equipment.

– N –

National Interagency Incident Management System (NIIMS) An NWCG-developed program consisting of five major subsystems which collectively provide a total systems approach to all-risk incident management. The subsystems are: The Incident Command System, Training, Qualifications and Certification, Supporting Technologies, and Publications Management.

National Wildfire Coordinating Group (NWCG) A group formed under the direction of the Secretaries of the Interior and Agriculture to improve the coordination and effectiveness of wildland fire activities, and provide a forum to discuss, recommend appropriate action, or resolve issues and problems of substantive nature. The NWCG has been a primary supporter of ICS development and training.

– O –

Officer The ICS title for the personnel responsible for the Command Staff positions of Safety, Liaison, and Information.

Operational Period The period of time scheduled for execution of a given set of operation actions as specified in the Incident Action Plan. Operational Periods can be of various lengths, although usually not over 24 hours.

Operations Section The Section responsible for all tactical operations at the incident. Includes Branches, Divisions and/or Groups, Task Forces, Strike Teams, Single Resources, and Staging Areas.

Out-of-Service Resources Resources assigned to an incident but unable to respond for mechanical, rest, or personnel reasons.

Overhead Personnel Personnel who are assigned to supervisory positions which include Incident Commander, Command Staff, General Staff, Directors, Supervisors, and Unit Leaders.

– P –

Planning Meeting A meeting held as needed throughout the duration of an incident, to select specific strategies and tactics for incident control operations, and for service and support planning. On larger incidents, the planning meeting is a major element in the development of the Incident Action Plan.

Planning Section Responsible for the collection, evaluation, and dissemination of tactical information related to the incident, and for the preparation and documentation of Incident Action Plans. The Section also maintains information on the current and forecasted situation, and on the status of resources assigned to the incident. Includes the Situation, Resource, Documentation, and Demobilization Units, as well as Technical Specialists.

Procurement Unit Functional unit within the Finance/ Administration Section responsible for financial matters involving vendor contracts.

– R –

Radio Cache A supply of radios stored in a pre-determined location for assignment to incidents.

Recorders Individuals within ICS organizational units who are responsible for recording information. Recorders may be found in Planning, Logistics, and Finance/Administration Units.

Reinforced Response Those resources requested in addition to the initial response.

Reporting Locations Location or facilities where incoming resources can check-in at the incident. (See Check-in.)

Resources Unit Functional unit within the Planning Section responsible for recording the status of resources committed to the incident. The Unit also evaluates resources currently committed to the incident, the impact that additional responding resources will have on the incident, and anticipated resource needs.

Resources Personnel and equipment available, or potentially available, for assignment to incidents. Resources are described by kind and type, e.g., ground, water, air, etc., and may be used in tactical support or overhead capacities at an incident.

– S –

Safety Officer A member of the Command Staff responsible for monitoring and assessing safety hazards or unsafe situations, and for developing measures for ensuring personnel safety. The Safety Officer may have assistants.

Section That organization level with responsibility for a major functional area of the incident, e.g., Operations, Planning, Logistics, Finance/Administration. The Section is organizationally between Branch and Incident Commander.

Sector Term used in some applications to describe an organizational level similar to an ICS Division or Group. Sector is not a part of ICS terminology.

Segment A geographical area in which a task force/strike team leader or supervisor of a single resource is assigned authority and responsibility for the coordination of resources and implementation of planned tactics. A segment may be a portion of a division or an area inside or outside the perimeter of an incident. Segments are identified with Arabic numbers.

Service Branch A Branch within the Logistics Section responsible for service activities at the incident. Includes the Communications, Medical, and Food Units.

Single Resource An individual, a piece of equipment and its personnel complement, or a crew or team of individuals with an identified work supervisor that can be used on an incident.

Situation Unit Functional unit within the Planning Section responsible for the collection, organization, and analysis of incident status information, and for analysis of the situation as it progresses. Reports to the Planning Section Chief.

Span of control The supervisory ratio of from three-to-seven individuals, with five-to-one being established as optimum.

Staging Area Staging Areas are locations set up at an incident where resources can be placed while awaiting a tactical assignment. Staging Areas are managed by the Operations Section.

Strategy The general plan or direction selected to accomplish incident objectives.

Strike Team Specified combinations of the same kind and type of resources, with common communications and a leader.

Supervisor The ICS title for individuals responsible for command of a Division or Group.

Supply Unit Functional unit within the Support Branch of the Logistics Section responsible for ordering equipment and supplies required for incident operations.

Support Branch A Branch within the Logistics Section responsible for providing personnel, equipment, and supplies to support incident operations. Includes the Supply, Facilities, and Ground Support Units.

Supporting Materials Refers to the several attachments that may be included with an Incident Action Plan, e.g., communications plan, map, safety plan, traffic plan, and medical plan.

Support Resources Non-tactical resources under the supervision of the Logistics, Planning, Finance/Administration Sections, or the Command Staff.

– T –

Tactical Direction Direction given by the Operations Section Chief which includes the tactics appropriate for the selected strategy, the selection and assignment of resources, tactics implementation, and performance monitoring for each operational period.

Task Force A combination of single resources assembled for a particular tactical need, with common communications and a leader.

Team (See Single Resource.)

Technical Specialists Personnel with special skills that can be used anywhere within the ICS organization.

Temporary Flight Restrictions (TFR) Temporary airspace restrictions for non-emergency aircraft in the incident area. TFRs are established by the FAA to ensure aircraft safety, and are normally limited to a five-nautical-mile radius and 2000 feet in altitude.

Time Unit Functional unit within the Finance/Administration Section responsible for recording time for incident personnel and hired equipment.

Type Refers to resource capability. A Type 1 resource provides a greater overall capability due to power, size, capacity, etc., than would be found in a Type 2 resource. Resource typing provides managers with additional information in selecting the best resource for the task.

– U –

Unified Area Command A Unified Area Command is established when incidents under an Area Command are multijurisdictional. (See Area Command and Unified Command.)

Unified Command In ICS, Unified Command is a unified team effort which allows all agencies with responsibility for the incident, either geographical or functional, to manage an incident by establishing a common set of incident objectives and strategies. This is accomplished without losing or abdicating agency authority, responsibility, or accountability.

Unit The organizational element having functional responsibility for a specific incident planning, logistics, or finance/administration activity.

Unity of Command The concept by which each person within an organization reports to one and only one designated person.

INDEX